HEGEMONY AND DEMOCRACY

Hegemony and Democracy is constructed around the question of whether hegemony is sustainable, especially when the hegemon is a democratic state. The book draws on earlier publications over Bruce Russett's long career and features new chapters that show the continuing relevance of his scholarship. In examining hegemony during and after the Cold War, it addresses:

- The importance of domestic politics in the formulation of foreign policy;
- The benefits and costs of seeking security through military power at the expense of expanding networks of shared national and transnational institutions;
- The incentives of other states to bandwagon with a strong but unthreatening hegemon and "free-ride" on benefits it may provide rather than to balance against a powerful hegemon;
- The degree to which hegemony and democracy undermine or support each other.

By applying theories of collective action and foreign policy, Russett explores the development of American hegemony and the prospects for a democratic hegemon to retain its influence during the coming decades. This collection is an essential volume for students and scholars of International Relations, American Politics, and US Foreign Policy.

Bruce Russett is Dean Acheson Professor of International Politics at Yale, and edited the *Journal of Conflict Resolution* from 1972 to 2009. His book with John Oneal, *Triangulating Peace*, won the International Studies Association prize for Best Book of the Decade. This is his twenty-seventh book.

Security and Governance Series

Edited by

Fiona B. Adamson, *School of Oriental and African Studies, University of London*

Roland Paris, *University of Ottawa*

Stefan Wolff, *University of Nottingham*

This series reflects the broadening conceptions of security and the growing nexus between the study of governance issues and security issues. The topics covered in the series range from issues relating to the management of terrorism and political violence, nonstate actors, transnational security threats, migration, borders, and "homeland security" to questions surrounding weak and failing states, post-conflict reconstruction, the evolution of regional and international security institutions, energy and environmental security, and the proliferation of WMD. Particular emphasis is placed on publishing theoretically informed scholarship that elucidates the governance mechanisms, actors, and processes available for managing issues in the new security environment.

Rethinking Japanese Security
Peter J. Katzenstein

State Building and International Intervention in Bosnia
Roberto Belloni

The UN Security Council and the Politics of International Authority
Edited by Bruce Cronin and Ian Hurd

The Dilemmas of Statebuilding
Confronting the contradictions of postwar peace operations
Edited by Roland Paris and Timothy D. Sisk

Protest, Repression and Political Regimes
An empirical analysis of Latin-America and sub-saharan Africa
Sabine C. Carey

The International Humanitarian Order
Michael N. Barnett

The International Politics of Mass Atrocities
The case of Darfur
Edited by David R. Black and Paul D. Williams

Truth Commissions and Transitional Societies
The impact on human rights and democracy
Eric Wiebelhaus-Brahm

Emerging Transnational (In)Security Governance
A statist-transnationalist approach
Edited by Ersel Aydinli

Peacebuilding and Rule of Law in Africa
Just peace?
Edited by Chandra Lekha Sriram, Olga Martin-Ortega and Johanna Herman

Hegemony and Democracy
Bruce Russett

HEGEMONY AND DEMOCRACY

Bruce Russett

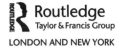

LONDON AND NEW YORK

First published 2011
by Routledge
2 Park Square, Milton Park, Abingdon, Oxon, OX14 4RN

Simultaneously published in the USA and Canada
by Routledge
711 Third Avenue, New York, NY 10017

Routledge is an imprint of the Taylor & Francis Group, an informa business

Typeset in Bembo and ITC Stone Sans by
Florence Production Ltd, Stoodleigh, Devon

British Library Cataloguing in Publication Data
A catalogue record for this book is available from the British Library

Library of Congress Cataloging-in-Publication Data
Russett, Bruce M.
   Hegemony and democracy/Bruce Russett
      p. cm.—(Security and governance series)
   Includes bibliographical references and index.
   1. United States—Foreign relations—21st century.
   2. Hegemony—United States.   3. Democracy.   I. Title.
JZ1480.R87 2011
327.73—dc22   2010036350

ISBN13: 978-0-415-57570-6 (hbk)
ISBN13: 978-0-415-57571-3 (pbk)
ISBN13: 978-0-203-82994-3 (ebk)

There is, has been, and will always be a certain group of people . . . who've consciously chosen their calling and do their job with love and imagination. It may include doctors, teachers, gardeners—and I could list a hundred more professions. Their work becomes one continuous adventure as long as they manage to keep discovering new challenges in it. Difficulties and setbacks never quell their curiosity. A swarm of new questions emerges from every problem they solve. Whatever inspiration is, it's born from a continuous "I don't know."

Wislawa Szymborska, Award Lecture for
Nobel Prize in Literature, 1996

CONTENTS

FIGURES

TABLES

ACKNOWLEDGMENTS

The author and publishers would like to thank the following for granting permission to reproduce material in this work:

Bruce Russett, "Democracy, War, and Expansion Through Historical Lenses," *European Journal of International Relations* 15:1 (March 2009), 9–36.

Bruce Russett, "Dimensions of Resource Dependence: Some Elements of Rigor in Concept and Policy Analysis," *International Organization* 38:3 (Summer 1984), 481–499. © 1984 World Peace Foundation and the Massachusetts Institute of Technology.

Bruce Russett, "US Hegemony: Gone or Merely Diminished, and How Does it Matter?" in Takashi Inoguchi and Daniel Okimoto, Eds., *The Political Economy of Japan: Vol. 2: The Changing International Context* (Stanford, CA: Stanford University Press, 1988), pp. 83–107. Copyright © 1988 by the Board of Trustees of the Leland Stanford Jr. University. Used with permission of Stanford University Press.

Bruce Russett, "The Real Decline in Nuclear Hegemony," in Ernst-Otto Czempiel and James Rosenau, Eds., *Global Changes and Theoretical Challenges: Approaches to World Politics for the 1990s* (Lexington, MA: Lexington Books, 1989), pp. 177–194.

James Lee Ray and Bruce Russett, "The Future as Arbiter of Theoretical Controversies: The Scientific Study of Politics and Predictions," *British Journal of Political Science* 26:4 (October 1996), 441–470, reprinted by permission of Cambridge University Press.

Bruce Russett and Allan C. Stam, "Courting Disaster: An Expanded NATO versus Russia and China," *Political Science Quarterly* 113:3 (Fall 1998), 361–382. Reprinted by permission from *Political Science Quarterly*.

Bruce Russett, "A Neo-Kantian Perspective: Democracy, Interdependence and International Organizations in Building Security Communities," in Emanuel Adler and Michael Barnett, Eds., *Security Communities* (Cambridge: Cambridge University Press, 1998), pp. 368–394, reprinted by permission of Cambridge University Press.

Jon Pevehouse and Bruce Russett, "Democratic Intergovernmental Organizations Promote Peace," *International Organization* 60:4 (Fall 2006), 969–1000, reprinted by permission of Cambridge University Press.

Bruce Russett, "Security Council Expansion: Can't and Shouldn't," in Ernesto Zedillo, ed., *Reforming the United Nations for Peace and Security* (New Haven, CT: Yale Center for the Study of Globalization, 2005), pp. 153–166.

Bruce Russett, *No Clear and Present Danger: A Skeptical View of the United States Entry into World War II*, prefaces from the 1972 edition (New York: Harper & Row) and the 1997 edition (Boulder, CO: Westview). Copyright © 1997 Bruce M. Russett. Reprinted by permission of Westview Press, a member of the Perseus Books Group.

Bruce Russett, "Liberalism," in Tim Dunne, Milja Kurki, and Steve Smith, Eds., *International Relations Theories*, 2nd edition (Oxford: Oxford University Press, 2010). By permission of Oxford University Press.

Every effort has been made to contact copyright holders for their permission to reprint material in this book. The publishers would be grateful to hear from any copyright holder who is not here acknowledged and will undertake to rectify any errors or omissions in future editions of this book.

1

A DEMOCRATIC HEGEMON?

The age of American hegemony

Dominance is a condition never reached without effort. Achieving superiority over others requires strength, skill, determination, and luck. Even if it comes when a primary opponent collapses, it can be retained only by repeated acts of will—in sport or in the supreme contest of international politics. A hegemon may be honored, respected, feared, perhaps even loved, but its victory must be reconfirmed each day. And, like all other achievements, it will ultimately pass away.

The English word hegemony comes from the ancient Greek term *hegemonia*, meaning leadership or supremacy. The Greeks applied it to their interstate system as the exercise of predominant influence by one state over others. In contemporary discourse *hegemony* typically implies something tougher than the benign term "leadership," instead conveying a dominance in part exercised as overt or at least implicit coercion.

Those under hegemony may welcome its leadership or protection, or may chafe under it, or both. In international politics it is not too far in meaning from the more pejorative *empire*, but without that term's connotations of a formal emperor or sovereign rule over far-flung territory. As a descriptor of an international system, hegemony lies somewhere between empire and *unipolarity*, with the latter more a characterization of a distribution of power rather than behavior, in which one state greatly surpasses any other state. Unipolar dominance is typically measured by material resources, but may also be based on cultural or ideological sources of influence. Empires are usually imposed by overt force on at least some parts of the territory and population, though peace may be the outcome, as in Pax Romana or Pax Britannica. Unipolarity does not carry quite the same implication about its founding, but advocates of preserving it often justify it as promoting peace, largely because the power disparity is so big that potential challengers will be deterred from provocation.

All three terms represent an emphasis on some kind of strong hierarchy in the international system, modifying the common assumption that the international system is anarchic ("without a ruler"). Unipolarity implies equal sovereignty with shared benefits though not equal power; empire implies no real independence and exploitation of the imperial periphery by its center (Jervis 2009: 190–191). Hegemony retains sovereignty and is noncommittal about the distribution of benefits. In this book I mostly use hegemony in the in-between sense of something less formal and perhaps less oppressive than empire, but with more emphasis on expecting cooperative behavior than the mere distribution of unipolar power may carry.

Some observers call the period from the end of the cold war (datable roughly from the fall of the Berlin Wall in 1989) the American hegemonic age. Others more skeptically talk about a hegemonic or unipolar moment (Layne 2006). Indeed, the high point may well have been the George W. Bush administration's confident attack on Iraq in 2003, expecting that it could move immediately from the demise of Saddam Hussein's rule to a similar thrust against Iran. That never happened, as US military forces became stuck in Iraq and the Iranian target was manifestly bigger and tougher. Events showed that regime change was harder than the Bush administration believed, and it could be even harder to provide security and control politics once a regime had been changed.

Yet the United States remains by any criterion the strongest military power in the world, in 2008 accounting for about 43 percent of all global military expenditures (Perlo-Freeman et al. 2010: 203). The margin over any of the others is truly overwhelming: China is second, with an estimated 6.6 percent. This degree of dominance is unmatched in any period of the Westphalian state system. It is not extreme to say that, with its spending and technological superiority, the United States largely controls the global commons, meaning the sea, air, and space.[2] It has global reach in unprecedented ways, and this is accepted willingly by the American population and, with less enthusiasm, by other nations. Control of the commons, however, does not necessarily imply an ability to dominate the world's land masses, where political rule requires boots on the ground and where asymmetric warfare skills can empower quite small insurgent or terrorist groups. The global economic downturn weakened most of the large powers, though China and India lost the least. American relative strength against most rival powers has not suffered much, but its absolute strength to conduct expensive and prolonged land interventions has dropped, while many of the nonstate actors with which it contends may even have been strengthened by economic desperation in the groups they wish to recruit.

In its land-power overreach the United States bumps up against the same imperatives that hobbled previous aspirants to empire. Napoleon certainly had greater ambitions—to absorb the territory, change the domestic political institutions, or extinguish the sovereignty of rival states. So did Germany's leaders in what has been called "the thirty-year (1914–1945) war for German hegemony." The strategic threat they posed from and to the European heartland virtually compelled the emergence of "balancing" coalitions against them, despite all the problems of coordinating such large and diverse alliances. That was expected in traditional realist balance-of-power analysis. By contrast, imperial Britain was not so threatening. As an island state offshore Europe, building a global empire dependent on sea power, it had limited ability to engage great continental land armies by itself. It was a case of a whale against an elephant, with neither able to inflict much damage on the other. Britain was at best a quasi-hegemon, maybe the biggest economic and industrial power but not in a position to dominate. As such it seemed to its European rivals less dangerous than Germany, Russia, or France were to each other. Consequently British quasi-hegemony lasted longer, and its eventual decline was due less to an emerging coalition than to the loss of its economic dynamism to Germany. The United States, not primarily a land power and without imperial claims to territory or formal sovereignty over others, can also try to be a relatively nonthreatening hegemon. Historically, great sea powers have been less likely than land powers to provoke other states into balancing against them, and their interests in promoting commerce may benefit from a liberal economic and political ideology (Levy and Thompson 2010).

For a hegemon, bilateral diplomacy may seem the easiest road to influence by providing an opportunity to do deals cheaply with weaker states. The larger and most relevant actors can often be bought off, and the rest pushed around or ignored. American hegemony, however, lacks that kind of raw dominance and commonly needs a multilateral structure of bargaining and negotiation. That requires it to rely more on international institutions that constrain itself as well as others, and on the legitimacy derived from the "soft power" of its economic, political, and social culture. Soft power is the ability to get others to do what one wants through attraction rather than coercion or payment (Nye 2003). Themes of influence and persuasion are common to theories about when states may "bandwagon" with a potential or actual hegemon rather than balance against it. Even the balancing against may be "soft," with no threat or intention of using military force against the hegemon. The goal of soft balancing is to create space for the balancing states to pursue some interests that may diverge from the hegemon's, and to distance themselves from hegemonic military actions that might entangle them in conflicts for which they have neither the capability nor the will.

Balancing, whether hard or soft, is hobbled by the problems of coordinating collective action, especially by large groups. Some analysts (e.g., Posen 2006) see the European Security and Defense Policy (ESDP) as a soft balancer, but it is difficult to find any widespread intention to undertake military actions that would be opposed to US interests. Even if there were, ESDP can act only by unanimity, a tough feat for an organization of twenty-seven countries with no clear leader or institutional structure to coordinate policy (Howorth and Menon 2009).[3] The problem of collective action to provide public goods is well recognized in economics and political science, and it will appear frequently in this book.

Realist analysis of states' behavior has tried to establish principles for predicting when states will balance against a threat, but bandwagon with a relatively non-threatening power. Part of the answer is that military power (the ability to control by threat or use of force) declines with the increasing costs of exercising power over great distance; hence in the cold war Western Europe supposedly felt less threatened by the United States than by the nearer and greater land power of the Soviet Union (Walt 1987). Yet that answer is incomplete without considering also the much greater threat to European political and economic values posed by Soviet military power as commanded by communist rule and ideology. The prospect of Nazi rule made German hegemony especially unattractive during World War II. So a purely material understanding of power cannot give strong predictions without taking into account the diverse cultures and institutions within and between the states that make up the international system. That "liberal" theme— the importance especially of democratic and capitalist institutions—drives much of the analysis of this book, and is highly important to understanding the prospects for continuing any kind of global hegemony. A central issue concerns the degree to which democracy and free markets empower or hamper a hegemon.

The structure of the book

The book is constructed around the question of whether hegemony is sustainable, especially when the hegemon is a democratic state. Various propositions about the causal relationship between hegemony and democracy find some theoretical and empirical support, with possible causation going both ways. For example:

- Democracy can hold leaders responsible when they begin costly, unnecessary, and unsuccessful hegemonic wars. Leaders can anticipate being held responsible. But wartime leaders may constrain democratic liberties.
- Democracy may help or hinder the financing of wars. If hegemonic wars benefit the broad populace democracy may not restrain leaders, and may increase warfighting effectiveness.
- A relatively nonthreatening democratic hegemon may find it easier to sustain an international coalition, but harder to get wartime allies to bear significant costs.
- The net effect of these and other propositions is unpredictable, inhibiting confident generalizations.

This introduction, and the conclusion, are new. Of the chapters in between, five were originally journal articles and five were in edited books that are not as readily available as most journal articles. (One chapter comprises the prefaces to two editions of a book by me.) I have not previously reprinted any of them. The selections are republished largely in their original form, save for updating some references, correcting printing errors, and providing a common formatting. There is some duplication of passages from one chapter to another, but in the interest of maintaining the integrity of each selection I have not eliminated it. The substance remains unchanged. Principal topics include the relative influence of domestic politics as contrasted with an alleged national interest in the formulation of foreign policy; the benefits and costs of seeking security through military power at the expense of expanding networks of shared national and international institutions; and the incentives of other states to balance against a potential hegemon rather than to "free-ride" on the benefits it may provide. Here is an outline of the subsequent chapters, with commentary on each item considering both circumstances at the time of its original publication and its claim to continued interest.

Chapter 2, "Democracy, war, and expansion through historical lenses," is a recent article that sets many of the themes for the whole book, notably many aspects of the democratic peace (what it is and what it isn't); the more general Kantian peace; and how democratic politics may encourage or constrain expansionary foreign policies. I wrote it as an update of recent research and my own thinking, and directed it especially to a European audience. It takes off from my understanding of Thucydides and other writers on the ancient Greek city-state system, asking what aspects of that system offer evidence or at least ideas about contemporary international relations. It argues that the democratic peace proposition applies largely to relations between democracies, rather than to whether democracies are in general more or less war-prone than other states. In particular, it contends that great powers are more war-prone in general than are less powerful states. That leaves indeterminate the question of whether and how great power democracies may differ from their autocratic rivals in overall participation in war. In weaving between ancient and contemporary times it begins to ask questions about the relationship between democracy and hegemony. For example, are democracy and hegemony compatible? Does democracy promote or restrain hegemony? Does hegemony strengthen or weaken democracy in the hegemonic state?[4]

The next three chapters were originally published much earlier. They concentrate on issues of hegemony, largely from a realist perspective that considers the conditions of hegemony and the degree to which some of the basic underpinnings of US dominance in the international system were sustainable or declining.

Chapter 3, "Dimensions of resource dependence: some elements of rigor in concept and policy analysis," is the first of three chapters written during the cold war, examining the role of ideas and theories in justifying an expansive foreign policy. It is an analytical essay on the United States' dependence on "strategic" raw materials from abroad, and its implications for a national interest in an activist foreign policy to ensure access. I wrote it at a time when fears of a serious decline in US economic and military capabilities were common (but see the next chapter's contrary view that the degree of US hegemony actually remained high, and secure). Following the oil shocks to the economy in the 1970s, these worries expanded to economically and militarily important metals. Such concerns frequently formed the basis for allegations that the US needed a Rapid Deployment Force to intervene if supplies to America from a key supplier country should be endangered by its political instability or hostility. To evaluate them this article proposes economic and political indicators for various dimensions of economic vulnerability or dependence, and shows those indicators for each of several allegedly vulnerable metals were considerably lower than for petroleum. Even petroleum did not score very high by most criteria. And better policy options for addressing most vulnerabilities that did exist would be increasing domestic production and stockpiling rather than resorting to military intervention. Of course, "strategic" arguments for intervention are still made whether or not such objective measures support them. They remain prominent, and not least for oil in the run-up to the two US wars against Iraq.[5]

Chapter 4, "US hegemony: gone or merely diminished, and how does it matter?" extends a previous and better-known analysis (Russett 1985) contending that American hegemony was alive and well throughout the cold war. This version gives special attention to Japan and its potential as a challenger, a supposed threat that received great attention in scholarly and popular writing at the time.[6] The analysis addresses the military and economic components of relative Japanese and US power, but also gives special attention to ideological or cultural "soft" power as initially conceived of by Antonio Gramsci. In addition, it draws heavily on a theoretical model for the provision of collective goods by the hegemonic power, which will appear in some following chapters and will be developed further in the conclusion to this book. The debates from this earlier period have important implications for the more recent fears about the rise of Chinese economic and ultimately military power as a challenge to US hegemony.

Chapter 5, "The real decline in nuclear hegemony," was written near the end of the cold war. Even then it was apparent that nuclear weapons had never been used since 1945, and that credible threats to use them had become rare. Over time, and now quite evidently so, threats to use them first, for offensive purposes, are not regarded as credible. Threats to use them for defense of the nuclear state's homeland can be more credible, but only in response to a nuclear attack or, *in extremis*, by a state whose territory and sovereignty could not otherwise be preserved (Israel, Iran, North Korea?). During the cold war, implicit or explicit threats to use nuclear weapons to defend allies from conventional attack were common, but once both sides had developed secure second-strike capabilities the threat became one to commit suicide to defend the ally, with the paradox that a rational actor would not deliberately do that. So the threat effectively morphed into one that the defender's escalation to using nuclear weapons might occur accidentally, or without authorization, in the fog of conventional war. Doing that, or preparing to do that, was not very credible either. Many serious analysts now contend that nuclear weapons are both useless and subject to a normative taboo (most importantly Schelling 2005; also Tannenwald 2008; Paul 2009) or simply useless, a waste of money and scientific talent (Mueller 2009).

In earlier decades nuclear weapons, and promises by powerful states to use them, helped reinforce hierarchies of centralized power globally, within alliances, and even within states. They enhanced American military hegemony, by deterring other powers and by having its allies largely controllable. It is no longer so clear that they do so, especially as a response to terrorism. If there were a WMD attack by some nonterrorist group, even one loosely associated with an Islamic state, what would be the appropriate nuclear target? Perhaps a military base if it could be reliably identified, but an attack on a civilian target would not diminish the terrorists' capability, and would likely only encourage more attacks. The proliferation of nuclear weapons to small states further undermines great powers' dominance and control. Under these circumstances, the endorsement by four realist US statesmen (Schultz et al. 2007) of complete nuclear disarmament as being in the interest of the United States makes the task look less utopian, though still very difficult.[7] Limited moves in that direction appear in President Obama's 2010 agreement with Russia to cut the number of nuclear weapons and delivery vehicles (Blair et al. 2010), in his declaration that the United States will not use nuclear weapons against states that do not themselves have nuclear weapons or try to acquire them, and in efforts to strengthen conventional means to perform tasks of deterrence and retaliation currently programmed for nuclear weapons.

The next two chapters in part consider the legacy of the cold war and its role in sustaining an expansionary foreign policy. In different ways, both consider how understanding the sources of Soviet/Russian foreign policy can offer policy options for incorporating potentially adversarial states into a cooperative international system. As such they continue the theme of hegemony, but modify the previous realist emphasis with substantial attention to the Kantian themes, especially that of democracy but also giving attention to the role of economic interdependence and international organizations.

Chapter 6, "The future as arbiter of theoretical controversies: predictions, explanations, and the end of the cold war" is an essay co-authored with James Lee Ray, assessing the possibility of explanation and contingent prediction in social science. It responds to complaints that political scientists totally failed, ex ante, to predict the peaceful end of the cold war. That nonviolent ending marked the extension and deepening of American global hegemony, and the demise of its rival even as a regional hegemon. It was predicted by extremely few analysts, and by virtually no one who focused on the material bases of the international system. Jim Ray and I contend here not only that it was explicable ex post, but that prediction was possible, and that a few analysts did provide a basis for predicting the cold war's end before the fact. Such analyses focused on domestic political forces demanding economic and political liberalization, forces that seemed unlikely to be released. But once they were, they produced economic and political policy changes within the Soviet Union that destroyed its ability to survive as a unified state powerful enough to rule its neighbors.

Chapter 7, "Courting disaster: NATO vs. Russia and China," co-authored with Allan Stam, discusses the question of expanding NATO into former communist states in Eastern Europe, and its likely consequence of alienating what during the 1990s was a somewhat democratic and not hostile Russia under Boris Yeltsin. At that time NATO membership for Czechoslovakia, Hungary, and Poland was assured, and plans were well under way to bring in other states, including Estonia, Latvia, and Lithuania, which had been part of the former Soviet Union. We understood that eastward expansion promised to strengthen liberal governments there, to discourage violent conflict between them, and to provide assurance against any resurgence of Russian efforts to control them. Yet we argued that at the same time it would stoke fear in Russia that the United States and NATO were expanding their hegemony into what had formerly been the Soviet sphere, right up to the borders of the new Russian state. So we raised the alternative of also seeking Russia's admission into NATO, so as to integrate it into the Western liberal political economy, relieve fears that expansion was a hostile move against Russia, and prevent the possibility that Russia would turn to China as an ally.

We did not imagine that integrating Russia (formerly NATO's reason for existence) would be easy, but that it should be tried. Moreover, doing so might serve as an example for engagement with China in the event of greater economic and especially political liberalization there. But the historic moment passed with Yeltsin's presidency. While some observers still think NATO membership is possible (for example, Kupchan 2010), it would mean admitting a nondemocratic state to an alliance that explicitly specifies democratic government as a condition of membership. As a former US ambassador to Russia and advisor to Ronald Reagan asserts, the recent Russian leadership does regard the United States as a hegemonic threat (Matlock 2010). Russian arms sales to China flourish, and in 2001 China, Russia, and four former Soviet republics from central Asia formed their own regional international governmental organization (IGO), the Shanghai Cooperation Organization.

The next three chapters focus on the role of international organizations in such a system, moving from international organizations in general, to the often greater effectiveness of IGOs comprised primarily of democratic states, and finally to the composition of the UN Security Council as both enabling and restraining a hegemon.

Chapter 8, "A neo-Kantian perspective: democracy, interdependence, and international organizations in building security communities," explores aspects of the large Kantian Peace project. Many aspects of that appear in various articles both previous to my book with John Oneal (Russett and Oneal 2001) and subsequently. Other parts of the discussion, however, do not appear elsewhere. It is keyed to Karl Deutsch *et al.*'s (1957) concept of security community, especially pluralistic security communities of sovereign states rather than amalgamated ones no longer with multiple sovereign members. Deutsch had experienced the forceful amalgamations of east and central Europe. His pluralistic version is much closer to Kant, who feared the "soulless despotism" of a world state and wanted only a (con)federation. In addition to the basic outline of a contemporary Kantian system, the chapter focuses primarily on the role of international organizations. It devotes much of its attention to the United Nations, partly with its rather weak coercive powers concentrated in the Security Council but also to various other parts of the UN system for promoting economic development and interdependence and also for protecting human rights. It also delves into the question of how "democratic" international organizations—especially global ones—can be in their institutional processes and still be both effective and regarded as legitimate. In doing so it touches on the advantages of having a strong if not hegemonic power to lead it, and the dangers of hegemony.

In *Chapter 9, "Democratic intergovernmental organizations promote peace,"* Jon Pevehouse and I extend the Kantian Peace empirical program, which produced less consistent statistical results for the peace-promoting effect of IGOs than for shared democracy or international trade. While differences among statistical models partially account for varying results, we attribute the problem largely to a failure of theory to conceptualize and measure different kinds of IGOs. The article originated in a conversation at Yale, after Jon had presented his work that found IGOs comprised largely of democratic countries are particularly effective in promoting democracy. We had an "aha!" moment with the insight that the same kind of "densely democratic" IGOs should be more effective than others in promoting peace among their members. So our article develops and illustrates several reasons why they might prevent or resolve conflict. We hypothesize that such IGOs are especially helpful in enabling their constituent democratic governments to make credible long-term commitments to peaceful behavior, in providing an institutional commitment to the peaceful settlement of disputes among their members, and in socializing their members to the norms of peaceful settlement. The results of our statistical analysis confirm a strong influence for this combination of democracy and IGOs on both the initiation and escalation of militarized disputes, in addition to the separate pacific influences of democratic governments and other kinds of international organizations. Some readers will find it helpful to revisit this chapter after reading the nontechnical discussion of our basic statistical analysis in Chapter 11.

Chapter 10, "Security Council expansion: can't and shouldn't" returns to the analysis of the UN begun in Chapter 9, concentrating here on the constitution and functioning of the Security Council. This essay was written in the context of the last major effort, led by Secretary General Kofi Annan, to reform UN institutions. It contends, with some regret, that efforts to change the composition of the Security Council will continue to fail. Such efforts confront two incompatible goals held in different degree by various proponents. One is to make the Council more effective (readier and more able to enforce its decisions), and the other is to make its decisions more "democratically" representative of emerging states in the post-colonial and post-cold war eras, and thus presumably more legitimate in the eyes of global opinion. The former requires satisfying the powerful states, especially the hegemon, who hold the capability of enforcing its decisions. The latter strongly implies restraining those very states' ability to act through the Council, resulting either in a failure to act or encouraging action outside of its control. Many coalitions formed around various plans to expand the Security Council's membership and change its voting rules. But to enact any particular plan required widespread support, and still could be defeated by a coalition of states who agreed on little more than that for very different reasons they preferred the status quo. More pointedly, the chapter argues that any change intended to dilute the voting power of the United States in the name of democracy would reduce US support for many UN operations without restraining its hegemony.

Chapter 11, "Liberalism," was written as a chapter for a collectively authored introductory international relations textbook edited by European scholars. As such it is particularly directed to an international audience. I have made a few additions, and some deletions of material that were more suitable for a textbook—such as a list of questions for discussion, and suggestions for further reading that are now integrated with other references. It serves first to bring together various aspects of the Kantian peace project and to return to some of the relationships between realist hegemony and the Kantian influences.

After opening with a brief overview of Kant's perspective on international relations, it shows, contrary to some academic analyses and widespread popular impression, that the number of deaths in violent conflicts—civil and international—declined sharply following the two World Wars, and again after the end of the cold war. The decline is especially striking when the number of battle deaths is divided by the rapidly growing number of people in the world. Then it moves to an empirical presentation of trends in the three Kantian variables since 1950, as proposed explanations for the decline in violent conflict, particularly in international conflicts. From there it goes into a nontechnical discussion of the kind of statistical method and evidence deployed in Chapter 9, and shows the basis for concluding that there is a strong and plausibly causal association between the rise of the Kantian influences and the drop in international violence. I then discuss the possibility of a self-reinforcing system of peace-promoting influences, as exhibited most strongly in late-twentieth-century Europe but to a lesser degree in the much wider international system. I conclude by referring to some of the themes identified in the introduction to this book, about the problem of collective action, hegemony, and the desirability of tempering hegemony with behavior according to Kantian principles. In doing so, the chapter bridges to the further development of these themes in the book's new concluding essay.

Chapter 12, "No clear and present danger," is from prefaces to the two editions of my revisionist book on World War II (Russett 1972, 1997b). The first edition challenged the intellectual and emotional legacy of that war. It proposed the notion that American participation in World War II had less effect on the essential structure of international politics thereafter than many thought, and did little to make the nation secure from foreign military threats—the presumed goal of a "realist" foreign policy. (By structure I meant the basic balance of forces in the world, regardless of which particular nations were powerful vis-à-vis the United States.) Rather, it suggested that most Americans might have been no worse off, and probably a little better, if the United States had never become a belligerent. Because it did, the Soviet Union replaced Germany as the great threat to European security. In effect, some lessons mistakenly drawn from the World War II experience had remained, in distorted form, as justifications for an interventionist foreign policy. The book was widely read and highly controversial, and I refined my interpretations over the subsequent quarter century as expressed in the preface to the 1997 edition. Even so, parts of it still seem relevant to considering the roots and trajectory of American hegemony. The five questions from page 108 of the book itself, referred to near the end of the second preface, were these:

1.   How bad an outcome, by whatever criteria, really is likely if American intervention does not occur?
2.   How likely—highly probable or only a long shot—is it that such a bad outcome will in fact happen?
3.   What favorable outcome is likely as a result of the contemplated intervention?
4.   How likely is it that such a good outcome will in fact be produced?
5.   At what cost—political, material, and moral—would the outcome probably be achieved? Would success be worth the price?

Chapter 13, "Democracy, hegemony, and collective action," the conclusion, expresses my developed conviction that major elements of both the principal theoretical schools—realist and liberal—are essential to understanding international relations. Relative power matters greatly, but so too do all the influences that affect how voters and elites make foreign policy choices based on very different perceptions of the national interest and of their own interests and values.

The first section of the chapter, entitled "Is hegemony sustainable internationally?" explores the consequences, for peace and deterrence, of a balance of power vs. a preponderance of power. It shows how a predominance of power within an alliance may provide security to its members even though the costs and benefits may not be shared equally and they may not entirely agree on all its goals and methods. It also discusses the role of economic power and capitalism as a source of "soft" power. The second section, "Is hegemony sustainable domestically?" continues the discussion of economics, notably the problem of hegemonic overstretch, and why some countries spend more on the military than do others. It then turns to the advantages and disadvantages of democracies in choosing and fighting wars. Democracies are sensitive to incurring substantial casualties in battle, and that in turn affects their strategies of combat and their ability to sustain long struggles.

The final section poses the biggest question: How long can a state remain both hegemonic and democratic? That question defies confident prediction but nevertheless is unavoidable. In the real world it is not a hypothetical question, but an existential one. One can plausibly imagine outcomes like a successful democratic hegemony, or its degradation into an empire, or the chaos from a failed hegemony.

The chapters between Chapters 2 and 12 follow a roughly chronological order, and the reader may discern some shifts in my evaluation of global conditions. During the cold war I was somewhat pessimistic about the chances that the world would avoid a horrible nuclear war.[8] With the end of the cold war I became more optimistic, believing that most of the world might manage to restructure its expectations and institutions so as to shackle what John Mearsheimer (2001) calls the tragedy of great power politics. Then, too much of that opportunity was squandered, first by missed opportunities in the 1990s and then by the conduct of two wars that leave Islamic extremism stronger than before. (Yes, leaders do matter.) I am left still hopeful but uncertain, beyond either pessimism or optimism.

Notes

1 Therefore I use the term American hegemony rather than American empire, unlike quite a few recent books using the concepts and behavior differently. Some (Colas 2007; Münkler 2007) find elements of both; Eland (2004) and Sylvan and Majeski (2009) come down squarely on the side of empire. Walt (2005: 31) refers to American primacy rather than hegemony, defining the latter as physical control to compel behavior. I prefer to use hegemony as a relationship maintained by some varying mix of hard and soft power.

2 Aircraft carriers are an instrument for controlling all three of these domains. The United States maintains twice as many carriers as all other countries combined, and they are much larger, with their combined flight decks covering about 70 acres as compared with 15 acres for the rest of the world's carriers (www.globalsecurity.org/military/world/carriers.htm). Strong navies serve as a means to secure and protect both commercial and security interests (Levy and Thompson 2010; Reuveny and Thompson 2004).

3 The few military actions undertaken by the EU, rather than by NATO under US leadership, have been operations intended to lead to post-conflict peacebuilding, with the approval of the United States.

4 For much new material on these themes, notably that democratic institutions and culture both benefited from and strengthened Athens' hegemonic capabilities see Ober (2008) and Pritchard (2010).

5 Nordhaus (2010) makes a trenchant analytical argument that an integrated global market for oil precludes the need for subsidizing domestic production, stockpiling, or preparing for military intervention.

6 A carefully nuanced but still alarmist evaluation of the implications of the Japanese "economic miracle" at that time is Kennedy (1987).

7 I have struggled for years with these questions, both normatively and empirically (e.g., Russett 1983, 2006, chs. 9-12).

8 Apparently the situation was even more dangerous than I thought. See Hoffman (2009).

2

DEMOCRACY, WAR, AND EXPANSION THROUGH HISTORICAL LENSES[1]

This chapter addresses some puzzles about the contemporary democratic peace, stimulated in part by two great classics of International Relations, Thucydides' *History of the Peloponnesian War*, and Immanuel Kant's *Perpetual Peace*. In very different ways, both these voices from the past can tell us important things about the present. When linked with contemporary social science research they can illuminate important influences on peace, war, and expansion both in the interstate system of classical Greece and in the contemporary world system.

The analysis begins with some general comments on what contemporary theory and evidence about the democratic peace (DP) most centrally claim, and then discusses how they apply to two questions that must be kept separate: Are democracies peaceful in general? Or are they peaceful only toward one another? In discussing both these questions I consider how well the reasoning and evidence for each apply to both the ancient and modern periods, with some reference also to their implications for understanding imperial expansion. I consider some of the most recent theory and research on democracies' international behavior to ask why some democracies, notably powerful ones, may engage in much international conflict. The presentation requires clarifying what we mean by democracy in both eras, and how democracy motivates decisions for war and peace. I contend that of all the differences between ancient and modern democracy, the most important to this discussion concerns the degree to which institutions can enforce accountability on those who make and execute the great decisions. These institutions were lacking in ancient Greece, and vary in effectiveness even now. I move back and forth between the two eras to illustrate points, and conclude with a partial analogy between ancient and contemporary events. The presentation requires examining a combination of realist power variables at the systemic and state levels, state institutions (not just a simple contrast of democracy and autocracy), and individual behavior.

Thucydides writes about a time and place that fit the realist definition of anarchy, a good Greek word meaning "without a ruler." That does not mean chaos or the absence of some order, but rather that no legal or military power is capable of enforcing laws to provide basic security to all the member units. States ultimately must rely on their own power to survive in a fiercely competitive environment. Acts undertaken for defensive motives may be seen by others as posing an offensive threat whatever the intention. Yet Thucydides neither creates nor fits a rigid realist paradigm. He is deeply concerned with individual behavior, and how it reflects self-interest. Most importantly, Thucydides does not concur with the realist assumption that states can be considered as rational unitary actors, carefully calculating the costs and benefits of alternative actions.[2] Changes in relative power provide the source of states' insecurity, but the perception of relative power, and choice about how to address it, form the heart of his story.[3] For Thucydides, domestic politics matters greatly: democracies and demagogues, passions and perceptions.

As for Kant, among other subjects he taught anthropology and geography at the University of Königsberg, and knew more about other countries than did most of his contemporary philosophers. Moreover, he describes phenomena that have recently emerged in some parts of the world, notably but not exclusively in Europe (Habermas 2007: ch. 8). States with republican constitutions, substantial commercial exchange, and ties of international law and institutions—Kant's three articles of perpetual peace—do not fight each other or expect to do so.[4] Law (within republics, and commercial and international law between them) in a "pacific federation" of sovereign states creates norms constraining citizens and leaders. Equally, institutions establish mutual interests so that citizens and leaders need not be angels guided solely by Kantian norms. Rather, constraints of interest make even self-seeking devils well-behaved "so long as they possess understanding" (Kant [1795] 1970: 112). Like Hobbes, Kant acknowledges the competitive and insecure elements of human nature, but provides an analytical solution for expectations of reciprocity. With this great innovation he breaks the security dilemma of potential war of all against all. In the daylight we can see the Hobbesian realist vision as the nightmare it is, and Kant's vision as the partial reality it has become.

A probabilistic theory about behavior between pairs of states

Despite great progress in refining the theoretical arguments and empirical evidence for democratic peace theory, the effort remains a work in progress. Just because the theory is likely to be challenged in this historical moment, continuing the progress is important, and that means fully understanding its implications for both ancient and contemporary peoples. To do so requires asking precisely what would constitute evidence for or against DP theory.

It is essential to recognize the probabilistic aspect of democratic peace theory. Virtually all social and political phenomena are too complex to support a law-like claim.[5] Inherent in any probabilistic understanding is that all the variance cannot be accounted for, and not just because of imperfect data. Chance, complex interactions, and nonlinearities will always modify the generalizations in ways that are impossible to grasp fully with statistical models (Lagazio and Russett 2004).[6] The goal of theory is to develop and apply general concepts, not just proper names such as the United States or George W. Bush, to explain some of the poorly predicted cases (see King 2001). Thus a close examination of prominent counter-examples is essential. Moreover, the other two Kantian articles reinforce joint democracy as a force for peace,[7] and such elements of realist theory as relative power and alliances, as well as personal perceptions, can weaken it. It is complicated enough to compute the probabilities for the modern era, and much harder for the Greek world where we have hardly any information about the characteristics and behavior of many states, or even of many states' existence. Certainly Thucydides does not have a full ledger on all the wars and states in the system. He focuses on a particular set of relationships, and especially wars, central to his narrative.

Though critics dispute about the reasons, there is now scholarly near-consensus for the basic empirical claim that rarely over the past century or two have democracies fought one another. Depending on how one defines key terms, full-scale war between pairs (dyads) of established democracies is somewhere between extremely rare and completely absent. Militarized disputes ranging in severity from purely diplomatic threats to small-scale violence falling short of a thousand war deaths are more common between democracies, but still much less so than between nondemocratic dyads.[8]

Democracy and autocracy are best conceptualized not as a dichotomy, but as a scale on which states may fall in the middle or at different various points toward either end. This point applies both within a particular historical context and between such contexts. The major component of DP theory is the dyadic proposition that the more democratic any two states are, the less frequent and less severe will be any militarized disputes between them.

In terms of a theory employed in some discussions below, Bueno de Mesquita et al. (2003: 42–43) characterize political systems in part by the size of their *selectorate*, "those who meet the polity's criteria for enfranchisement or . . . citizenship," and "whose endowments include the qualities or characteristics institutionally required to choose the government's leadership and necessary for gaining access to private benefits doled out by the government's leadership." These twin privileges— participation in choosing the leaders, and the consequent access to benefits—are essential to their theory. Segments of the nominal selectorate who produce low turnout in elections, or who are in one way or another disfranchised, are likely to be given fewer benefits. Of course, being in the selectorate matters only if there is free competition for votes.

The selectorate is typically a majority of the adult population in modern democracies, though it was not so in ancient Greece. Athens at the start of the war, with an enfranchised citizenry amounting to about 10 percent (40,000 men; not slaves or foreigners) of the population, has been labeled a "radical" democracy by the standards of its day (Boegehold 1996: 579). If all attended the assembly, a winning coalition would have been 20,000, but in practice it was much less.

By contrast, Spartan rule was at the top of a pyramid whose big base was a subjugated class of helots, in near-slavery. During the Peloponnesian War era the peak of that pyramid would have been fewer than 4,000 land-owning male citizens (Woodruff 1993: xiii) in a total population of roughly 200,000. With a winning coalition under 2,000, it might best be called a militarized oligarchy, but short of the end characterized by tyrannies of the time.

For the nineteenth through twenty-first centuries, the Polity 21-point composite scale measures competitiveness of political participation, openness and competitiveness of executive recruitment, and institutional constraints on executive power (www.cidcm.umd.edu/polity/). Most European democracies rate +10 on that scale, and the toughest dictatorships -10. The standards for a full democratic franchise rise from the nineteenth century to the twentieth. Before 1990, the South African "democracy for whites only" rated as a mixed regime at +4, perhaps looking rather like Athens on the criterion of full popular participation.[9] Comparisons between Greek and modern systems of democracy are nevertheless very difficult, as will be apparent subsequently.

Are democracies peaceful in general?

Unlike Kant, Thucydides certainly does not see democracies as more peaceful than autocracies, and regards different elements of politics as making democracies either more or less effective in preserving their security. While I suggest (Russett 1993: ch. 3) that there is *some* evidence that pairs of democratically ruled Greek states were *somewhat* less likely to fight one another than pairs composed of only one or no democracies,[10] I will not push that rather weak claim here. In the contemporary world the dyadic principle (democracies rarely fight each other) finds much support. But in neither arena is there strong and robust evidence that democracies are especially peaceful monadically (more peaceful in general). The question then becomes why we see little evidence for the dyadic proposition in the Greek world, and what theoretical implications we can draw regarding the weakness of the monadic claim in both arenas. To answer that requires close examination of theory and evidence from both historical periods.

The sweeping claim that democracies are peaceful in general fails to address the dangers democracies face in the realm of power politics in an incompletely Kantian world. The evidence varies with the empirical domain, what variables are included in the analysis, and how the variables are defined and measured. This should not be surprising. As I show below, the dyadic claim by definition includes both the dynamics of domestic political interactions between leader and potential opposition and the interactions between one independent state and another. The monadic claim completely ignores the latter. So by relegating all such influences to the error term, a consistent monadic claim about democratic war-proneness is harder to support.

One important refinement of the simple relationship arises as follows. Suppose that highly democratic states comprise only a small minority of states in the entire system. That was in fact true of the nineteenth and twentieth centuries until after the end of the cold war when democracies became a slight majority (Russett and Oneal 2001), and even more so of the Greek city-state system (Russett 1993: ch. 3). Add to that the strong evidence that the most peaceful dyads are democracies with each other, with autocratic dyads being more conflict-prone and mixed dyads (democracies–autocracies) even more conflict-prone. That also was true of the nineteenth and twentieth centuries, and has become stronger since the end of the cold war (Oneal 2006: 240–243). The combination of many mixed dyads in the system and greatest hostility between mixed dyads means that the average difference in total conflict involvement by democracies and autocracies may appear slight. Perhaps we might see a stronger monadic effect in a system where democracies were a strong majority (Gleditsch and Hegre 1997). We do know that geographical neighborhoods in which democracy is the predominant form of government are especially peaceful (Gleditsch 2002a).

Another major qualification concerns which side starts or escalates the fight, moving a substantially peaceful diplomatic dispute up to the level of a militarized one, and a low-level militarized dispute up to full-scale war. On this the evidence is stronger: even when democracies are involved in diplomatic disputes with dictatorships they are less likely than the dictators to initiate the use of violence (Reiter and Stam 2003; Rousseau 2005; Oneal 2006; Boehmer 2008), and less likely to escalate any violence to a high level (Huth and Allee 2002; Caprioli and Trumbore 2006; Oneal and Tir 2006).[11] In other words, it is the dictator's action that tends to produce the fight.

While this qualification keeps aspects of a monadic version of the DP alive empirically, it does not help with the problem of democratic powers who claim a right to "preemptive" (more correctly, preventive) military action.[12] So some further theoretical points are required to dispel an expectation of finding it applicable to specific cases either in the contemporary world or in ancient Greece.

A very big refinement is that all great powers are war-prone. Great powers may defend or coerce smaller states, but must rely on their own power to protect themselves (Jervis 2005: 35). At the same time, their power gives them choices and opportunities not available to smaller states (as the Athenian delegation reminded the citizens of Melos). A big state can usually defeat a small one, and big states' leaders have more latitude to make mistakes without suffering catastrophic results. Whether democratic or autocratic, their widespread interests and intervention capabilities allow them to be militarily effective beyond their geographical neighborhoods, and so they are more likely than small states to get into conflict (Russett and Oneal 2001).[13] That was true of the United States and the Soviet Union, and of Athens and Sparta. Moreover, great powers usually lack strong Kantian constraints of trade and intergovernmental organizations (IGOs).[14] So the difference in simple conflict involvement between democratic and autocratic great powers may be minimal. Weede (2005: 44–46), an advocate for the DP and what he calls the capitalist peace (the evidence for which is sometimes exaggerated),[15] supports the view that democratic great powers are not monadically peaceful. Müller

(2004) agrees that democracies behave peacefully toward each other, but makes several arguments about why theories to explain dyadic peace do not necessarily tell us why democracies in general often fight wars with nondemocracies. Part of the answer surely lies with the great power phenomenon, where just five countries—the United States, the United Kingdom, France, along with regional powers India, and Israel—account for nearly 80 percent of the violent conflicts by democracies. A similar pattern emerges for dictatorships, with the Soviet Union and China at the very high end.

Great powers' distinctive behavior also manifests itself in decisions about whether to come to the defense of smaller allies. The principle of collective action shows that small or weak states individually can contribute little to the probability that a strong state will win in wartime. Thus small states have great incentive to free-ride on or "hide" from the big state's military efforts, even when they have stakes in those efforts. A big state, by contrast, can make all the difference for the survival of a weak one.[16] Free-riding (or band-wagoning) may nevertheless become an unstable equilibrium if the great power seems to lose the ability to defend its allies, or appears likely to drag them into otherwise avoidable conflicts.

Yet another qualification concerns the institutions by which democratic leaders are held accountable for their actions, and can be removed for acts that damage the interests of a majority of the population. A simple but powerful argument focuses on the difference between parliamentary and presidential systems. To stay in power the prime minister is dependent on the support of a majority in the parliament; she is always subject to a possible vote of no-confidence, and especially so if she relies on a multi-party coalition to remain in office. Losing a vote of confidence means either replacement by a new coalition and probably a new leader, or having to contest a general election. Knowing that a no-confidence vote may be called can restrain her short of experiencing the vote itself. A president's hold on institutional power, by contrast, is not directly dependent on maintaining a majority in the parliament. She even may continue to govern effectively through years of divided government, during which one or both legislative houses is controlled by the opposition. Short of the next regularly scheduled election, she can be removed only by extraordinary legal means like impeachment, or by violence. Thus a key mechanism to ensure executive responsibility for the general welfare is missing (Stepan and Skatch 1993; Aurswald 2000 gives a more complex typology).

Finally, one should not forget, as Thucydides surely does not, the influence of particular leaders' personalities and perspectives, such as a "we-versus-them" attitude (Keller 2005) or a conviction that peace is served by forcibly transforming other states' regimes (Saunders 2011). The ability of long-standing democratic institutions to restrain leaders may vary with both the configuration of domestic political power and characteristics of individual leaders. Random and chaotic elements, such as the 2000 election in the United States, affect the ascent to leadership and encourage counterfactual "subjunctive" history.[17]

Untangling this complex interplay of influences is necessary to comprehend why a monadic democratic peace may be hard to identify in a world that still contains many autocracies. It is so contingent on other influences at the systemic, dyadic, and national and sub-national levels of analysis that its appearance will often seem weak or variable. Nevertheless, understanding those contingencies should prove enlightening about some questions of imperialism and democratic foreign policy in many eras.

Culture and motivation

A major line of research develops the proposition that democracies are generally more successful in war than are autocracies. This too is a well-established fact for the nineteenth and twentieth centuries, during which democracies won nearly 80 percent of their wars (all but possibly one or two of them against autocracies). Autocracies lose more than half of all their wars (half of those fought against other autocracies, and more than half of those against democracies). Democracies are more likely to win when they start the conflict because they are likely to choose their uses of force more carefully. They select better, generally choosing to fight wars they can win quickly and easily, not running up costs in blood and treasure that will turn voters against the leadership. Their choices may also benefit from freer circulation of ideas and information. Democracies won more than 90 percent of the wars they initiated, but little more than half of those they did not start. (Examples such as Athens against Syracuse and recent events do not disprove the generalization.) Autocracies, by contrast, won only about 60 percent even of those they initiated.

Modern democracies also may be able to fight more effectively because they can deploy a better motivated and educated fighting force, with troops and commanders capable of taking initiative in battle (Reiter and Stam 2002: ch. 2). Military and civilian morale is likely to decline, however, in wars of choice that drag on with increased casualties and declining prospects of victory (Eichenberg and Stoll 2006; Voeten and Brewer 2006). This decline in democratic support is less evident in wars of state survival or other vital national interests (Horowitz *et al.* 2007).

In the Greek world, Thucydides recounts the funeral oration of Pericles, whom he admires. Pericles (2.37–40) praises the culture of Athenian democracy as the source of Athenian greatness. Its institutions are for "the many and not for the few"; "everyone has equal access to the law." The culture of Sparta relies on discipline, "painfully training" its young men, whereas education into the culture of Athens trusts "less to our equipment and guile than to our personal courage in action." Athenians are "especially daring in our analysis and performance of whatever we undertake."[18]

In oligarchic Sparta the elite hoplites were renowned for their discipline and motivation, but not for their initiative. Sparta's greater weakness, however, was in the helots, who could not be relied on to fight except under compulsion. Indeed, Spartan generals often were reluctant to extend their forces too far from home lest the helots take that as an opportunity to rebel (Cartledge 1996). In the Athenian democracy all free citizens were enfranchised and had a stake in the political and economic system. They could settle as colonists (cleruchs) on islands seized from defeated enemies (Russett 1993: 49). Free soldiers formed a much larger proportion of the population than in Sparta, and were better educated. Athens, with its greater population base, could motivate a much larger number as well as proportion of its citizens than Sparta, without imposing such great sacrifices on them. There was nothing in Athens like the Spartan upbringing of its soldiers. Not only was Athens a great power, it was the richest of all Greek states. The navy was essential for maintaining and expanding trade and the empire (Cornford 1907).[19] That, plus changing the obligation of Delian League members from providing ships to money tribute, allowed Athens to pay its own sailors well. Its navy was manned not by galley slaves subject to the lash, but by free men who rowed willingly and could be depended on to fight vigorously in the hand-to-hand combat characterizing much of naval warfare.[20] They could take remarkable initiatives, as after the landing on Pylos reported by Thucydides (4.4). The Athenian position was exposed to Spartan attack. The officers did nothing, so the rower-soldiers, unable to remain idle, took it upon themselves to build a strong defensive wall, at great effort without proper tools.[21]

Thucydides (6.20) has Nicias warning Athens about the Syracusans' readiness to fight for their democracy. Since then many writers have asserted that soldiers warring on behalf of popular governments (perhaps democracies, or at least where the soldiers predominantly accept the official ideology) will fight more willingly and more effectively than for regimes with less popular legitimacy. A variant of this would be the claim that soldiers may fight for democracy, or even a king, but not much for the institution of monarchy. Democratic governments typically provide more public goods for their citizens than do most autocracies (Russett and Oneal 2001: 56). By contrast, it is said that the primary motivation for fighting hard is troops' loyalty to their comrades in arms in small tightly knit units, rather than to a particular regime or ideology which may seem irrelevant to their opportunities for honor and survival.

Reiter and Stam (2002: ch. 5) explore in a contemporary context several variants of a contention that democratic armies will be more effective. They consider troops' morale, the willingness of soldiers to take initiative on the battlefield (the Athenian claim), and the possibility that officers in democratic armies may be chosen more for competence, whereas a dictator who must always worry about being betrayed by his underlings will value personal loyalty more. Their analysis suggests that hypotheses about better military morale in democracies are not supported, but those about greater initiative and better leadership are. An extreme example of the last two phenomena is Iraq under Saddam Hussein, a corrupt dictator and corrupted institutions. His advisors and military commanders were chosen for personal loyalty to him rather than competence (some were chosen because of their incompetence to act independently), and feared for their lives if they offered the slightest doubt or criticism (Woods *et al.* 2006; Rosen 2007: ch. 5; also 96–97 re. tyrants in general). Democratic leaders don't kill the bringer of bad news, but nevertheless may not encourage or believe it; e.g., insisting three years after the invasion of Iraq that WMDs had really been present (Draper 2007).

Institutions and expansion

Kant makes some arguments about the culture of republican government, but his central one is about political institutions. He contends that in states with republican constitutions the enfranchised masses, both bearing the costs of wars and making the decisions about whether to fight, would be more reluctant to go to war than would the leaders of an oligarchy. Leaders of oligarchies, by contrast, could keep most of any benefits of war to themselves but make the masses pay most of the costs. Some of the benefits can be used to pay off key members of the oligarchy and the state security forces on which they depend for their rule. So dictators may fight more wars, including ones which they do not have great expectations of winning.

Contemporary democracies may be more able and willing to mobilize their economic resources in wartime (Friedberg 2000). Citizens and foreigners may be readier to lend to a democratic state in wartime or extended periods of international tension like the cold war, because their chances of getting paid back are better than with an autocracy (Schultz and Weingast 2003). The general populace will support the war effort if they can expect a significant share of any winnings. This is the heart of the Bueno de Mesquita et al. (2003) theory which expands and systematizes an institutional argument that democracies and autocracies go to war, and succeed, for different reasons. Consequently, democracies may be able to spend relatively more on military forces in war than can most of their autocratic counterparts. Bueno de Mesquita et al. control for relative power, and predict wars by democracies that can expect to win easily. Reiter and Stam (2002, 2007) dispute this claim, and particularly the later claim by Bueno de Mesquita et al. (2004) that democracies increase their ability to mobilize resources more over the course of a long war than can autocracies. Yet Bueno de Mesquita et al. distinguish between wars for specific goals and wars for survival of the state or its regime (also see Goemans 2000). In the relatively rare but dire situation of a war for survival, such as World War II, a coercive dictatorship like the Soviet Union becomes highly motivated to sustain a high rate of extracting resources from the civilian population throughout the war.

While the question of whether democracies or autocracies can successfully demand greater sacrifice from their populations remains unsettled, it nevertheless misses a key point. Whatever the reasons for a democracy's military success, that success may then prime it for further efforts to exert its military power. Great power democracies, with an especially high probability of winning, may be especially conflict-prone in general, even while remaining at peace with other democracies. This leads to the matter of democratic military expansion, which cannot be ignored in ancient Athens, in the history of Western colonialism, or in the present day. A wide franchise may restrain the impetus to start wars that seem likely to be long and costly, but for shorter and easier wars that wide franchise may enable democracies to mobilize human and material resources well. Indeed, Bueno de Mesquita *et al*. (2003: 252) argue that democracies are even more likely than autocracies to fight colonial wars, often against weak nondemocratic states. A war to acquire a colony usually does not require major mobilization of resources. The new colony's government can be replaced by a leader who will be dependent on the victor and who, though he may not be very democratic, has a large enough base to sustain the postwar settlement (451–454).[22] Bueno de Mesquita and Smith (2007) also contend that donor countries use foreign aid to autocrats in poor countries to buy policy concessions rather than to promote development. This reflects a common contemporary critique of foreign aid programs.

Although other Greek democracies had some of the mobilizing advantages that Athens had, none had remotely the level of resources available to it as a large state with a vast empire. Athens' overall mobilizational advantage gave it incentives for expansionist or imperialist wars, raising both the probability of winning and the expected benefits to both elites and wider population. Ferejohn and Rosenbluth (2008) develop this theoretical argument with illustrations from ancient Greece, Rome, Renaissance Italy, and more recent history.[23] A theme of the combination of democracy and imperialism as cause of Athens' downfall is prominent in Thucydides (Ober 1998: ch. 2).

Unlike the weak monadic effect of democracy, having an economy heavily dependent on foreign trade (a high ratio of trade to GDP) usually exerts a monadic influence on peacefulness as well as a dyadic effect in reducing conflict with primary trading partners (Russett and Oneal 2001: 146). Nevertheless, a very powerful trading state with many potential export markets and suppliers of imports may be more able than a smaller one to afford the "luxury" of fighting a political adversary or imposing economic sanctions on it. Recent work (Dorussen and Ward 2008a, 2008b) is showing that the pacific effects of trade and international organizations manifest themselves especially in networks that encourage third-party mediation.

For Greek democracies with less wealth and power than Athens, and sometimes different in culture, the net economic cost and benefit to leaders and peoples could be different, and the number of other democracies available for generalization is not large. Then as now, most democracies are not imperialist, though some are, at some times. That in turn leads to further questions: Are expansionist democracies expansionist because a particular kind of democracy feeds expansionism, or because expansionism promotes and supports a particular kind of democracy? Or is it simply that most great powers, democratic or not, are expansionist in certain periods of their history? Or does becoming a great power merely signify a *successful* policy of expansionism?[24]

The dyadic democratic peace: why so little in ancient Greece?

Focusing on the dyadic democratic peace makes clearer the need to control for many other influences that affect war and peace decisions in the ancient world or the contemporary one. Only great powers can fight unaided at great distance. Other distant states usually lack both the capability and the incentive to fight each other. So both distance and relative power should be included in any dyadic analysis. This has not been done in systematic analyses of the Greek city-state system, and it should be before reaching conclusions either way. Distance is easily measured, but a reliable index of relative power may be much harder to acquire. Athens frequently fought allies who wanted greater autonomy, and alliances have not proven to be a robust restraint on fatal disputes in the contemporary system (Bennett and Stam 2004). In principle, it would be important to add the rest of Kant's prescription (commercial ties and international law/organizations) to a multivariate analysis of the ancient world. Yet in the Greek system international organizations other than the Delian League (under Athenian hegemony) did not exist, and data on system-wide trade patterns are not available.

A fuller understanding of why we see little evidence for the dyadic DP in Thucydides' time, however, emerges from looking more closely at the causal explanatory "mechanisms" posited for the contemporary democratic peace. Theories often distinguish, somewhat arbitrarily to be sure, between cultural/normative explanations and structural/institutional ones (Maoz and Russett 1993). Normative explanations generally say that leaders and citizens of democratic states expect political conflicts of interest to be settled largely without violence by means of negotiation, mediation, and arbitration. Democratic peoples have a cultural aversion to violence, and prefer to settle international conflicts by similar means. When they see other states whose regimes are founded on similar principles, they can expect conflicts of interest between their states similarly to be subject to peaceful settlement rather than the use or threat to use military force. By contrast, they expect states governed by autocratic principles not to share a cultural preference for peace and so behave more assertively in their interactions with such states.[25]

Democratic norms provided only weak restraints on interstate behavior in the Greek system. I also am coming to the view that, while shared democratic culture and norms provide a significant influence on peace between democracies in the modern era of international relations, their effect is not as powerful as are the structural explanations that stress the importance of democratic institutions.

Most institutional theories emphasize deliberative institutions and a separation of powers with checks and balances. They put great weight on open political competition in keeping decision-makers accountable to a wide electorate. Many writers (e.g. Bueno de Mesquita et al. 2003; Rousseau 2005; Reiter and Stam 2002; myself) regard this conceptualization as the most compelling explanation of the DP.[26] By this interpretation what matters is the "invention" of institutions of representative government constrained by free elections. That means institutions, which produce elections that matter—in a wide quasi-universal franchise, and truly competitive elections that the incumbent can actually lose. In a long or losing war, large parts of the electorate will pay severe costs in money and blood. If that happens, the democratic leader and party can expect to be thrown out of office, especially if it was a "war of choice" rather than resisting a clear attack. So a wise democratic leader will anticipate such an electoral response and avoid starting a war in the first place.[27] In presidential systems, this constraint is likely to be more effective when at least one branch of the legislature is controlled by the opposition party, giving it a more informed and credible platform if it chooses to oppose the use of military force (Howell and Pevehouse 2007). Conversely, a president may be emboldened when fully in control of the legislative branch.[28]

The character of domestic political institutions provides the basis for a theory of strategic interaction, as two states' leaders contemplate the incentives and constraints on each other's choices. A democratic leader will especially avoid starting a war with another democracy, since she knows that other democracies, if attacked, can motivate their populations for long and effective resistance.[29] Autocratic leaders, however, have much less fear of being driven from office if the wars they start go badly, and whether or not they succeed in war they may be able to make the general populace pay most of the costs and retain enough gains to hold the loyalty of their narrow base of supporters in the oligarchy and the domestic security forces. Much systematic evidence supports that theory as a probabilistic statement, even though one may find exceptions where democratic leaders are not wise and still may be not be driven from office.[30]

Comparisons even among modern forms of government run many hazards, not least the notion that all democracies have equally accountable executives and all autocracies are equally unaccountable (Gleditsch and Ward 1997; Tsebelis 2002; Gandhi and Przeworski 2006; Weeks 2008). Freedom of the press is highly correlated with democracy, and probably contributes importantly to democratic accountability (Van Belle 2000).[31] But the degree of press freedom varies within contemporary democracies and autocracies, and so may its effect on foreign policy. Other institutions and competitive practices vary notably across democracies and autocracies. Such differences can suggest where and when the democratic peace may not operate so effectively. Voting turnout varies widely among democracies. If benefits are distributed disproportionately to those members of the populace who are anticipated to vote, war costs may be shifted to low-voting groups. In the Woodruff translation, Thucydides (2.44), quotes Pericles, "It is not possible for people to give fair and just advice to the state, if they are not exposing their own children to the same danger when they advance a risky policy."[32]

While there is little evidence of a general autocratic peace, we know that certain types of autocracies get along better with each other than do other types (Peceny and Beer 2002). Institutional distinctions among autocracies and democracies are complex and hardest to make in the mid-range of the scale (Vreeland 2008). Correspondingly, the effect of regime type on behavior is weakest there, and much stronger for the more uniform types at the highest and lowest ends of the scale (Lagazio and Russett 2004). That gives all the more reason for caution in generalizing about the equally great variation within any binary scale of democracy and autocracy in the Greek world, or about similarities between ancient and modern eras.

Using interpretations such as these, the failure to observe much democratic peace in the different conditions of ancient Greece should not be surprising. One reason could be that the Athenians had many slaves (hardly a modern democratic norm), and only men voted in what was by our standards a narrow electorate. More important, however, may have been the lack of institutional constraints in the form of separation of powers and representatives subject to periodic and regular electoral removal. The assembly of citizens met on at least 40 days per year. There was no higher authority than the assembly, and its decisions were final. Only it could reverse its own decisions (as it did hastily reverse its initial hasty decision to slaughter the Mytilenians). Generals and treasurers were elected, but the nine chief administrative officers (archons) were chosen by lot without any requirement of special capacity or training. So too was a Council of 500, whose members each served for a year. Its executive committee changed composition ten times a year (Boegehold 1996: 579–581). There was no professional bureaucracy to resist rash action or be held responsible, nor representative institutions to consider action more deliberately than the assembly. The free citizens of the assembly, with their stake in retaining and expanding the system, were not especially pacifist. That they, rather than their elected representatives, took the decision to go to war made it harder to blame leaders (even demagogues) as responsible.[33]

Kant expects citizens of a republic to hesitate greatly before taking on a dangerous enterprise like war, for that "would mean calling down on themselves all the miseries of war, such as doing the fighting themselves, supplying the costs of the war from their own resources," and carrying the burden of debt. But he distinguishes a republic, where "the executive power is separated from the legislative power," from the possible despotism of "badly organized constitutions of ancient and modern times" (i.e., of democracies without a system of representation).[34] The combination of Athenian citizens who had the potential to gain from war and the lack of representative institutions meant a citizenry with neither pacific preferences nor constraint.

Analogies between the ancient Greek city-state system and the modern international system are necessarily imperfect, but the comparison helps us to understand both better. The comparison may lead us to be somewhat more hopeful about the contemporary world, with its wider democracy and more complex national political institutions, along with a much denser Kantian network of commerce and international organizations. It is nonetheless sobering to remember the Athenian expedition to Syracuse and subsequent developments which may have or develop contemporary parallels. Some of these may be applicable: Its motivation included commercial and strategic interests throughout the (Greek) world. Although Athenians feared that Syracuse might actively join the Spartan alliance, this was a preventive war (6.18) and a diversion from confronting their main enemy. It was urged on them by Alcibiades, an aristocrat by birth who played a man of the people, appealing to fear and ambition. They underestimated the possible costs and risks of failure. They thought, or at least hoped—with very little information—that the democratic faction in Syracuse would revolt in their favor. But all the Syracusans fought to defeat the Athenians, killing many of them. Hearing of this, Athens sent out a second expedition, which also was defeated. Ultimately their navy was destroyed, and the Athenians retreated into Attica, where the Spartans put them under siege. Athens was forced to surrender, and its democracy fell to an oligarchy. Athenian independence and democracy were later restored, but the war had irreparably weakened both sides. Athens' golden age was then over, for ever.

Notes

1 For comments I thank Karina Cendon Boveda, Bruce Bueno de Mesquita, Fred Chernoff, Ted Couloumbis, Allan Dafoe, Daniela Donno, Benjamin Fordham, Jolyon Howorth, Richard Ned Lebow, Andrew Mack, Nikolay Marinov, William Odom, John Oneal, Frances Rosenbluth, Nicholas Sambanis, Elizabeth Saunders, Arlene Saxonhouse, and audiences in Dresden, Germany and at the Alexander Onassis Foundation in Athens.

2 Keohane (1983: 508) gives the basic realist model, exemplified in the modern era by Waltz (1979) who substantially channels Hobbes' seventeenth-century world of monarchical autocracies for which some form of unitary actor assumption is fairly accurate. Gilpin (1988), though a realist emphasizing structural power balance, also incorporates domestic regimes, including for ancient Athens its commercial imperialism. Mearsheimer and Walt (2007) are acutely aware of what they see as the Israel lobby's influence on American foreign policy, but interpret it as a distortion of a policy reflecting some consensual national interest. See Payne (2007), also Morgenthau (1960: 4–11).

3 Most famous is Thucydides (1.23), in the Crawley translation used by Strassler (1996: 16), "the growth of the power of Athens, and the alarm which this inspired in Sparta, made war inevitable." In Blanco's words (Blanco and Roberts 1998: 11–12), this is "the truest explanation for the war is that Sparta was forced into it because of her apprehensions over the growing power of Athens." Woodruff (1993: xxx–xxxii, 16) translates it as "the growth of Athenian power, which put fear into the Lacedaemonians and so compelled them into war." He interprets compulsion as involving subjective human agency rather than objective necessity. Either way, alarm/fear/apprehension suggests a role for perception and emotion rather than fated inevitability. The meaning of inevitability here depends on far more than the translation. Kagan (1969) says the war "was caused by men who made bad decisions in difficult circumstances. Neither the circumstances nor the decisions were inevitable." Other examples include Lebow (2003), who holds that war was not strictly inevitable and that Thucydides did not believe it to be; Welch (2003), who warns against making Thucydides fit any contemporary schema or event; and the 'Interpretations' in Blanco and Roberts (1998: 405–522). (Unless otherwise noted I use Blanco's translation for all quotations.)

4 To adapt John F. Kennedy's famous 1969 statement in Berlin, "We are all Königsbergers," in my presentation in Dresden I added, "Under the threat of attack, we are all Dresdeners."

5 Weart (1998) makes such a claim for the Greek world; Robinson (2001) refutes it.

6 Many models for explaining international conflict share a problem with those doing structural analysis to explain civil conflict: they can predict with some success where conflicts will arise, but not when. Part of the problem for both enterprises lies in the crude fit between concept and measurement, and errors in measurement, and try as we do with the data the limits are inherent, and serious. The "error term" includes many nonstructural reasons, or "accidents" that may convert structural tensions into fatal disputes at particular times. Some of these are things we simply haven't thought about and probably won't. Many others are factors we cannot consistently measure across time and space, but certainly are not random since we do have some theory about them. Major examples are characteristics of particular leaders, misperceptions of relative power or intent, and processes of strategic interaction. Others are events, like the assassination of the Austrian archduke, that succeed partly because of accident and are not very predictable. These

are not easily put into our equations, but each may become important under circumstances of high international tension; i.e., preceded by some period (often months, or a year or more) of tension and threats. Despite their limitations, predictions derived from formal statistical analyses often perform better than experts. Among experts, fame and extensive media work militate against success, and foxes (generalists) do better than hedgehogs (specialists). See Tetlock (2005).

7 This reinforcement can be additive (two independent effects) or interactive (synergistic). For an interesting argument that democracy and international institutions are synergistic see Hasenclever and Weiffen (2006). Claims that the causal chain is predominantly one of conflict reducing trade and IGO linkages are not supported (Pevehouse and Russett 2006; Hegre et al. 2010).

8 For conclusions that theory and evidence support this claim see Chernoff (2004); Rousseau (2005); Gleditsch (2008); and Kinsella (2005), in dispute with Rosato (2003, 2005). Mansfield and Snyder (2005) contend that autocracies undergoing partial liberalization are more likely to engage in militarized international conflicts, but that claim vanishes when liberalization moves into the range of truly democratic institutions or when one looks at which side first used force (Oneal et al. 2003; Rousseau 2005: ch. 6; Bennett 2006; Russett 2006).

9 Even within the modern era there is some variation in the Kantian peace over different periods. Not surprisingly, the effect of democracy emerges clearly only in the twentieth century, coincident with the widening franchise, strengthens between the World Wars, and then remains strong during the cold war and afterwards. The pacific effects of trade, though weakest before 1914, are discernible throughout the past century and a quarter, but IGOs had little effect between the World Wars (Russett and Oneal 2001: 194; Oneal and Russett 2006, 242–243). Lagazio and Russett (2004) found substantial continuity using a model that derived its parameters from the pre-World War II era for an out-of-sample test in the post-World War II years.

10 This statement is based on a compilation from Thucydides and many other ancient and modern sources. It covers 232 political units, of which 33 were democratic at some or all times during the Peloponnesian War.

11 MacMillan (2003) cites normative arguments that democracies may be generally peaceful if one controls for the contexts and conditions of decisions to go to war.

12 See Levy (2008). Preemption is a cold war term for self-defense when a massive nuclear attack is believed virtually certain, imminent in hours or minutes, and could not effectively be defended against. Preventive war is to confront a rising power months or years before it can equal or surpass one's own capability. For a contemporary analysis see Doyle (2008).

13 Sometimes a state joins an existing conflict less because of past hostility to its new adversary than because of its relationship with an ally. A small state may be dragged in by a bigger one, or a big one may be dragged in by a small state, which is important to its own material status or reputation. Such triadic relationships do not fit the usual dyadic analyses, and require some form of network analysis. This links to a methodological dispute about whether even to include joiners when predicting multi-state conflicts. If the joiner shares structural characteristics (e.g., economic links or similar institutions) with one of the initial combatants, standard models may work well, but not when the joiner and its wartime ally come together for other reasons.

14 Russett and Oneal (2001) focus on the degree to which mutual trade in a dyad constrains the political system of the "weak link" larger state for which that trade by definition amounts to a smaller percentage of its GNP. For example, Japan–US trade amounts to three times as large a share of Japan's GDP as of the US economy, and US–Guatemala trade is a 500 times larger share of Guatemala's GDP than of the US economy. Great powers join most of the "universal" organizations, but do not embed themselves in as many regional or functional IGOs as do many middle and smaller states, which are more dependent on trade and on allies for security.

15 Mousseau *et al.* (2003) report that poor democracies are more likely to fight each other. But the income level it applies to is just one percent of democratic dyads in 2000 (Oneal and Russett 2005: 305–306). An attempt to replace democracy with capitalism alone as a cause of peace (Gartzke 2007) has been rebutted. Though Gartzke's finding that capitalist variables correlate with peace is robust, his dismissal of the democratic peace is driven by a bias in his sample—dyads without data on capitalist variables are dropped—and is sensitive to changing two other aspects of his model specification: regional dummies and incorrectly implemented temporal controls (Dafoe 2011). Weede (1992) showed great integrity in acknowledging quickly that the rarity of violence between democracies is better explained by democracy than by his previous interpretation of extended deterrence by superpower alliance and subordination of other states (Weede 1989).

16 Free-riding is also common in alliances during peacetime. In the big superpower alliances of the cold war era (NATO, Rio Pact, Warsaw Treaty Organization) most small members contributed much lower shares of their GDPs than did the big powers (Oneal and Whatley 1996).

17 The butterfly ballot in Florida mimicked Edward Lorenz's (1972) butterfly in the Amazon, producing the hurricane of George W. Bush's election. A comprehensive computer coding of unscripted remarks on Iraq by President Bush and six advisors (Armitage, Cheney, Powell, Rice, Rumsfeld, Wolfowitz) finds the "decider" scoring the highest on belief in ability to control events, distrust, ingroup bias, and need for power, and the lowest on self-confidence and task emphasis (Shannon and Keller 2007).

18 Machiavelli ([1512–1517] 1998: esp. II:2) says much the same about large citizen armies fighting for their own glory and interests in the Roman Republic.

19 The combination of Athenian size and wealth made possible the extravagance of its armada to Syracuse (6.30; also see Forde 1989: 52; Ober 1998: 114). An open economy with high levels of international trade and investment does not, however, serve as a marker for imperialism and increased conflict. On the contrary, contemporary states with open economies tend to be more peaceful in general, not just with other trading states (Russett and Oneal 2001: 148–149).

20 The contemporary equivalent might be the all-volunteer professional armed forces equipped with high-tech weaponry. Whether democratic or autocratic, states with armies of professional volunteers rather than conscripts have incentives to minimize their own casualties because they invest more heavily in the recruitment and training of their soldiers (Horowitz *et al.* 2007). Avant (2006) contends that democratic governments (notably the United States) which employ privatized security forces can evade some legislative restraints and transparency that might otherwise restrain them. Machiavelli ([1512–1517] 1998: II:20) also warns about uncontrolled mercenaries.

21 On the Athenian navy in particular, see Hirschfeld (1996) and Shaw (1993).

22 Also see Bueno de Mesquita and Downs (2006). Doyle (1997: 266–277) discusses liberal colonialism. Lintott (1982: ch. 3) argues that while Athens frequently installed democratic constitutions in its allied states, it exerted influence on policy through local dignitaries. For a view that democratic peace theory is perverted when claimed as a reason or excuse to spread democracy by force see Russett (2005). Raising Machiavelli's question about whether it is better to be loved or feared, Jervis (2005: 237–238) concludes that US unilateralism, especially after Iraq, has left it with neither. It squandered a unique Kantian opportunity to reshape international relations.

23 In the contemporary era, Fordham and Walker (2005) report that democracy is associated with lower military spending as a percentage of GDP (also see Goldsmith 2003) and possession of an empire with higher spending. But democracies with large empires spend more than autocracies (personal communication from Benjamin Fordham).

24 One must take care when using the term empire in the contemporary era. Kagan (1969) matches autocratic Sparta and democratic (but imperial) Athens with the Soviet Union and the United States, respectively, though he would not regard the latter as imperial. Doyle (1986a) defines an empire as controlling both internal and external policy of its subject units, whereas a hegemony allows internal autonomy and controls only external

policy. Athens often intervened in the domestic politics of its allies, and so qualifies as an empire. The United States has a mixed record: little concern with the domestic politics of many of its allies, but frequent military or political intervention to support a particular domestic order. Risse (2003) distinguishes a hegemonic leader who permits small states "voice opportunities" to keep their behavior within the accepted rules of order, from an imperial leader who plays by the rules only when it suits its interests. The Gramscian concept of self-constraint through the consensual development of ideological hegemony rather than overt imperial coercion is also relevant; e.g., Cox (1983). Münkler (2007) regards the distinction between empire and hegemony as fluid and inconsequential. Lake (2009) characterizes an empire as a negotiated relationship in which the weaker units are subordinate over a broad range of economic and security matters. Vast asymmetries of negotiating power cannot be ignored (Miller 2008).

25 Müller (2004; also Müller and Wolff 2006) distinguishes between pacifist democracies, which seek a modus vivendi with autocracies and may try to assist their transformation into democracies, and militant democracies which are fundamentally antagonistic to autocracies and may try to overthrow autocracies by force. He roots this in differences in norms, saying that the prevailing norm in a state may change with the ruling coalition and policy discourse, and external conditions. Schafer and Walker (2006) do a rigorous job of theory development and testing in comparing the attitudes of Bill Clinton and Tony Blair toward other states. They find evidence for a dyadic democratic peace in both leaders, but not for a monadic one. They characterize Blair as the more conflictual, reflecting his personal style of political action rather than differences in national culture or institutions. Neither study, of course, leads to confident predictions of which set of norms may prevail in a particular state and time.

26 Lake (1992), an early contributor to DP theory, attributes democracies' wartime success to the relative political weakness of rent-seeking expansionist leaders in democratic systems. His empirical analysis, however, tests only for victory in all wars, rather than their relative frequency of waging or winning expansionist wars.

27 A promising refinement by Jackson and Morelli (2007) proposes that the incentives of a state to go to war depend on how much the leader's risk/reward preference differs from that of the general populace. In the absence of cross-national data on preferences, however, democracy must serve as a reasonable though imperfect proxy for the institutions that would reduce such differences.

28 James Madison ([1793] 1857: 452), chief drafter of the Constitution, held that executive power to wage war is but co-equal with the legislature's, lest it be abused since, "In war, the honors and emoluments of office are to be multiplied; and it is the executive patronage under which they are to be enjoyed. It is in war, finally, that laurels are to be gathered; and it is the executive brow they are to encircle."

29 Thucydides (7.55) was well aware of the loss of the Athenians' mobilization advantage when they engaged democratic Syracuse.

30 We now see that George W. Bush and his advisor, Karl Rove, failed to construct by institutional and rhetorical means a "permanent" Republican majority able to resist the electoral mechanisms for punishing gross failure in a war of choice. They would have reduced democratic control at home while claiming to promote democracy abroad.

31 A related argument is that in the modern era the transparency of democracies' debates makes their diplomatic threats more credible when the opposition is united, and inhibits leaders from making threats when opinion is divided (Fearon 1994; Schultz 2001). Wars arising from misperceptions thus would be less likely. But I doubt this influence was very important in the Greek world, given the distance and barriers to "real-time" information on each other's intentions.

32 A list of competitive national elections in 140 countries from 1945 to 1998 ranks the United States 114th in turnout of voting age citizens (International Institute for Democracy and Electoral Assistance, www.idea.int/vt/survey/ voter_turnout_pop2-2. cfm, accessed 13 May 2008). US turnout is depressed by burdensome registration requirements, holding elections on workdays, and disfranchising felons. Of US Hispanic

men, one in every thirty-six is incarcerated as is one in every fifteen black men (Liptak 2008). The voting turnout rate would be even lower if resident noncitizens, legal and illegal, were included in the denominator. Together, noncitizens and felons amount to about 10 percent of the population (McDonald 2006). Some evidence (O'Toole and Stroble 1995) suggests that countries with compulsory voting (the opposite condition to voting restrictions) spend more public funds on housing and health and less on the military. African Americans, though generally far more opposed than whites to military action (Nincic and Nincic 2002), are under-represented in voting. Yet since the start of the all-volunteer military, minorities have been substantially over-represented in both the active duty and reserve forces, often induced by the benefits and possibilities for upward mobility. With the Iraq War and its casualties the attraction has waned, especially for African Americans, and the Army has resorted to paying large enlistment bonuses (Abruzzese 2007). Military recruitment now often focuses on high schools with many undocumented Latino immigrants who are given dubious promises of quick citizenship for themselves and their families (D. Davis 2007). Kriner and Shen (2010) report that US casualties in Iraq are not correlated with ethnicity per se, but even more than in previous wars they are concentrated at low levels of income and education, among groups that are less likely to vote.

33 In recounting Athenians' reaction to news of the final destruction of their forces at Syracuse, Thucydides (8.11) says, "When the truth sank in, the people raged at the politicians who had promoted the armada—as if they themselves had not voted for it!" Ober (1989: 336) contends that orators who tried to control the people were "never able to define a sphere of influence, authority, or power for themselves." Thucydides is himself not always consistent. When looking back on the Sicilian campaign elsewhere (2.65), he draws a more complex picture, blaming competing leaders for "surrender[ing] even policy-making to the whims of the people." Saxonhouse (2006) gives a nuanced discussion of this issue.

34 The quotations are from Kant ([1795] 1970: 100, 101, 123). Six members of both the EU and NATO require parliamentary approval before sending troops abroad, but none of the long-term global powers (France, Britain, and the United States) do so (Born and Hänggi 2005; also see Wagner 2006; Peters and Wagner 2009). Such a constraint may not be compatible with the activist foreign policy typically pursued by major powers.

3

DIMENSIONS OF RESOURCE DEPENDENCE

Some elements of rigor in concept and policy analysis[1]

Alarm over "dependence" on external sources of raw materials is not new. British opponents of changes in the Corn Laws warned in the 1840s that increased food imports would make the United Kingdom vulnerable to starvation in wartime—fears nearly realized by the German submarine campaigns of the two World Wars. Britain itself tried to block Germany's imports (especially of nitrates and petroleum) to bring that country to its knees. In the 1970s, oil dependence became an examplar of the dangers to economic and political stability posed to industrialized states from excessive reliance on a wide range of "strategic" raw materials, chiefly minerals. Such dependence, and perceived threats, became the primary rationale for preparing an American Rapid Deployment Force.

Many recent pronouncements are long on exhortation and short on analysis. They paint a bleak picture of dependence, often relying on percentages of US consumption of various metals imported in peacetime, perhaps with some examples of their military uses and the alleged unreliability of the chief producers. Thus, one often sees concern about American dependence on supplies of cobalt: 90 percent of US consumption in 1979 was imported, of which 41 percent came from Zaire, and cobalt seems to be essential to the manufacture of jet engines.

Such examples strongly appeal to the economic interests or ideology of particular listeners. High-cost domestic producers may be receptive to arguments about the need for tariffs or other protectionist measures and seek relaxation of environmental restrictions on production. Users may be anxious for government action to ensure reliable supplies or to bear the cost of maintaining a stockpile. Fervent anti-communists are receptive to images of a Soviet strategy of "resource war," and friends of South Africa see opportunities to promote a more conciliatory policy toward that state.

The harder it is to provide a rigorous concept and measures of raw material dependence, the easier it will be for these fears and appeals to find a ready audience, and the harder it will be to create a rational policy for dealing with whatever cases of dependence really exist.[2] In this article, I shall derive insights from the theoretical literature on complex interdependence, economic sanctions, and cartels, using them to establish a more rigorous set of dimensions by which to measure dependence and criteria for the importance of those dimensions. On the basis of these theory-based measures, we shall be able to establish whether the United States is as resource-dependent as alarmists contend. Only by such rigor can we hope to avoid confounding individual or group interests with vague and potentially dangerous appeals to national interests.

Robert Keohane and Joseph Nye's definition of dependence will suffice for my purposes: they term it "a state of being determined or significantly affected by external forces." (Keohane and Nye 1977: 8). By contrast with the term interdependence, "dependence" thus conveys an asymmetry, an imbalance, of costly effects. Dependence includes the phenomena typically included in dependency (or *dependencia*) theory, but it is certainly not limited to poor or weak states. Indeed, the impetus for this article comes from allegations that large, rich, industrialized economies also suffer from dependence. The degree to which that claim is true, or is balanced by other states' dependence (hence inter-dependence), or is made trivial by weaker partners' dependence, becomes an empirical question requiring a careful measurement strategy. Dependency theory typically concerns itself with the degree to which asymmetric relations lead to conditioning or control—power over decisions—in the dependent state (Caporaso 1978: 13–44). The concern with power is part of the issue with large industrialized states (most obviously in the effects of being subject to an embargo or boycott), but equally at issue are the effects of price increases or supply interruptions that external actors may impose without any political purpose or even involuntarily.

Keohane and Nye also distinguish between two elements of dependence, sensitivity and vulnerability. Sensitivity, they say,

> involves degrees of responsiveness within a policy framework—how quickly do changes in one country bring costly changes in another, and how great are the costly effects? It is measured not merely by the volume of flows across borders, but also by the costly effects of changes in transactions on the societies or governments.

Vulnerability, by contrast, is defined as "an actor's liability to suffer costs imposed by external events even after policies have been altered . . . Vulnerability dependence can be measured only by the costliness of making effective adjustments to a changed environment over a period of time." (Keohane and Nye 1977: 12–13). This distinction is not as clear as one might hope. Nevertheless, the two elements together point to a variety of considerations: the size, in volume or value, of flows; the impact of the flows on a country's economy (e.g., impact on production or on inflation rates); and the cost of adjustments by finding substitute suppliers or materials. Costs may be immediate or protracted, and they may reflect both market adjustments by economic actors and deliberate policy interventions by governments. A government may, for instance, establish a stockpile of raw materials to be drawn upon in a military or economic emergency. By meeting the costs of the stockpile, the government may substantially reduce the economy's dependence. In the event an interruption of supply occurs, the value of lost imports may be high. By drawing on the stockpile, however, the economy will not be vulnerable to the interruption in flow and thus to additional costs from inflation or from lost production of goods using the commodity.

Any measurement of dependence must be rooted in an awareness that fears of dependence in industrialized economies arise from several different economic and political possibilities. The first involves changes in market conditions that suppliers impose deliberately, for economic reasons: in effect, the possibility of significant price increases imposed by a single supplier or, more likely, by a cartel, in order to reap monopoly (or oligopoly) profits. Price increases imposed by bauxite producers in the 1970s provide an example, and the literature on international cartels is apposite.

A second possibility concerns changes in market conditions imposed deliberately, but for political reasons, by suppliers or hostile third parties. Here we refer chiefly to embargoes, boycotts, or trade sanctions, such as the American economic sanctions against the Soviet Union for its actions in Poland and Afghanistan or OPEC's ostensible embargo (rather than price-oriented cartel action) against Israel and its allies. Here, too, there is a substantial international political economy literature.

The third possibility includes changes in market conditions (price or availability of a commodity) that result from essentially uncontrollable events, such as weather, climatic change, or international conflict involving the production or shipping of an exporting nation. Particularly worrisome is political or social conflict within an exporting state that reduces the ability of that country to maintain its previous level of exports. Here we refer to involuntary actions of the exporter, as contrasted with deliberate decisions to raise prices or deny goods, and probably the most relevant literature is on the political stability of underdeveloped countries.

Measures of dependence

Since we are concerned with various threats, various responses, and both short-term and long-term effects, no single or simple measure of dependence can suffice. The difficulty is to devise a measurement strategy that avoids either becoming just a "laundry list" or (by summing together incommensurate elements with an arbitrary weighting scheme) producing the appearance of precision where the reality is utterly absent.[3] The result will necessarily be a multidimensional measure of dependence, but we can combine some elements and suggest circumstances under which particular elements may be important. Furthermore, we can identify some elements that constitute necessary, if not sufficient, conditions of dependence: if they are absent, no alarm over other elements is warranted.

1.   The most common measure of dependence is simply imports of a commodity
     as a percentage of a country's total consumption of that commodity. Using
     this measure, one can quickly accumulate a substantial list of commodities
     on which the United States is dependent, and a longer list for the European
     Community (EC) or Japan. But if an importer can choose among many possible
     suppliers of a commodity, in a reasonably competitive market, the importer
     can hardly be characterized as dependent in a politically or economically
     meaningful way, since the costs of dependence are minimal.

2.   If the problem is one of lack of diversity, or concentration, of supplier
     countries, then some measure of that concentration is appropriate. Better than
     simply the percentage imported from the largest supplier is a measure that takes
     into account the relative importance of several major suppliers. The classic
     instance in the economics literature is Hirschman's index of concentration; in
     writings on international politics, often Ray and Singer's CON (Hirschman
     1945 and Ray and Singer 1973: 403–437). These indices reflect the percentage
     share of goods coming from each supplier, normed in such a way that zero
     represents a country importing the commodity in question from many suppliers,
     all small, and 100 indicates a country taking all its imports of the good from
     a single supplier. A high index of concentration on one or a few suppliers,
     particularly in combination with a high ratio of imports to consumption, would
     seem a necessary condition of dependence. But it is hardly sufficient, for it says
     nothing about the reliability of those suppliers, possible alternative sources of
     supply, or the importance of the commodity.

3.   One crude way to tap the matter of importance is to measure the value of
     imports of the commodity as a percentage of the country's gross national pro-
     duct (GNP). By such a measure, oil is far more important than cobalt.

4.   The availability of alternative supplies of the commodity—supplies not limited
     to those available from current suppliers—is a crucial element in any evaluation.
     This category subsumes several different aspects of opportunity to find
     alternative supplies.

4a. The elasticity of supply from foreign and domestic producers is the percentage
     increase in additional supply that will be forthcoming in response to a given
     percentage increase in price paid by the consumer. In the short run, it is
     determined partly by the amount of idle productive capacity in the industry;
     in the long run, by worldwide reserves (in the ground) of the commodity.
     Reserves are a function of geological conditions, information about mineral
     deposits, technology, and price. Technological developments, such as new
     recovery techniques or deep-sea mining procedures, can make economically
     accessible reserves of what previously had been unexploitable deposits. Price
     increases can also turn previously uneconomic deposits into reserves worth
     mining. By common convention, short-term supply elasticities usually refer
     to at most a one-year period, and longer-term elasticities to a three-to-five
     year span. Longer-term elasticities are usually impossible to calculate with any

confidence. There is room for governments to make policy interventions, developing opportunities for long-term supply.

Several measures are relevant to computing short-term elasticities. They include domestic production as a share of consumption and the ratio of a country's imports to total world production, or possibly to total world trade in the commodity. But especially in the short run, the market structure of the industry matters—oligopolistic or cartelized producers may be able to extract substantial price increases even with idle capacity. Crude measures of concentration by producer companies or by all producer countries (not just of concentration by extant suppliers to the consuming country) thus give some indication, if but a very incomplete one, of relative supply elasticities. And in international trade, the political willingness of supplier countries may play some role, particularly when the initial damage stems from a boycott. Because of these uncertainties, it may be difficult to estimate even short-term supply elasticities to any satisfactory extent.

4b. Supplies may be expanded by means other than new production. Another major opportunity for policy intervention is the establishment of a government-owned or government-operated stockpile of the commodity, as, for example, the US strategic stockpile. Establishment of such a stockpile, however, does not imply easy decisions about the circumstances under which it is to be drawn upon. Should its holdings be made available only in response to a military threat to national security, or to any threat of severe economic dislocation? If economic difficulties are included, how much of a price increase should trigger release of the commodity? If the stockpile is drawn upon too soon and prices continue upward, the stockpile may be exhausted when it is most needed. If release from the stockpile is delayed, inflation or unemployment may already be severe by the time the commodity finally becomes available. Some allied countries may also have access to US stockpiles, and their needs must be considered.

Stockpiles may also be held privately, perhaps by producers or importers and, more commonly, by consumers, especially by fabricating industries for which the commodity constitutes an important component (e.g., chromium for the steel industry). Large stockpiles may even be held by speculators, like those who have developed a lively enterprise in assaying, stockpiling, and insuring holdings of "strategic" metals in Rotterdam. Private stockpile holders do not respond to the same cues as do the managers of government stockpiles. While the latter are supposed to be motivated by concerns for national interests—such as the effects of price and quantity on employment, income, and security—the former are primarily concerned with effects on their own profit margins. Interest rates are also very important to private stockpilers, since the funds required to finance purchase and storage must be diverted from profitable activities or borrowed.

The interests of private and public stockpilers not only differ, they frequently conflict. Private consumers, for instance, would naturally prefer that the government should bear the costs of stockpiling. If the government will not operate a stockpile, they may. But if the government does stockpile aggressively, private holders may draw down their own stockpiles, partly because the government is acting as the insurer and partly because they expect the government to release its stockpile at a price that will make private speculation unprofitable. Thus, public commodity holdings may be accorded excessive significance if their effects on private holdings are not taken into account (Wright and Williams 1982: 341–353; US Congress, Office of Technology Assessment 1976; 1983).

4c. Supplies of many raw materials may also be extended by recycling, with readiness to recycle being significantly affected by price increases. About 10 percent of US chromium consumption is currently provided by recycling, and the percentages for more valuable metals, like gold and platinum, are higher.

5a. Analogous to elasticity of supply is demand elasticity, defined as the percentage decrease in demand for a product associated with a given percentage increase in its price. The availability of substitutes is relevant both for the final product containing a commodity and substitutes for the commodity itself. In the latter case, we properly refer to cross-price elasticities for substitutes.

Elasticities depend on such factors as the nature of the demand for the final product (the demand for military hardware seems relatively insensitive to price considerations) and whether the commodity represents a significant component of total cost. Price increases may stimulate either direct substitution of a similar product or conservation. The latter is actually a form of substitution, though a more distant one: for example, if gasoline prices go too high, one may buy gasohol or conserve fuel by consuming more home entertainment. Conservation of home heating oil may be accomplished by "consuming" (installing) insulation. In the case of cobalt, however, demand proved quite inelastic in the short run after the 1977 price increases, partly because it was used in jet engines (military demand), partly because no substitute with adequate technical characteristics exists, and partly because even a fourfold increase in cobalt costs made only a very small difference in the total cost of the manufactured product.

Technological development as it would affect long-term price elasticities is, of course, difficult to anticipate. But even short- and medium-term elasticities can be very hard to estimate, particularly if the analyst has no experience with massive price increases on which to draw. Cobalt illustrates the difficulty. A report published in 1974 suggested that the short-run (1-year) price elasticity for that metal was −0.68, the longer term (3–5 years) elasticity −1.71 (quite high). A study just a few years later, however, drew on the experience of a sharp run-up of cobalt prices in 1977 to predict long-term price elasticity at only −0.32—half that of the *short*-term elasticity given in the earlier report! (Congressional testimony of James C. Burrows, reported in Tilton 1977: 66; and US Congress, Office of Technology Assessment 1982: 9).

5b. "Criticalness" of a material for an economy or for a state is a related but still separable aspect. The volume or dollar value of a commodity consumed may be quite trivial by some measure like imports/GNP. Demand may be very inelastic, but still the commodity's absence may not critically affect national security. For a component of major military hardware, however, the situation is quite different. In that case, a shortage may stimulate not only a sharp price increase but political demands to rectify the shortage, by drastic measures if necessary. There is no simple measure of criticalness. The price that should be paid for a given increment to national security always varies with the individual making the assessment, and the amount of additional security that can be bought with a given new expenditure is subject to notoriously subjective estimates. Ideology and political considerations weigh heavily. They may be kept in perspective with a measure of defense-related consumption as a percentage of total consumption.

Even the attempt to measure the economic effects of a shortage of supplies faces great difficulties. For example, moderate-sized shortages may be compensated for fairly easily by substitution of the material or of the final product, perhaps with the assistance of government controls to protect access to supplies for some "kernel" of critical industries. But at some point, the shortage will become so great that even these kernel industries cannot obtain enough, and the bottleneck will shut down large segments of the economy. Allied bombing, for instance, had little effect on essential German military production throughout most of World War II. By the spring of 1945, however, the destruction of German capacity had become so severe that major sectors "crashed." Some such effects show up in sophisticated input-output analysis (see, for example, Morgenstern *et al.* 1973: ch. 8). There is in this case, as with the estimation of elasticities, good reason to think the effects may be distinctly nonlinear. A crude measure of the contribution to GNP by industries that use a given commodity captures these effects very imperfectly.

6. Concern about "critical" raw materials available from only one or a few foreign sources will be serious only if those sources are regarded as unreliable suppliers. No source is usually deemed as reliable as one within the boundaries of one's own country, but neighbors (e.g., Mexico and Canada for the United States) may be regarded as good enough. "Unreliable" may be defined by a geopolitical analyst chiefly as "distant," particularly if the distance requires ocean transportation. More often, however, a Western analyst implies one or a combination of the following factors.

6a. Hostile sources. Reliance on the Soviet Union as principal supplier is thought to be especially unwise. Soviet-aligned or other Marxist governments may come under similar suspicion. In fact, there is very little historical experience of Marxist governments using economic sanctions against industrial states for political purposes, but it is of course easy to imagine. Western states have themselves used sanctions fairly extensively, if not very successfully.[4] One could obviously not rely on supplies from the Soviet Union in the event of a war with that country. Concern applies to possible alternative governments as well as to current ones. Iran turned from a reliable supplier of oil into a hostile, unreliable one. Much the same might happen with South Africa (particularly, ironically, if the United States is too closely identified with the current regime).

6b. Unstable regimes. Governments may be presently friendly and reliable, but their long-term future may be in considerable doubt (e.g., Saudi Arabia). This factor is not just a matter of potential regime hostility. A regime that is simply unable to preserve sufficient domestic order to maintain supplies poses an equivalent threat. Mines must be kept operating; electricity supplied; railroads, pipelines, and ports running. Faced with large-scale domestic terrorism or insurgency, the government of a less developed country (LDC) may not be able to provide these conditions. Indeed, its domestic opponents will see deprivation of export earnings as a highly effective means for over-turning the regime. Nor can a new, revolutionary regime necessarily depend on the quick reestablishment of former economic conditions. Post-revolutionary Iran's sharp reduction in oil exports in 1979 (from about 5.5 million barrels per day to about 2 million) stemmed less from any deliberate policy choice than from continued social and political chaos.

6c. Cartel-prone sources. Even if not seen as hostile or politically unstable, foreign suppliers may be regarded as likely to engage in cartel behavior: not denying supplies of an important raw material but raising its price substantially. The probability of large price increases depends in part on current market structure (whether an effective cartel already exists—it does not for most raw materials) and in part on elements we have already identified, such as concentration of suppliers and conditions affecting the elasticities of supply and demand. But cartel-proneness also depends on various other factors, many of them political. One is the closeness of ties between supplier and consumer states. For instance, Australia is a major source of bauxite on the world market, and that fact is often regarded (perhaps wishfully) as a restraint on price increases by LDC bauxite producers. Other factors include previous and current ties among the various producer states who are potential candidates for membership in a cartel. Again, the bauxite producers are thought to be culturally, and perhaps politically, more diverse than are members of OPEC and hence less likely to be able to cooperate effectively over a long period.

Other economic/political considerations include the producer economy or regime's dependence on export sales of the commodity. Even a hostile government is unlikely to cut off foreign sales of its country's product if a high proportion of national income, or of foreign-exchange earnings, or of government revenue, is derived from those sales. A cartel aims not to cut off sales to a particular customer entirely but to raise prices. Nevertheless, a cartel member has to balance the needs for current earnings against the possibility of future income. As with some OPEC members, governments with large, poor populations, relatively modest reserves of a commodity, and ambitious economic development programs may feel strong needs to maximize current earnings, even if large price increases stimulate substitution for their commodity in the long run. The financial reserves of the state, as well as its level and sources of current earnings, are relevant.[5] Some of the components of cartel-proneness are fairly easy to measure, but others are not. Combining them into some overall, composite indicator is extremely hard and cannot be done with any precision. Also very important is the variety of possible countermeasures available to the consumer should a producer take hostile or price-raising action. We must relax our implicit assumption of mere reactivity by consumers, and consider the various asymmetries which may give substantial countervailing power to purchasers.

7. *Symmetries* are especially significant where large, developed countries are dealing with smaller, poorer countries that produce raw materials—as is very often the case. If supplier countries are hostile or cartel-prone, what vulnerabilities do they have? One might respond by constructing corresponding measures of supplier countries' dependence on goods that they must import, with indicators of imports as a percentage of GNP, concentration of suppliers, and so forth, in key production and distribution facilities. Just as the commodity represents a given percentage of the importer's GNP, earnings from that commodity represent a percentage—usually a much larger one—of the exporter's GNP. But attention to international trade in goods misses almost the whole point about LDC "dependence" (penetration and asymmetrical control). Commodity dependence is but a pale shadow of the range of instruments of reverse control facing less developed countries, and here the large body of writing on dependency is most certainly relevant. A measurement strategy for addressing this issue has been outlined elsewhere (see Duvall *et al.* 1981). In the case of the United States and Saudi Arabia, the network of mutual ties (interdependence) is very strong, diverse, and weighted in favor of the United States. Consider, for example, military ties, cultural penetration, technological dependence, and, of course, Saudi deposits of capital in American financial institutions and Saudi needs for continued prosperity in the markets that import Saudi oil.

It is perhaps not hard to measure each of these asymmetrical elements of dependence individually, but it is very difficult to imagine how they can be combined into some meaningful composite index. This task is all the more formidable because reverse ties are so diverse and because so many are much less tangible than commodity transactions. The need to make some such assessment when considering potentially hostile or cartel-prone suppliers is obvious. But when we consider unstable states—whose reliability as suppliers is in question not because of matters under their own volition but because of conditions that may be quite beyond their governments' control—we find that the asymmetrical aspects of dependence matter much less. Whatever the degree to which its fate is bound to its export purchaser, an exporting government may be simply unable to maintain a reliable, low-cost supply of its country's product.

An illustration

Examples from four raw materials illustrate the varying relationships among these different components. One, bauxite and its intermediate product alumina, is the source of the metal aluminum. Bauxite/alumina is a component of the US strategic stockpile, though for several reasons most observers regard America as substantially less dependent on unreliable foreign sources for aluminum than for two other metals. Chromite (and its intermediate product ferrochrome) and the platinum-group metals (including palladium, iridium, and rhodium) usually appear on lists of materials whose users are dependent on foreign sources. For comparative purposes, I include petroleum, whose price and supply conditions first triggered widespread alarm about supplies of raw materials and which has now become the standard with which most other "strategic" materials are usually compared. The data in Table 3.1 are sometimes approximate but reasonably accurate for the years 1979–1980.

By the first two measures (imports as a percentage of consumption and concentration of import suppliers), the United States is more dependent on all three of the metals than on petroleum. Furthermore, while we have no direct estimates of the elasticity of supply, we can measure several of the contributions to that elasticity (high concentration of producing countries, US imports taking a large proportion of world production). Such factors are quite a bit more unfavorable for the metals than they are for oil, suggesting a highly inelastic supply.

These aspects of the metals markets are, however, mitigated by several countervailing considerations. Imports amount to only a very small percentage of GNP, suggesting a much lighter inflationary impact on the economy from a large price jump for metals than what occurred with oil. Petroleum once consumed offers no possibility for recycling, but for each of the metals, recycling makes a discernible contribution to US supplies. All three metals are also held extensively in private and government stockpiles, amounting in the first two cases to 2 and 3.5 years' supplies, and to 0.75 of a year's supply even for the platinum group. Some minimal inventories must, of course, be maintained in private hands simply to maintain orderly supplies and production, but the same proposition is also true of oil (the pipelines must be kept filled), and the safety margin represented by extant supplies is very much larger than with either private holdings of oil or the Strategic Petroleum Reserve, which in 1979–1980 was especially small.

Estimates of demand elasticity contain, as noted, a great potential for error. Nevertheless, what estimates we have indicate that US demand for these metals is much more responsive to price increases than is the US demand for oil. Whatever the talk about some metals, chiefly chromium and the platinum group, being vital to high-technology weapons systems for national defense, the fact is that the defense industry uses only a very small fraction of total consumption of these metals. Needs (inelastic demand) in the defense industry might prevent substitution there, but the overall fairly high elasticities and the small defense share of consumption suggest that adequate substitutability exists in other industries. Problems might arise if the

TABLE 3.1 Some aspects of US dependence on selected raw materials, 1979–1980

	Bauxite/alumina	Chromite/ferrochrome	Platinum-group metals	Petroleum
1. Imports as % of consumption	70[a]	90	89	46
2. Concentration of import suppliers (CON)	53	51	69[b]	31
3. Imports as % of GNP	0.05	0.01	0.05	3
4a. Elasticity of supply-components				
Concentration of countries by production (CON)	40	48	69[b]	33
Imports as % of world production	25	14	50	13
Domestic production as % of consumption	5[a]	0	1	54
4b. Government stockpile as % of annual consumption	100[a]	250	50	1.5
Private stockpiles as % of annual consumption	100[a]	100	25	15
4c. Recycling as % of consumption	25[a]	10	12	0
5a. Elasticity of demand: 1 year	−0.13	−0.1	−0.05	−0.05
3–5 years	−0.80	−1.0	−0.65	−0.5
5b. Criticalness				
% of consumption used in defense	3.8	6.8	3.1	8
Commodity-using industries as % of GNP	8	16	2.5	75
6. Reliability of foreign sources major supplier countries, with % of imports	Jamaica 33 Australia 27 Guinea 15 Suriname 14	South Africa 44 Soviet Union 12 Zimbabwe 8 Turkey 8	South Africa 50(62)[b] Soviet Union 22 United Kingdom (12)	Saudi Arabia 22 Nigeria 18 Venezuela 15 Libya 10
6a. Hostility of suppliers (in order on scale of 1–5)[c]	2,1,3,3 (2)	1,5,2,1 (2)	1,5,1 (2)	2,2,2,5 (2)
6b. Instability of supplier regimes (1–5)[c]	2,1,2,4 (2)	2,1,2,2 (2)	2,1,1 (2)	3,3,2,2 (3)
6c. Cartel-proneness (1–5)[c]	(3)	(1)	(2)	(5)
7. Symmetry (suppliers' invulnerability to nonmilitary countermeasures [1–5])	1,3,3,3 (2)	4,5,3,3 (4)	4,5,3 (4)	2,4,3,5 (3)

a. Data on bauxite/alumina sometimes include aluminum metal. Thus imports are approximately 94 percent of bauxite/alumina consumption by value, but 25 percent of US consumption of aluminum is derived from recycled aluminum rather than from bauxite or alumina. Thus import reliance (row 1) is given as only 70 percent. Similarly, "private stockpiles" refers to both aluminum metal and bauxite and alumina stocks as related to total aluminum consumption.

b. Imports of platinum-group metals are derived almost exclusively from South Africa, so import concentration is computed as if South Africa directly supplied the share coming indirectly through the United Kingdom.

c. Entries in parentheses give weighted average of individual countries.

Sources: US Department of Commerce, Bureau of the Census (1981); *Commodity Yearbook, 1982* (1982); Deese and Nye (1981). Demand elasticity estimates from Hogan (1981: 296), and congressional testimony as reported in Tilton (1977).

United States tried to fight a large-scale war calling for a vastly expanded military effort over several years, but that is not a likely event. Otherwise, the nation's defense will not collapse from a shortage of these metals, none of which is as important to other industries as is virtually ubiquitous petroleum. The possibility of economic bottlenecks should not be exaggerated.

Finally, the reliability of relevant foreign sources for these metals seems at least as high as or higher than for oil. About half of US foreign suppliers of bauxite/ alumina are nearby, in the Caribbean. The other suppliers are more distant, but their governments seem no more hostile and in political terms are probably more stable than those of the oil-supplying states. The judgments embodied in these codings are necessarily subjective and disputable, but I doubt they are worse than those that either a crude count of previous events (e.g., past irregular government changes) or even theory-based quantitative indicators of potential instability and hostility would produce.[6] Of the major metal-supplying governments, only the Soviet Union sits at the extreme of bad political relations. For bauxite/alumina, Australia is a politically close and stable ally. The current Seaga government in Jamaica is trying to attract American investment with a favorable business climate, and despite sporadic violence, the country has a history of orderly, democratic elections and power transfers. Guinea is a Marxist state but not a Soviet satellite, and the regime has been stable through twenty-five years of independence. Suriname had seemed stable until the overthrow of its government in 1982. Its stability and political orientation are now questionable, but it is the least important of America's four chief suppliers of bauxite and alumina.

The situation may be a little harder to estimate for the other two metals, but it is not really unfavorable. The major supplier of both, South Africa, is the subject of some official (and much greater private) censure for its apartheid policies, but such censure does not significantly affect South African policy toward the United States. (The South African government must retain cordial relations toward the United States, and knows it.) Zimbabwe is governed by an ostensibly Marxist leader but has tried to retain a favorable environment for business and foreign investment. Even were Zimbabwe's "hostility" score revised up to 3, the preponderant role of South Africa as a chromium producer and supplier would keep the weighted average score at about 2. Turkey is a NATO ally; while it has witnessed many irregular changes of government in the past decades, the regime's basically pro-Western orientation has never been in question. South Africa's form of government seems stable. While there is always the possibility of an explosive change, it is surely no more volatile than Saudi Arabia. A social upheaval in South Africa would cause an immediate interruption in supplies, but in the long run, a black-dominated government would be likely to return to normal economic activities much as those in Angola and Zimbabwe have done.

Cartel-proneness is also difficult to judge. OPEC is surely the most successful major commodity cartel so far, and even it has looked rather shaky in recent years. By comparison, the International Bauxite Association has achieved only moderate success (approximately doubling prices between 1973 and 1976, and no more since), as might be inferred from the diversity of its producer countries. The chances of an effective chromium cartel being formed by three such different regimes as South Africa, Zimbabwe, and the Soviet Union seem very small—though they would doubtless increase if a black government ever came to power in South Africa. The likelihood of Soviet-South African cooperation on a platinum cartel is no higher, but I have coded cartel-proneness for that metal at 2 in deference to South Africa's near-dominance of the market. Nevertheless, the current South African government depends heavily on its image as a reliable source of raw materials and "friend of the West"; to be perceived as a price-gouger would be very dangerous for it. Large-scale price-raising or embargo-like behavior is also inhibited, in the case of bauxite/ alumina, by the susceptibility of small, poor economies to American counter-action. (Australia is less economically vulnerable but very dependent on the United States for its military security.) The relative invulnerability of the major producers of the other metals (South Africa, Soviet Union), however, is surely much greater for those fairly autarchic states than for Saudi Arabia with its many aspects of dependence on the United States. These last elements, reliability and symmetry, can be buttressed by the (admittedly also very subjective) estimates by several authorities of major interruptions in supply.[7] The important point is that all the estimates for strategic metals do not, by comparison with those for oil, appear very high.

The balance sheet

All of the data in the table would benefit from further discussion and refinement, but they are sufficient for us now to make some summary points about conceptual clarity and measurement of raw material dependence. Four elements constitute necessary but not sufficient conditions for an accurate judgment that a country is "dependent" on external commodity supplies. All four of those conditions must be satisfied to justify such a judgment. In addition, at least one of a set of further conditions must also be present. But even all of these together are not sufficient for a final judgment of "dependence," for a set of mitigating conditions can, if sufficiently powerful, vitiate the judgment.

The necessary but not sufficient conditions are items 1, 2, 4a, and 6. Imports as a percentage of consumption (item 1) and concentration of import suppliers (2) are almost surely necessary conditions for any judgment of high dependence. If imports do not constitute a "large" share of consumption, or there are many alternative external suppliers, international supply disruptions from one or a few countries need not be much feared.

Supply from other sources must be relatively inelastic (4a). If additional supplies can be obtained at little additional cost from unused or underused foreign sources, or from new domestic production, dependence is again not serious. The same applies to a determination that the largest foreign suppliers are in some way unreliable (6). If not, then the political and economic consequences of dependence are likely to be minimal. But not even when all four of these conditions are satisfied can a judgment of meaningful "dependence" be sustained.

Conditions of which at least one is necessary but not sufficient are items 3, 5a, and 5b. In addition to constituting a large share of consumption, imports of the commodity must have real importance to the health of the economy—not just to minor consumption goods or luxuries. One possibility is that imports constitute a large percentage of the importing country's GNP (3), with the implication of severe potential effects on the general level of prices or employment. Similar, but not identical, concerns apply to other aspects of demand for the material: that the demand be quite inelastic (5a), perhaps because the commodity is "critical" (5b) to the defense industry or is a major component in production in very large segments of the economy. At least one of these aspects is necessary, though in practice they (especially 3 and 5b) are likely to go together anyway.

Lastly, several conditions (4b, 4c, and 7) may sharply mitigate what otherwise looks like a situation of high dependence. One is a relatively favorable opportunity for recycling (4c), which is a way for "domestic production" to assume greater prominence. Another, quite different, is a symmetry (or even a positive asymmetry) of vulnerabilities with foreign suppliers (7). If the suppliers are vulnerable to counter-measures, the chances of deterring deliberate hostility or vigorous cartel-like behavior are greater (though the chances of a regime becoming unstable are not affected.)

Perhaps most important—chiefly because it is the most open to policy choice and deliberate control—is the matter of stockpiles (4b).[8] A government can protect its economy by building up national stockpiles of critical materials, or by encouraging expansion of privately held stockpiles by government subsidy, tax incentives, or legal fiat. Stockpiling is particularly appropriate for strategic metals because of the ease of storing them, their high value per unit of volume, and resistance to deterioration. If the stockpiles are large enough (perhaps as much as several years' worth of consumption), the threat from external dependence can be made minimal even when *none* of the other conditions are favorable. Not even all of them together will suffice.

These points illustrate the folly of simply compiling a laundry list of elements of vulnerability, or of constructing a summary index by awarding points to each element. One must think in terms of necessary, sufficient, and mitigating conditions. The need emerges clearly from Table 3.2, which gives some summary judgments to the numerical estimates of Table 3.1.[9]

By the first set of "all necessary, but not sufficient" conditions, the three metals generally rank high and well above oil. (Estimated reliability of major suppliers is the sole exception.) These conditions alone seem to justify fears about assured access to foreign supplies. Such fears become more remote, however, when we look at the next set of conditions, of which at least one must be present in addition to those in the first set. Save for the inelastic demand for platinum, the situation for the metals looks more favorable than for oil, and the metals meet none of the conditions at a high level. Finally, they look even better on the mitigating conditions (where the scale is reversed, and "High" indicates *non*dependence). Some resources can be provided by recycling, and the bauxite/alumina producers are

TABLE 3.2 Summary judgments of aspects of US dependence

Conditions	Bauxite/ alumina	Chromite/ ferrochrome	Platinum group	Petroleum
All necessary, but not sufficient				
1. Imports/consumption	H	H	H	M
2. Import concentration	H	H	H	M
4a. Inelastic supply	M–H	M–H	H	L–M
6. Unreliable	M	L–M	L–M	M–H
At least one necessary, but not even all sufficient				
3. Imports/GNP	L	L	L	H
5a. Inelastic demand	M	M	H	H
5b. Criticalness	L	M	L	H
Mitigating				
4b. Stockpiles	H	H	M	L
4c. Recycling	M	L–M	L–M	Nil
7. Symmetry	H	L	L	M

Note: L is low, M medium, and H high.

very vulnerable to counterpressures. Most pertinent of all are the government strategic stockpile and its private counterparts, which provide very substantial insurance against supply interruptions or rapid price jumps.[10] These large stockpiles, together with domestic production and reasonable shifting of consumption from inessential (more elastic) to essential demand, give great protection against serious harm to the economy or the national security of the United States. The interests of particular firms may be endangered, and those firms may be politically influential. But their interests should not be confused with national interests.

Doubtless the analysis needs to be refined and extended to other commodities. It also needs to be applied to other industrialized countries, like Japan and the members of the European Community. For those countries, the numerical results often would look less favorable,[11] though the potential strength of those states might enable them to take more effective domestic countermeasures. In any case, the logic and measurement strategy employed here makes it clear that American access to raw materials should not be exaggerated. In consequence, one should be skeptical about allegations of a need for intervention by a Rapid Deployment Force to assure supplies of those materials.

Notes

1   I thank the General Service Foundation for support of this research; Michio Halada for research assistance; and Thomas Biersteker, Paul Bracken, Jim Lindsay, Miroslav Nincic, H. Bradford Westerfield, and Brian Wright for comments.

2   Examples of such a mixture of rhetoric and policy recommendations can be found in Council on Economics and National Security (1981), and Miller *et al.* (1981). Similar

considerations have repeatedly been voiced by members of the Reagan administration and by Alexander Haig when president of United Technologies Inc. Magdoff (1969: ch. 2), made many of the same points earlier, from a critical perspective.

3 Two examples of a laundry list converted to a single index by equal weighting of all elements (compounded by extremely subjective "measures" of many elements) are King (1977), and Suprowicz (1981: ch. 15). More general, and much better, attempts to devise measurements of dependence are Caporaso (1974), and especially Richardson (1981).

4 The literature on economic sanctions is vast. Two recent contributions are Renwick (1981); and Nincic and Wallensteen (1984).

5 The most complete political and economic theoretical statement on cartels is probably Bobrow and Kudrle (1976: 3–56). Other treatments include Bergsten et al. (1978: ch. 3); Doran (1977); and Krasner (1974: 68–83). The more recent decline in OPEC's effectiveness has diminished most observers' expectations that other producers' cartels could have marked, sustained impact on prices.

6 One who disagrees might, alternatively, measure hostility by the COPDAB or WEIS indicators of conflict and cooperation, though they suffer serious reliability problems. See, for example, Howell et al. (1983). For 1976 both Australia and South Africa had COPDAB cooperation/conflict scores toward the United States of over 10, while the Soviet Union showed a score of –4.

7 One appraisal of chromium supply prospects put the chances of a medium shortage (10–50 percent of supply for more than six months) of chromite/ferrochrome at about 20 percent over the period 1980–1985, and the chances of a larger shortage (over 50 percent shortfall for more than six months) at under 10 percent. The main contributor to these likelihoods was the author's estimate of the chance of major violence in South Africa. He made no estimates for platinum, but with much the same players, the chances would presumably be about the same. By contrast, he put the odds for similar disruptions of bauxite/alumina supply at under 10 percent to nil. For further comparison, a 1980 US government study of the chances of a major oil supply shortfall from foreign action was using ranges of 5–20 percent for a one-year interruption of one-third of American oil consumption at some time during the decade. This appraisal is of the same order of magnitude as the estimates for chromium and much higher than that for bauxite/aluminum. Metals estimates are by Fischman (1980: 500, 512); petroleum estimates are reported in Hogan (1981: 298).

8 Tilton and Landsberg (1983) support this conclusion.

9 Note that the scale is essentially limited by the commodities listed in the table. If we were to add some other domestically produced commodity, like wheat, the lower (favorable) end of the scales would drop substantially. The upper end also lacks a firm anchor, since we cannot definitively say how much "dependence" justifies a particular response like military intervention.

10 In 1975 the Office of Minerals Policy Development, US Department of the Interior, estimated the optimal size of the strategic chromium stockpile. On the assumption of a 20 percent chance of an embargo lasting four years, the office's optimum stockpile was just under 1.3 million tons, which happens to be the actual holdings of the stockpile in 1981. On the same probability estimate, the same size stockpile would be optimal for containing serious cartel-induced price increases for more than three years. Reported in US Congress, Office of Technology Assessment (1976).

11 See the comparisons in Landsberg and Tilton (1982: 75, 100).

4

US HEGEMONY

Gone or merely diminished, and how does it matter?[1]

Prognoses for stability and cooperation in the international political economy depend heavily on assessments of changes in the relative power of the United States, Japan, and other major powers. Has US hegemony declined greatly over recent years? Much of the recent literature on "hegemonic stability" has been devoted to explaining the effects of a decline in US hegemony on the international system since the highpoint of US dominance immediately after 1945. In a variant of the theme, scholars have searched for ways to maintain the international regime established during that hegemony. Others have perceived an ethnocentric bias in some of this angst (for example, Strange 1982a).

The premise of a major decline in US hegemony has, however, gone largely unexamined, and it rests at the heart of any consideration of Japan's role in the international system. I suspect that my Japanese colleagues, especially, will give some credence to my conclusion that the decline in US hegemony is easily exaggerated. If so, I further suspect that will in part be because of the great sensitivity of Japanese (and other non-American analysts) to the dual and interlinked domains of international political economy and security.

In this chapter I make the familiar but crucial distinction between power base and power as control over outcomes. I am much readier to concede decline in the former—though it, too, can be exaggerated, especially by selecting an unusual baseline for evaluating later developments—than in the latter. Simple power variants of hegemonic stability theory predict that power base and control over outcomes would decay simultaneously. For reasons made clear below, collective goods theory —a key component of the hegemonic stability literature—seems to predict both that the achievement of these goods will decline and that they will be achieved only to suboptimal degree. Turning then to control over outcomes—the achievement of various goods in the global system and the regimes by which those goods are achieved—I distinguish between security goods and economic goods. A sensitivity to demands and achievements in the domain of international security helps to temper assessments, based primarily on political economy, that the decline has been great. I evaluate the degree to which achievement of those goods has in fact declined in the past three or four decades, and I try to develop some assessment, against some reasonably explicit baseline, of the degree to which the results can be judged suboptimal. I conclude that the decline has been substantially less than would be expected if those goods had been collective ones, and less than many variants of hegemonic stability theory would predict.

This substantial continuity of outcomes must be explained. First, I acknowledge the variants of hegemonic stability theory that emphasize institutionalization as a partial explanation. But I then argue (1) that many of the gains from hegemony have been less collective goods than private ones, accruing primarily to the hegemon and thus helping maintain its hegemony; (2) that this applies to short-term as well as to long-term gains; (3) that the costs of achieving these goods (both collective and private) have not been borne so unequally, by the hegemon, as might be the case had they been relatively pure collective goods; and (4) that one important gain—cultural hegemony—has proved a major resource to the hegemon in maintaining its more general hegemony. These gains have helped the United States both to maintain its power base in ways not readily measured by standard indicators and to continue to control outcomes. Specifically, the international system was structurally transformed, largely by the United States. The transformation of preferences and expectations continues to produce the goods (for example, free trade) needed by the United States and the dominant elements of the rest of the world (especially the other industrialized noncommunist states) to maintain a compatible international system. Thus, the United States does not have to exert such *overt* control over *others* to maintain control over *outcomes*. In the conclusion, I attempt a balanced evaluation of the nature and degree to which US hegemony has really declined and speculate about its implications for the international system in general and Japanese–American relations in particular.

Power base and control

The perception of a significant decline in US power over the past two decades is widespread, indeed virtually universal. Many observers, writing from diverse perspectives, characterize the decline in strong terms. Richard Rosecrance, for example, says the US "role as maintainer of the system is at an end"; Kenneth Oye speaks of "the end of American hegemony"; and George Liska repeatedly applies the word "dissolution" to the state of the "American empire" (see Rosecrance 1976: 1; Liska 1978: ch. 10; Oye 1979: 4–5). People on the left applaud the decline; many on the right lament it. The perception of a US decline is particularly common, however, in the literature on international regimes; that part of the literature identified with "hegemonic stability" theory is the most straightforward. Strong characterizations of that decline are frequently associated with Robert Gilpin, Stephen Krasner, Charles Kindleberger, and even Robert Keohane.[2]

To be sure, most of these characterizations are nuanced and change as the world and theorizing about it change. Nearly everyone recognizes that the United States retains great power in the economic sphere; at least, it is a greater power than any other state. These same writers typically carefully note a continuing degree of US preeminence. The decline is relative to past US power or perhaps to the amount necessary for a hegemon to maintain essential elements of the world economic order; the United States has not declined to a position of utter impotence. My purpose in this chapter is not to criticize individual authors, but to point out the assumptions and consequences of emphasizing the decline rather than the continuity and to show that there is still much to be said for continuity.

The standards used to measure the decline are seldom clear. Part of the difficulty stems from the lack of agreement on how much power is necessary to produce hegemony. Unless there is some rather sharp stepwise jump at which hegemony comes into existence or is lost (and what that level may be has never been specified), one is necessarily talking about a continuous distribution of relative power, and there is always room for argument about whether a given degree of superiority is enough to produce particular (and also rarely well-specified) results. This is a basic theoretical problem.

A second and related difficulty is a lack of agreement on the relevant dimensions and indicators of power. In some amorphous manner, of course, our senses do not deceive us. The United States' power, as measured by various power base indicators, surely has declined. The litany is too familiar to require full recitation, and some examples will suffice: loss of strategic nuclear predominance; decline in conventional military capabilities relative to the USSR, especially for intervention, and in military capability generally (with effects compounded by perceptions of "helplessness" in the Vietnam and Iran traumas); diminished economic size (relative GNP), productivity, competitiveness in foreign markets, value of the dollar on foreign exchange markets, and terms of trade with some commodity producers (principally oil until recently); the loss of a reliable majority over the unruly in the UN; and the loss of assured scientific preeminence in the "knowledge industries" at the "cutting edge" and even in the numerical and financial base that enabled US scholars to dominate global social science.

Even with the power base indicators, however, it is not quite a case where "all the instruments agree" that it is a dark, cold day. President Reagan's rhetoric about "a definite margin of superiority for the Soviet Union" had to be corrected the next day by the director of the Bureau of Politico-Military Affairs at the State Department and his remarks about a "window of vulnerability" by the Scowcroft Commission. Reasonable (if, on both sides, rather ideological) people can debate the relative importance of warheads versus throw-weights versus "kill ratios," the proper exchange rates for comparing Soviet and US military expenditures, and the true balance of conventional forces between NATO and the Warsaw Pact. The United States' economic and industrial predominance in the world looks slightly less impressive if one considers its share of world GNP rather than its share of world manufacturing production. Although virtually all of these as well as other power base measures would show a clear decline in US predominance over the past forty years, they do not reveal an equal rate or depth of decline. A few would show the United States slipping to second place; more would merely show a shrunken lead.[3]

It also makes a great difference where in time one begins measuring the power base indicators. If one begins with 1945, all of them show a significant, though never precipitous, decline in the US power base over the subsequent four decades. That much is not really arguable.[4] But 1945 represents the summit of US relative strength. The old powers—Europe and Japan—were physically and economically devastated, and the United States unscathed. That situation could not continue. Indeed, the United States hastened its passing, and by 1955 the former powers had recovered significantly. The first postwar decade, the era of the sharpest decline in US predominance, represented a substantial return to normalcy. The immediate postwar years look even more peculiar if one starts the series in 1938 or earlier years. The United States' military preeminence dates, without question, only from World War II. Its military predominance in 1945 over all other states (even, at that point, the Soviet Union) was unprecedented for any power at least since the time of Napoleon. Since then, the Soviet Union has achieved parity, but the Soviet and US dominance over all other powers, including those of the Western alliance, remains. The name of the Soviet-US military game is duopoly. A long-term perspective on economic power makes clear the unusual degree of US superiority in that power base as well.

Table 4.1 provides a historical perspective on hegemons' ability to dominate three of the most common dimensions of a national power base. GNP is the most fungible of resources, usable for many kinds of influence efforts; it also represents market size, whose attraction can give important advantages in international trade negotiations. It represents the basis of structural power; that is, the ability to define the context within which others must make decisions. Military expenditures give a good if hardly perfect indication of relative military strength. Manufacturing production is a basic source of both economic and military strength.

Several facts are apparent from these data. First, the United Kingdom was *never*, even at its peak in the nineteenth century, the dominant power as measured by either GNP or military expenditures. The wealth provided by its industrial strength was always overwhelmed in GNP terms by the demographic base of its sometimes less wealthy but more populous chief competitors; its military expenditures were always markedly below those of one or more of its continental rivals. Only in manufacturing production, and for that matter only rather briefly, did it lead the world. (For purposes of this analysis, however, we probably should discount the surprising manufacturing capacity of China and India since they were hardly great powers in the world system.) These data should encourage a cautious interpretation of Britain's hegemonic power during this era. Britain's commercial power (which would be reflected in trade or financial indicators) was not evident in other important

TABLE 4.1 Four leading powers indexed to "hegemon," 1830–1984: gross national product, military expenditures, and manufacturing production

Year	Country and percentage of "hegemon's" value							
	Largest		2nd largest		3rd largest		4th largest	
Gross national product								
1984	US	100	USSR	51	Japan	34	W. Germany	17
1950	US	100	USSR	29	UK	19	France	13
1938	US	100	Germany	37	USSR	37	UK	27
1913	US	306	Russia	123	Germany	113	UK	100
1870	US	117	Russia	117	UK	100	France	86
1830	Russia	132	France	105	UK	100	Austria-Hungary	87
Military expenditures								
1984	US	100	USSR	100	China	18	UK	15
1950	USSR	106	US	100	China	18	UK	16
1938[a]	Germany	657	USSR	481	UK	161	Japan	154
1913	Germany	129	Russia	125	UK	100	France	99
1872[b]	Russia	127	France	119	UK	100	Germany	68
1830	France	148	UK	100	Russia	92	Austria-Hungary	54
Manufacturing production								
1983	US	100	USSR	52	Japan	30	W. Germany	16
1950	US	100	USSR	24	UK	19	W. Germany	13
1938	US	100	Germany	40	UK	34	USSR	29
1913	US	235	Germany	109	UK	100	Russia	26
1870	UK	100	China	75	US	51	France	37
1830	China	319	India	185	UK	100	Russia	59

Notes: The "hegemon" of the time is underlined; there was no hegemon in 1938, but I have arbitrarily used the US values as the base.

a. The United States ranked fifth.
b. Data for 1872 were used since the figures for French and German (Prussian) military spending were inflated in 1870 and 1871 by the Franco-Prussian War.

Sources: 1984 GNP data from OECD, *Main Economic Indicators* (May 1985); USSR total is estimated. Other GNP data from Bairoch (1976); and US Bureau of the Census (1975). 1984 military expenditures from World Armaments and Disarmament (1985). SIPRI lists Soviet military expenses as 71 percent of the US figures, but US government sources (CIA and DIA) give Soviet expenditures as exceeding those of the United States. I have set the two countries as equal. The estimate for China, given by SIPRI and used here, may be somewhat low. Military expenditure data for previous years are from the Correlates of War national capabilities data provided by Professor J. David Singer. Manufacturing production data from Bairoch (1982). Data for 1870 are interpolated from Bairoch's figures for 1860 and 1880. 1983 data from *UN Monthly Bulletin of Statistics* figures applied to Bairoch's 1980 data.

power base indicators. Second, despite slippage since filling the immediate post-World War II void, the United States retains, on all these indicators, a degree of dominance not reached by the United Kingdom at any point and comparing well with the US position in 1938. (US military expenditures for 1950, not yet reflecting the Korean war, are artificially low for the cold war period.) The basis of US hegemony may have declined, but it has hardly vanished.

Other indicators are imaginable, but many of the data are not available for a long time span, and that length of historical perspective is essential to the argument. Moreover, the meaning of some potential indicators is not entirely clear; for example, does a large volume of foreign trade indicate market dominance or vulnerability?[5] Nevertheless, any truly scientific assessment requires more, and more rigorous, measurement than Table 4.1 provides, as well as some agreement on appropriate baselines for temporal comparison. With conceptual and theoretical clarity, one could establish appropriate rules for measuring a decline in a power base. Until that time, it would be well to remember Galileo's experiment with falling bodies: to explain their velocity, one must first determine the velocity. In this instance, to be persuasive, the hegemonic stability literature demands better measurements.

The more important question, however, is "so what?" In what ways has this decline produced (been reflected in?) a decline in US power as control over outcomes; that is, in the "ability to prevail in conflict and overcome obstacles" (Deutsch 1978)? Surely it is control over outcomes that really interests us. The *Oxford English Dictionary* defines *hegemonic* as "capable of command, leading," and *hegemony* as "leadership" as well as "predominance, preponderance." If we are to have a question worth investigating, we must at least identify hegemony with success in determining and maintaining the essential rules, not merely with power base or resource share. Like Robert Keohane and Joseph Nye, we must see hegemony as a condition in which "one state is powerful enough to maintain the essential rules governing interstate relations, and willing to do so." We must avoid making a tautology out of Stephen Krasner's statement that "the theory of hegemonic leadership suggests that under conditions of declining hegemony there will be a weakening of regimes" (Keohane and Nye 1977: 44; Krasner 1982: 199).

Rather, we should ask, under conditions of declining power base predominance, is there either a weakening of the basic regime (the network of rules, norms, and so forth) or of the ability of the preponderant state to determine those rules? Weakening of the network is difficult to investigate empirically with precision, although good efforts have been made, especially with aspects of the trade regime. Here, however, I address the influence of the preponderant state and emphasize the distribution of *desired outcomes* as a result of the rules, in conformity with Krasner's formulation of a causal chain from "basic causal factors" to regimes to outcomes and behaviors.

It is widely acknowledged that the United States occupied a position of hegemony in the international system immediately after World War II. Its enemies were defeated and its allies exhausted. The productive base of the US economy alone escaped wartime devastation; indeed, it was enormously expanded by the war effort. The United States was the world's foremost military power, and it alone had the nuclear "winning weapon." Although the United States' preponderance was not so overwhelming as to enable it to set all the rules for the entire world system, its power did permit it to establish the basic principles for the new economic order in the over 80 percent of the world economy controlled by the capitalist states and to organize a system of collective security to maintain political and economic control over that 80 percent. Although its power fell short of that necessary in an ideal case of hegemony, virtually all analysts of the regimes school agree that the United States circa 1946 came closer to meeting the criteria of global hegemony than has any other state in world history. Indeed, to quote Timothy McKeown and Robert Keohane, one should have important reservations about the "supposed hegemonic leadership" of nineteenth-century Britain and wonder whether Britain was hegemonic in any meaningful sense (McKeown 1983: 73–97; Keohane 1984a: 37).

One can also have some reservations about the scientific status of a "theory" of hegemonic stability derived in large part from a single case that attempts to explain behavior in that same case. (Proponents of this theory frequently acknowledge the problem, but I shall not be greatly concerned with it here.) One can appropriately, as many have done, seek to extend insights and test propositions by looking at various "issue-area" regimes within the overall set of rules and by looking at the behavior and outcomes of actors in various arenas (for example, in small groups or in shifting coalitions within organizations) where degrees of hegemony may be examined, compared, and even manipulated. Empirical tests of the theory of collective goods have been made in just such arenas, and with care their findings can be extended to the global situation. The questions addressed are important and should not be evaded because the set of cases is small or problematic. Nevertheless, the necessity to make extensions from arenas where global conditions are but crudely approximated should force the analyst to look closely at such key assumptions as whether the goods provided by a regime truly meet the definition of collective goods (Snidal 1979), of behavior by unitary actors (Krasner 1975; Ruggie 1980), and of "fairness" in the distribution of costs and benefits (Oppenheimer 1979).

Achievements, goods, and regimes

In the years immediately following World War II, the United States emerged as a hegemonic power, perhaps following the path George Modelski characterizes as occurring at roughly hundred-year intervals (Modelski 1978). The United States provided the world with a variety of goods (some of them collective goods), including security, international organization, and a framework for international economic relations. The idea of a hegemon providing collective goods to permit peace and prosperity within a wider area is an old one; in fact, Karl Deutsch's work on integration anticipated much of what emerged in the regimes literature of the 1970s (Deutsch et al. 1957).

Another perspective on the provision of goods in the postwar international system is a radical one. It recognizes the existence of a Pax Americana and identifies the following achievements (not necessarily identified as collective goods):

> The pacification of capitalist interstate relations and the imperial guarantee against nationalization created a reliable world legal framework which reduced the risks of transnational expansion; decolonization opened up the entire periphery to primary transnational expansion based on comparative advantage rather than on the monopolistic privileges and restrictions with which rival metropolitan states had increasingly enmeshed their colonial possessions; the gold–dollar standard restored the possibility of capitalist accounting on a world scale, thus enhancing secondary transnational expansion, which depends decisively upon reliable calculations of the cost advantages of alternative locations of production.
>
> (Arrighi 1982: 77)

Two kinds of achievements or goods are encountered in this quotation from Giovanni Arrighi: security (peace) and economy (prosperity). Each can be broken down further, and we can ask what conditions or regime made possible those achievements.[6]

In the passage quoted above, Arrighi speaks of the "pacification" of relations among capitalist states. At least since 1945, there have been no wars between the developed (capitalist) industrial states. Whether this is attributable more to the spread of advanced industrial capitalism or to the spread of representative democracy in the world is hard to say because the two potential explanatory variables are so closely correlated. All the correlations may be spurious, although various arguments do not necessarily agree on the direction of causality (see Russett and Starr 1981: ch. 15; Doyle 1983).

Nevertheless, the fact of no interstate war is indisputable. Moreover, by fairly early in the postwar era, even the preparation for, and expectation of, war among these states quickly diminished nearly to the vanishing point. By the end of the 1950s, one could say with reasonable confidence that a "security community" or "stable peace" had been established nearly everywhere in the OECD states, even between traditional enemies.[7] Nor have there been any civil wars (1,000 or more deaths) within any of the advanced capitalist countries or any serious expectation of such. (There has been fear that the violence in Northern Ireland and the Spanish Basque country could escalate above this threshold.)

One could argue that the absence of war between democracies has been a fact of life for the almost two centuries since the end of the Napoleonic era (see Singer and Small 1976), but the recent extension of stable democracy and (therefore?) of a "zone of peace" to various industrialized countries where it was previously fragile (for example, Germany, Italy, Japan) is surely a major achievement. It is, moreover, an achievement that can be credited in some degree to the United States, either as a result of enforced suppression of hostilities[8] or, in Arrighi's terms, by provision of a "cohesive political and ideological framework."

Stable peace has not, however, been achieved in the Third World and its capitalist states. Virtually all post-1945 wars have been fought on the territories of Third World states, between or within Third World states or between Third World states and intervening First or Second World states. Open insurgency was often avoided only because of the threat of direct foreign intervention or the establishment of powerful coercive states within Third World countries, usually with strong external support. It is all too often a "peace" based on threat, either mutual (deterrence) or one-sided (dominance).

From the point of view of Third World peoples, the achievement of stable peace is doubtless suboptimal. From the viewpoint of the United States, however, the judgment must be less certain. The wars have been fought in Third World countries and the civilian casualties incurred there. The costs of maintaining coercive states have been largely borne by Third World peoples. The result has been sufficient pacification to provide a reliable legal framework for transnational corporate expansion and to discourage most large-scale nationalization without "fair" compensation. Parts (some countries, some classes) of the Third World have shared fully in the resulting prosperity; others have not. But overall by historic standards (even compared with the colonial era of direct control), the results show not a bad ratio of costs and benefits for the United States.

If *stable peace* has been achieved among and within many capitalist countries, it surely has not been achieved between capitalist and communist countries. Instead, we can speak only of *containment* or deterrence and the ability of US hegemony to achieve stable boundaries between the capitalist and communist spheres. The United States was able to erect, in the first decade after the war, a *cordon sanitaire* around the Soviet Union that held from the "loss" of China to the accession of Castro, with some breaches thereafter. It is a "peace" maintained by deterrence, initially somewhat one-sided (the US nuclear monopoly, though compensated by Soviet conventional superiority in Europe) and becoming increasingly based on a system of mutual threat. Although there are many flaws and dangers in this system, the facts of substantial success for containment and the avoidance of superpower war should not be dismissed.

Other goods or achievements relate to the economy and are embodied in various regimes.[9] The second gain Arrighi identifies from establishment of the Pax Americana is decolonization and consequent entry of the United States into previously closed trade and raw materials markets. As the price of US assistance for postwar reconstruction, the former colonial powers were required to accede to the demands of their colonial peoples for independence. Clear-cut examples include (but are hardly limited to) the experience in 1949 when the threat of a cutoff in US economic aid halted the Dutch military operation to restore control over the Dutch East Indies (Indonesia), US pressure in 1962 that helped impel the Dutch effectively to cede West New Guinea (Irian Jaya) to Indonesia, and the

US refusal to approve an urgent IMF loan that forced the British and French to retreat from their effort to reoccupy the Suez Canal in 1956 (see Lijphart 1966: ch. 11; and Hoopes 1973: 384).

The US goal was more than mere nominal independence for the colonies. Dismantling of the formal and informal barriers that had largely restricted colonies' trade to their former metropoles was to follow. Britain, for instance, was strongly pressured to give up the structures of Commonwealth Preference and the Sterling Area, which had provided it with a relatively closed, secure market. Britain was also required, most notably as part of the settlement of the Anglo-Iranian oil nationalization in 1953, to give US-based multinationals a dominant share of Middle Eastern oil supplies. Decolonization as an ideology was attractive to Americans; it cost them almost nothing (the only American colony was the Philippines) and created enormous economic opportunities. With its then-dominant technology and industrial organization, the United States was in position to move into these hitherto closed markets. Decolonization meant acceleration of the introduction of advanced capitalism into the Third World—and the United States was the most efficient capitalist. The postwar international trade and finance regimes brought worldwide prosperity, not least to the United States.

Continuity and distribution of gains

These achievements, often embodied in regimes, are important products of US hegemony. Moreover, they represent a continued achievement of outcomes desired by the United States, even at a time of a discernible decline in standard power base indicators. If one shifts perspective from narrow issue-area regimes to broader aspects of the post-World War II international environment, one has to be impressed by the degree to which perceived US interests, not just the interests of other states, were served. One also should be impressed by the strong elements of continuity, of sustained reward, characteristic of these achievements. These two elements—the fact of important gains to the United States itself and their continuity—are interlinked.

First, the matter of continuity. Over the past decade we have seen a breakdown in détente, by which we mean a breakdown in the rules and norms governing Soviet-US behavior. "Prompt hard-target kill" weapons have been acquired, in numbers and capabilities formerly avoided; troops have crossed some of the implicit boundaries between East and West; and continued adherence to formal agreements like SALT and the ABM treaty is in doubt. Yet the rules and norms, built up over the decades, have not entirely been abandoned. Some vestige of a regime in East-West relations remains.

More dubious is the continuity of containment, but even there I suggest that the argument of drastic decline is readily exaggerated. The United States' strategic nuclear predominance is gone, forever in my opinion. (Members of the Reagan administration may disagree about the "forever.") Most of us feel less secure about maintenance of the balance of terror than we did, especially about the risks of a low-level political or military conflict spiraling into something like Armageddon. But the risks of deliberate Soviet nuclear attack still seem remote and are likely to remain so indefinitely, barring either gross US provocation or gross US negligence in providing a secure nuclear deterrent.

Despite some breaches, the *cordon sanitaire* around the Soviet Union still looks quite effective. Counterbalancing the effects of Soviet gains in Afghanistan, Vietnam, and Africa has been the Soviet loss of China, once its foremost ally. By any standards of resources or population, the reentry of China into the world economy and the reorientation of Chinese foreign policy more than compensate for "free world" losses elsewhere. The United States' losses in the Middle East have by no means been translated into Soviet gains (witness Iran) (see Khalilzad 1984). The biggest switch in that part of the world (Egypt) was from "them" to "us." Soviet penetration of Latin America since Cuba still remains more of a threat than a major reality (and the Soviet accession of Cuba occurred despite US nuclear predominance at that time).

Continuity also applies to the United States' relations with the industrialized countries. The hegemonic stability literature does not give sharp predictions on whether and, particularly, how much the achievement of goals will decline as the relative power base of the hegemon declines. Except as a "crude theory," (Keohane 1984a: 34) it emphasizes the mediating and conditioning roles of, for example, international institutions and the characteristics of domestic political systems. Nevertheless, some decline, particularly in light of the sharp decline in US military power, might be expected. But it has not happened. By no reasonable criterion has there been any decline in the achievement of stable peace among the advanced capitalist countries. They hardly are able to solve all their common problems, but— and this is no small achievement—war among them is now less thinkable than ever. War among them became no more thinkable during the 1970s era of détente when their apparent common threat, the Soviet Union, became less threatening. And although wars in the Third World remain common, there is no discernible trend toward greater frequency (Small and Singer 1982: 134).

If US predominance (hegemony) vis-à-vis the Soviet Union is gone, US nuclear predominance (hegemony) over all other states remains and is perhaps stronger than ever. There is little sign that it will erode in the future. Europe seems unable to put together a substantial deterrent of its own. In a nuclear world, US military hegemony over its allies may never end. And that kind of hegemony provides the United States with some fungible resources for maintaining a degree of hegemony in other areas. ("Open up your domestic market more, or Congress may tire of keeping our military commitment.")

In the economic realm, the structure of a relatively open world economy (GATT, the various rounds of trade liberalization, and so forth) remains substantially intact. Despite the spread of some measures like "voluntary" export restraints and many observers' anticipation of a major relapse into protectionism, the sky has not fallen.

It is significant that world trade fell only in 1982, and then by only 1 percent, after a decade of increased protectionist efforts. The inflation-adjusted increase in world trade between 1973 and 1983 was between 6 and 7 percent, as contrasted with a 28 percent drop from 1926 to 1935. Progress in opening up the biggest protected capitalist economy outside the United States (Japan's) continues to creep forward.[10] Currencies remain convertible. The United States can use the attractiveness of its financial markets and its high interest rates to finance its military buildup with other people's money (especially Japanese money).

It would be perverse to deny that there has been some demonstrable (if less easily measurable) decline in the United States' ability to get others to do as it wished in recent decades. That decline has been well documented in the regimes literature, although I consider the decline often to have been exaggerated. Since I have quoted Arrighi to illustrate the gains achieved by the United States by its world predominance, it is only fair to quote a long passage where he considers both the persistence and the decay of those gains:

> In general, the US government has simply exploited, in the pursuance of national interests, the core position that the US national economy still retains in the world-economy. Its internal reserves of energy and other natural resources, the sheer size of its internal market, and the density and complexity of its linkages with the rest of the capitalist world imply a basic asymmetry in the relation of the US economy to other national economies: conditions within the US state's boundaries influence, much more than they are influenced by, conditions within the boundaries of any other national economy. This asymmetrical relation, though independently eroded by other factors, has not yet been significantly affected by the undoing of the US imperial order. What has been affected is the *use* made by the US state of its world economic power: while in the 1950s and 1960s the national interest was often subordinated to the establishment and reproduction of a world capitalist order, in the middle and late 1970s the reproduction of such an order has been subordinated to the pursuit of the national interest as expressed in efforts to increase domestic economic growth.
>
> In such a sense, this redeployment of US world political-economic power in the pursuit of national interests has been a major symptom of, and factor explaining, the state of anarchy that has characterized international economic relations since 1973. It is important to realize, however, that at least insofar as the advanced capitalist countries are concerned, this state of anarchy in interstate relations has been strictly limited to monetary and budgetary policies and that it has yet to undermine the two main "products" of formal US hegemony: the unity of the world market and the transnational expansion of capital. These substantive aspects of US hegemony have survived the downfall of the US imperial order; and their operating reach throughout the world capitalist economy has, if anything, been continually extended.
>
> (Arrighi 1982: 65)[11]

As will shortly be apparent, I disagree on several counts with Arrighi's assessment. I contend that the US national interest was served, not subordinated, even in the short run, by the policies of the 1950s. I also regard his characterization of a "state of anarchy"—even as applied only to monetary and budgetary policies—as much too strong. A literal "absence of government" is not necessarily synonymous with chaos, as Hedley Bull and others have urged (Bull 1977). (It is worth emphasizing that, once the world capitalist order was established, the tasks of maintaining and reproducing it became far easier.) The strengths of Arrighi's argument, however, include its emphasis on asymmetries (versus simplistic uses of "interdependence") and hence the remaining power of the United States to influence others and its emphasis on the substantive aspects that remain.

If the fact of significant continuity is accepted, then it must be explained. The institutions for political and economic cooperation have themselves been maintained. Keohane rightly stresses the role of institutions as "arrangements permitting communication and therefore facilitating the exchange of information."[12] By providing reliable information and reducing transaction costs, institutions can permit cooperation to continue even after erosion of a hegemon's influence. Institutions facilitate opportunities for commitment and for observing whether others keep their commitments. Such opportunities are virtually essential to cooperation in non-zero-sum situations, as explicit attention to gaming experiments demonstrates (Axelrod 1984). Declining hegemony and stagnant (but not decaying) institutions may therefore be consistent with stable provision of desired outcomes, although the ability to promote new levels of cooperation to deal with new problems (for example, energy supplies or environmental protection) is more problematic. The institutions provide a part of the necessary explanation.

Collective or private goods?

The nature of the institutions themselves must be examined. They were shaped, in the years immediately after World War II, by the United States. They, and the regimes of which they are a part, have significantly endured. The US willingness to establish those regimes and their institutions is sometimes explained in terms of the theory of collective goods. It is commonplace in the regimes literature to argue that the United States, in so doing, was providing not only private goods for its own benefit, but also (especially?) collective goods desired by, and for the benefit of, other capitalist states (nations?—but one should be particularly careful here in equating state interest with "national" interest). Thus, not only was the United States protecting its own territory and commercial enterprises, it was also providing desired military protection for some fifty allies and almost as many neutrals. Not only was it ensuring a liberal, open, near-global economy for its own prosperity, it was providing the basis for the prosperity of all capitalist states (and even for those states organized on noncapitalist principles willing to abide by the basic rules established to govern international trade and finance). Although it would not be quite accurate to describe such behavior as self-less or altruistic, certainly the benefits—however distributed by class, state, or region—did accrue to far more peoples than just to Americans. Coupled with this is the implication that the United States paid substantial costs in the immediate postwar period to set in place the basis for the accrual of long-term benefits for itself and others.[13]

If this were a case of provision of a collective good, several conclusions would follow. First, collective goods theory predicts that, in the absence of a strong central authority able to coerce members to pay appropriate contributions, the collective good will be supplied only to a suboptimal degree. Second, the costs of providing the good will be borne unequally and by the hegemon. Implicit in the assessment of *inequality* in burden sharing is usually an assumption of *inequity* or unfairness; that is, the ratio of costs to benefits weighs against the hegemon, implying that although the hegemon bears disproportionate costs, the nonhegemonic powers desire the good as much as, or almost as much as, the hegemon does. (This proposition should make us critical of the prior assumption, and its consequent normative implications, that the principal goods provided truly are collective ones. If the goods are largely private goods for the benefit, and at the desire, of the hegemon, then it is hardly fair to berate the smaller states for an unwillingness to pay an equal share of the costs.)

A corollary is a serious doubt about the willingness, and even the ability, of the hegemon to continue to pay the costs. It is argued that the short-term costs were so heavy, and the benefits distributed so widely to those who never paid the costs, that a weakening of the United States, and loss of its hegemony, was thus inevitable. So, too, except as it could be retarded by such factors as institutionalization, was a weakening of the regimes that the United States had established and sustained.

As so applied, collective goods theory would predict the very weakening whose existence I have contested. Yet paradoxically, the absence of that weakening can, in fact, be understood by a different application of collective goods theory. It requires a careful examination of the goods provided and an awareness of the degree to which they were not collective but private. To the degree that they were private goods—benefits to the United States itself—they have brought important if sometimes obscured resources to the United States, resources that help it to maintain regimes and to obtain for itself a variety of private goods.

A collective good must meet the two standard criteria of nonrivalness and non-exclusiveness. By the first is meant that one's enjoyment or consumption of the good does not diminish the amount of the good available to anyone else; by the second, that it is not possible to exclude any party from enjoyment of the good, as a result of which many actors may be "free-riders" unwilling to pay any of the costs for providing the good. Few goods ever fit these criteria perfectly; one can usually find some possibilities of rivalness and exclusion,[14] but judgments of less and more are perfectly feasible. I argue, on the basis of an examination of each of the major goods identified above, that they do not primarily meet the criteria for collective goods, but that in many ways they represent private goods accruing heavily to the United States. If that judgment is accepted, the conclusion that the exercise of hegemony necessarily weakened the United States does not follow. And if the

United States has not been severely weakened, we need not be surprised at its continued willingness, and ability, to secure these goods.

The first of the goods at issue is "stable peace," particularly among the industrialized states. It probably satisfies the criterion of nonrivalness, although some radical critics contend that peace within and among the industrialized states is achieved only at the price of exploiting (through dominance, military threats, and military intervention) the Third World. Whatever one thinks of that assessment, clearly peace does not meet the criterion of nonexclusiveness. It certainly is feasible to exclude various countries or areas from stable peace with oneself if one so wishes—by attacking or invading—and even for "peace" by dominance one can choose boundaries to the area one pacifies.

Many Western observers would probably judge containment to be largely a collective good. It was desired by *most* of the citizens of all the countries protected, not just by the United States. The unanimity of this desire has weakened recently, however, as many of its beneficiaries, notably in Western Europe, increasingly doubt the reality of a Soviet military threat to their security or way of life. Containment is achieved both by deterrence and a willingness to defend. It is neither entirely nonrival or nonexclusive. As the distinction in the alliance literature makes clear, deterrence satisfies the criterion of nonrivalness well and that of nonexclusiveness reasonably well, but defense is another matter (Russett 1970: ch. 4).

Fortifying one area may, by requiring the adversary to concentrate troops there, actually enhance the defense of other areas. Or, by drawing the hegemon's resources away from other areas, it may indeed prove to be "rival" by leaving weak spots elsewhere in the perimeter. (In the Korean war, many American analysts feared too great involvement there would divert needed forces from the European theater.) One may attempt to exclude "unimportant" countries or uncooperative governments from one's defense or deterrent umbrella, although, as with South Korea in 1950, it is not always possible to stick to one's resolve to exclude them. Since defense is significantly a private good, there are strong incentives for small or large states to provide substantial military capabilities of their own. Other important goods can be derived from military forces, such as technological knowledge, prestige, and internal security.[15]

Prosperity, as provided by an open world economy, is also somewhere on the continuum between a private and a collective good. It is partly nonrival and partly rival. General gains accrue from prosperous and expanding markets, yet a capitalist economy lives by competition. One sells at the expense of a competitor. (The mixed-motive game characterization is appropriate.) As the Soviet Union has been, states can be formally excluded from the most-favored-nation system, the system that provides much of the basis of international prosperity (Stein 1984).[16] Within the system, the rules of the international trade and finance game prohibit many kinds of discrimination (exclusion from benefits), but many loopholes can be found, for example, the various preferences, restrictions, and common-market arrangements.

I have already argued that the United States was well positioned, in the immediate postwar years, to reap *at least* a proportionate share of the collective and private gains that were obtainable from the prosperity induced by decolonization and a more open world market. Of course, there were costs. Postwar reconstruction entailed immediate costs in the high military expenditure the United States carried in the interests of containment, in the Marshall Plan, and the trade concessions to Japan, which largely substituted for heavy grant assistance to that country. The United States, in accordance with the liberal free-trade regime it was sponsoring, had to open its own previously protected markets. But these costs were, during the first decades after World War II, recouped many times over from the general prosperity stimulated by a relatively open world market, and specifically by US access to others' previously closed markets. These, of course, included the metropolitan countries of Europe as well as markets in the Third World. The United States mitigated EEC discrimination against US trade by insisting that EEC trade and investment barriers be low, and save for agricultural products, it succeeded in gaining access on terms not much worse than those accorded to intra-EEC enterprises.

The gains from an open global economy surely exceeded the costs to the United States. Despite what ultimately proved to be important burdens shouldered by the United States to maintain that open economy, when compared with the costs other powers accepted in decolonization, the balance sheet for Americans does not look at all bad. (For example, the costs associated with maintaining the dollar at a fixed price in gold eventually became too great, but for a long time they were substantially balanced by the gains from seigniorage and autonomy.) Indeed, the gains from decolonization helped shield the United States from what might have been a *rapid* deterioration of its relative and absolute economic position. The two defeated powers, Germany and Japan, did quickly close much of the per capita economic gap between them and the United States—as a consequence of the deliberate US policy to build strong pillars of containment on either end of the Soviet Union. But the major power whose decolonization occurred *after* the war—Great Britain—was in no way able to close the gap.

The United States had a large surplus productive capacity after World War II, making the costs of overseas economic assistance not very onerous. Furthermore, given that excess capacity, the postwar US prosperity was dependent on foreign economic expansion in a climate of worldwide prosperity. Had the European or former colonial economies been allowed to stagnate, almost surely the US economy would have done likewise. Most major currencies became convertible with the dollar by the mid-1950s, at stable exchange rates, thus in Arrighi's terms "reducing the risks to capital of, and so favoring, the expansion of international trade and investment."[17] Again, the United States was superbly positioned to capture its full share of those gains. It is also worth remembering that although this open world economy did not, especially in the first decades, include the communist countries, when those states did seek partial global economic integration (Eastern Europe beginning in the 1960s, the Soviet Union and China somewhat later), the terms were largely set by the initial US specifications, for example, most-favored-nation status.

Nor is it any more correct to describe the costs of obtaining noneconomic goods as disproportionately borne by the United States. This can be seen even in the instance most often cited, the cost of containment. In purely economic terms (share of GNP, a cost that the wealthy United States could most easily bear), the burden sharing has been skewed so as to fall more heavily on Americans. But non-Americans have consistently provided the real estate and the personnel. For example, the United States' formal allies in Europe and Asia have maintained twice as many soldiers under arms as has the United States. They did so immediately after the war as well as in recent years, many of them with compulsory national service.

Thus, a careful toting up of costs and benefits to all parties, coupled with a rigorous application of the criteria for collective goods, casts much doubt on the proposition that the United States provided disproportionate benefits to others. Most of the major goods provided by the postwar US hegemony ("stable peace" within much of the noncommunist world; a *cordon sanitaire* around the major perceived security threat; a relatively open, expanding, and largely predictable world economy) were obtained in degrees that were not markedly suboptimal from the US point of view. The burdens were not distributed in such a way as to be grossly unfair to the United States, relative either to the gains of the United States or to the burdens borne by many other noncommunist countries. Indeed, by many radical and even liberal perspectives, US aid and rearmament expenditures—both in themselves and as a stimulus for a wider, and more open, world economy— prevented a postwar repetition of the Great Depression. It was the ideal outcome; the United States did well by doing good.

Cultural hegemony

How do we explain the United States' ability to achieve and maintain a rather favorable balance sheet of costs and benefits? An answer, found in a few versions of the hegemonic stability literature, asserts that in the early years, at least, the United States was such a powerful hegemon that it could skew the division of private goods in its favor and *enforce* "adequate" burden sharing for the collective goods on other noncommunist states. By this interpretation, the United States in effect provided something functionally equivalent to the coercive mechanism of central government that ensures the provision of collective goods within nation-states.[18] In this sense, the US hegemonic regime (or regimes, as one prefers) was essentially imposed and maintained by politico-economic coercion and not largely by the threat or fact of physical violence. I would not dispute that other countries' bargaining position and ability to resist US demands in the immediate postwar era were weak, and I acknowledged that—at least in comparison with the period before World War II— relatively strong international institutions, dominated by the United States, were created. But the qualification of "strong relative to what went before" is an important one, and I find it hard to believe that the institutions provided the basis for the coercive, tax-collecting power necessary to enforce near-optimal (from the US point of view) provision of collective goods at a distribution of costs that was not, overall, unfair to the United States. Coercive hegemony is at best challengeable (Keohane 1984a), and another answer must be sought.

Another major gain to the United States from the Pax Americana, perhaps less widely appreciated, nevertheless proved of great significance in the short as well as the long term: the pervasive global cultural influence of the United States. By *culture*, I mean, following Clifford Geertz, a set of symbols that conveys meaning about the beliefs, values, and aspirations of a group of people (Geertz 1973). This dimension of the power base is often neglected. After World War II, the authoritarian political cultures of Europe and Japan were utterly discredited, and the liberal-democratic elements of those cultures revivified. The revival was most extensive and deliberate in the occupied former Axis powers and especially Japan, where it was nurtured by imposing a democratic constitution, building democratic institutions, curbing the power of industrial trusts by decartelization, building trade unions, and imprisoning or discrediting most of the wartime leaders. Liberal ideas from the United States largely filled the cultural void. The effect was not so dramatic in the "victor" states, whose regimes were reaffirmed (Britain, the Low Countries, and Scandinavia), but even there the United States and its culture were widely admired. The upper classes often thought it too "commercial," but in many respects the spread of American mass-consumption culture was the most pervasive dimension of the United States' impact. American styles, tastes, and middle-class consumption patterns were widely imitated, in a process that has come to bear the label "coca-colonization."

Altogether, the near-global acceptance of so many aspects of American culture—consumption, democracy, language—quickly laid the basis for what Gramscians would call cultural hegemony (Hoare and Smith 1971).[19] It paid off in immediate benefits in markets and the willingness of many people to bear significant burdens to establish and maintain the *cordon sanitaire*. In longer-term ways, it shaped people's desires and perceptions of alternatives, so that their preferences for international politics and economics were concordant with those of Americans. (The rationalization of hegemony itself is part of this process.) The structure of pervasive American cultural influence was part of a structural transformation of the international system. It meant that in many cases Americans would be able to retain substantial control over essential outcomes without overtly exerting power over others.[20] Rather, others' values were already conditioned to be compatible with American wishes in ways that would benefit Americans as well as themselves (antiauthoritarianism and, with limits, acceptance of free-market economics).[21]

Gramscian ideas of influence are notoriously difficult to operationalize because by definition they leave no traces in events (overt persuasion, much less coercion, is usually unnecessary). But they should not be dismissed.[22] The mushrooming expansion of US television, film, and printed media in the world, often in spite of other governments' efforts to reinforce their cultural boundaries, supports a Gramscian kind of interpretation.[23] It is truly a worldwide phenomenon, not just one limited to the European and Japanese industrial states, and mightily facilitated by the use of English as an international language.[24] The internalization of Western (but especially American) norms by the rulers and middle classes of the Third World forms a constant theme in *dependencia* writing. It has not noticeably diminished over the years. To the contrary, a Mitterrand or a de Gaulle can offer but ineffectual resistance in an industrial country; only the draconian measures of Khomeini bring much success in an underdeveloped one.

The international institutionalization associated with regime building facilitates the spread of common cultural and political norms, especially among governing elites. This helps to achieve consensus on what problems must be solved, and how. Norm-creating institutions broaden individuals' self-images; institutions may change the "decision criteria—members may become *joint* maximizers rather than just self-maximizers" (Stein 1982).

The spread of American (democratic, capitalist, mass-consumption, anti-communist) culture has laid the basis for innumerable US economic and political gains. The spread of American culture has been a collective good in the sense of being nonrival. (More strongly: to the degree one state in the global system becomes more Americanized, others are influenced to become more, not less, so.) It also is a good not readily capable of exclusion. If one regards it normatively as a "good," then all parties are beneficiaries. But the private benefits to the United States itself can hardly be ignored, and since many would have liked to exclude American culture more than they were able to do, it was hardly to them an unalloyed "good." It was appropriate that the Americans—who have reaped so many gains from that dominance—should pay whatever extremely modest costs it may have entailed. It forms a structure of long-term influence that persists, deeply, to this day. It is among the primary reasons why a decline in material power-base dominance has not been reflected in an equivalent loss of control over outcomes.[25]

Conclusions for Japanese–American relations

These observations begin, I think, to untangle a central puzzle often posed in the hegemonic stability literature. Two empirical assumptions at the hard core of the hegemonic stability research program depart so far from reality as to have seriously misleading effects. First, the characterization of a hegemonic United States as predominantly supplying itself, and others, with collective goods is inaccurate, and for those goods that can correctly be called collective, the United States has not paid disproportionate costs. Second, the description of US hegemony as having declined is also a gross overstatement, particularly when one looks at the military and cultural, as well as economic, elements of hegemony.

Clarity about the past and present is essential to any comprehension of the future, although forecasting is hazardous even with the best of models and information. Having refuted more-sweeping claims about hegemonial decline, we now are in better position to evaluate soberly the effects of what deterioration has occurred. Although reports of the demise of US hegemony have been greatly exaggerated, surely some decline is unquestionable. The question is whether the decline represents a terminal illness or merely normal aging compounded by a few minor ailments.

It is useful to think of competing hegemonic systems (a US-led one and a Soviet-led one), but even so the degree of change in US dominance, and the importance of the Soviet Union, differs across military, cultural, and economic dimensions. The United States' *military* dominance over the Soviet Union is gone and will not return. But over the next decade or two, it is not likely that US decision-makers will allow "essential equivalence" to deteriorate. If anything, the Reagan administration's efforts will reverse the slow decline of the 1970s. The United States has the economic and technological base to do that, and its leaders seem to have the will. Only the United States and the USSR have the capacity for global power projection; China does not, nor, now, does even Britain. Barring true European unity, *only* the United States and the Soviet Union can run the nuclear race. Any Soviet and US success in constructing space-based antimissile systems will have the effect—and perhaps the intent—only of reinforcing their nuclear duopoly. A working superpower SDI would drastically reduce the effectiveness of small, less sophisticated missile forces. Moreover, if the Soviet Union had an effective SDI, the US nuclear umbrella, as a means of covering its allies, would be thoroughly degraded: a US threat of first use of nuclear weapons would lose its last shred of plausibility. No Japanese eminence in high-tech electronics or rocketry can, without truly enormous expense, allow Japan to compete in that league. At best, nonsuperpowers can produce some modest shifts in the conventional military balance in their areas; they cannot, in this century, hope to play the nuclear game against the leaders.

The United States' cultural hegemony is not amenable to the precise measures familiar in the strategic literature, but I fail to see powerful signs of its imminent decline. (The 1986 conference from which this volume resulted, conducted in English and centrally concerned with the concepts and hypotheses of American social science, attests to its continued vitality.) American culture will continue to assimilate the elements of other cultures and so will become more international, but the solid rooting of that culture in American political, social, and economic norms will remain.

The most substantial, though not precipitate, decline is likely to be in the realm of international economics. The United States is caught in a scissors between the growth in Soviet military might and the rise of Japan and the EC as economic competitors; the effect is to reduce US ability to pay the military costs. Ultimately an economic decline will erode the military and cultural dimensions as well. Conversely, the decay of US economic dominance is likely to be hastened by efforts to retain great military power. Military expenditures at 6 percent or more of US GNP (as compared with 1 percent for Japan) must sap US economic vitality by diverting funds from productive investment and scientific endeavor from the fields of high-technology civilian needs in which Japan can effectively compete.[26] The long-term unsustainability of such heavy US military expenditures makes it imperative, if Japanese-American cooperation is to be maintained, that Japan find some way of increasing its contribution to Western security. Perhaps that can be largely through development assistance if a much greater Japanese military role is not politically acceptable.

The Soviet Union has never quite been a top-level player in the economic realm. In fact, the impact of the United States' relative economic decline in the world at large has been cushioned by Soviet economic failures. The United States' hegemony has been too substantial for bipolarity or multipolarity to be an adequate representation of reality. Perhaps for this reason, cooperation among major states has been more apparent, and conflict more muted, than in the realm of military affairs. If so, a continued US decline may portend a greater increase in conflict. The decline cannot be so severe as to produce equality of Japanese and American GNPs until well into the twenty-first century, even at very disparate growth rates (for example, 5 percent per annum for Japan and 1 percent for the United States). But continuing disparate rates of economic growth, even if not dramatically different, would bring approximate equality of the two big capitalist economies.

At some stage, the continued decline of US hegemony will begin to have severe effects on the international system. There will be a lag in the relationship between declining power base and declining influence over outcomes because it is easier to maintain a system or regime than to establish it in the first place and because many elements of contemporary international regimes are quite robust.[27] Moreover, we do not know how the decline will be manifested or what the functional relationship will be. A smooth, relatively linear relationship between power base decline and influence decline would give decision-makers time to adjust and to try to construct alternative regimes or alternative means to sustain existing regimes. If, rather, there is a distinctly nonlinear relationship or a reasonably sharp inflection point, the results would be much more unsettling. Talk of the relationship between those two variables alone ignores the potential shocks from other kinds of international change. A regime that was weakened by a steadily changing power relationship could be thrown sharply into disarray by a shock it might earlier have absorbed. Such imaginable, if not likely, shocks include a close SinoSoviet rapprochement, a major US military intervention or political defeat somewhere in the world, and a severe disruption to Middle Eastern oil supplies at a time when oil is in short supply.

It becomes important, therefore, to ask how the effects of declining hegemony may be managed, both by the declining hegemon itself and by its nearest "challenger," Japan. In this context, the term *challenger* is not really appropriate. Japan may challenge the United States' economic leadership, but it is unlikely to challenge its military superiority. Japan and the United States do not have sufficient conflicts of interest for us to imagine them, in the foreseeable future, as military antagonists. Their interests converge more-than they conflict. Each has an enormous interest in maintaining an international order organized around liberal political and economic principles—democracy and free-market open-trading economics. They will not always interpret those principles identically, nor will their national systems converge totally. But the basic, and overwhelming, convergence of interests is apparent.

To say that they share great common interests is not to say that they necessarily will be able to cooperate enough to serve those interests. We have *some* theory and experience concerning the possibility of "power transitions" in international politics, but the notion of power transition has dubious relevance to this case. Most power transitions have come as the result of war, either from a challenger's defeating a hegemon or a new hegemon's arising when both former hegemon and former challenger are exhausted from war. Another Japanese-American war hardly seems likely, and if there should be a Soviet-US war, the matter of subsequent power transition would be of little interest—the destructiveness of such a war would make our concepts of the international system utterly obsolete.

Largely peaceful power transitions in international politics are rarer; even at the point early in this century when the United States passed Britain, that passage was assisted by the cost of British exertions in World War I. As I noted above, an exchange of first and second economic positions between Japan and the United States is less likely, in peacetime, than is an extended period of approximate parity marked by coexistence, muted though not absent competition, and some active cooperation in pursuit of shared goals. The historical precedents for such an experience are meager. (Soviet-US détente was stillborn; the Concert of Europe after 1815 was largely a multilateral rather than a bilateral détente.) The lack of fully appropriate models should be sobering; the situation has probably been rare because it is not easy to achieve and maintain.[28] Such a situation is poorly captured by terms like *leader* and *challenger* or by standard theories of multipolar systems. Cooperation is not anticipated by the usual "realist" theories of international relations. Collective goods theory and game theory emphasizing situations like the prisoners' dilemma also point to difficulties in the way of cooperation.

Yet there also are theoretical reasons not to dismiss the possibilities too readily. Constructive influences ignored in most "realist" analyses—like ties of communication and community—can be encouraged by deliberate effort. Game theoretic analyses stressing conditions of repeated interaction, and thus the strategic rationality of actors, give grounds for encouragement. States may anticipate that although free-riding may provide them with short-term gains, their noncooperation will induce collapse of the regime, and so they may continue to cooperate. Goods once provided by a large power who dominated all other powers may later be provided by collective action among the two or three largest members.[29] If, therefore, the decline in US hegemony results less from a markedly slow US growth rate than from a relatively rapid Japanese growth rate, the prospects for cooperation may be more promising. The potential benefits from cooperation are worth further theorizing, a search for relevant evidence, and planning.

Notes

1 I wrote this chapter while a fellow at the Netherlands Institute for Advanced Study and thank the staff and other fellows for making that such a pleasant and productive environment. I also thank the General Service Foundation and the Yale Center for International and Comparative Studies for financial support, and several colleagues—

especially Robert Keohane, Stephen Krasner, Jim Lindsay, Susan Strange, William R. Thompson, and H. Bradford Westerfield—for insightful comments on an earlier draft. A version of the first sections of this chapter appeared in Russett (1985).

2 See Gilpin (1975; 1981: 231), Krasner (1981), Kindleberger (1976), and also many of the contributions to the Spring 1982 special issue of *International Organization*. Keohane (1984a) represents a special case. His is the most sophisticated version of hegemonic stability theory and explicitly argues against equating a decline in power base with an equivalent decline in the characteristics of a regime. Nevertheless, he repeatedly uses phrases like "a post-hegemonic world" (216) and "the legacy of American hegemony" and "hegemony will not be restored in our lifetimes" (244), and the book is entitled *After Hegemony*. The only strong emphasis on the continuity of US power is Strange (1982b).

3 Keohane's *After Hegemony* identifies four criteria for identifying a hegemon in the world political economy: preponderance of material resources and raw materials, capital, markets, and production of highly valued goods. A broader view of hegemony, however, requires inclusion of military, scientific, and other resources.

4 This is true, for example, with Rupert and Rapkin (1985).

5 See, e.g., Waltz (1979: ch. 7); Waltz regards the United States as more autonomous, and hence stronger, than more internationally involved states.

6 Much of the hegemonic stability literature (for example, "founding father" Kindleberger's *The World in Depression* (1973)) is concerned with specific issue-areas and goods rather than with such broader achievements or goods as peace and prosperity. Focusing on narrow issue-areas makes the thesis of a decline in US hegemony more plausible—at least for those selected issue-areas. Nevertheless, the issue-areas are usually selected because they are assumed, implicitly or explicitly, to be symptomatic of a broad decline in US ability to maintain the conditions of global prosperity. Peace—harmony among the industrial capitalist powers and containment of the USSR—is one of those conditions. Thus, although some writing on hegemonic stability can escape the strictures of my critique, a general evaluation of the state of US hegemony and its consequences—an evaluation that is both common and necessary—must carry the discussion beyond the selected, rather narrow, issue-areas. Gilpin (*War and Change*) and many of the contributors to the Spring 1982 special issue of *International Organization* would surely agree.

7 The terms are, respectively, from Deutsch *et al.* (1957); and Boulding (1978).

8 To me, this is not the most persuasive explanation, but see Weede (1983).

9 I use the term *regime* in Krasner's sense: "principles, norms, and decision-making procedures around which actor expectations converge." See Krasner (1982: 85).

10 For the comparative data on trade, I am indebted to Strange (1985). Hughes and Wael-broeck (1983), reply that the increase in protectionism during the 1970s was small. There is some evidence that protectionism rises during periods of cyclical economic downturn, but these increases should not be mistaken for long-term trends. On the collapse of the Bretton Woods fixed exchange-rate system, see Patrick and Rosovsky (1983: 38): "In our view, despite excessively wide swings in real rates among currencies, the flexible exchange rate system was a way of maintaining the liberal international economic order rather than being a cause of its demise." See also Keohane (1984a: 213):

> Substantial erosion of the trade regime . . . has occurred, but . . . what is equally striking is the persistence of cooperation even if not always addressed to liberal ends. Trade wars have not taken place, despite economic distress. On the contrary, what we see are intensive efforts at cooperation, in response to discord in textiles, steel, electronics, and other areas.

On liberalization of the Japanese economy, see Vernon (1983); and Komiya and Itoh (1988).

11 One could quarrel with Arrighi's use of "national interest" and qualify it by reference to the interests of the ruling classes, but on the whole I am not inclined to do so—major qualification would require some near-heroic assumptions about false consciousness.

12 Keohane (1984b: 348). Keohane's discussion is reminiscent of Deutsch (1963).
13 The proposition that the burdens of empire almost inevitably outweigh its benefits is a
    common one. Note Elvin (1973: 19):

> The burdens of size consist mainly in the need to maintain a more extended
> bureaucracy with more intermediate layers, the growing difficulties of effective
> co-ordination as territorial area increases, and the heavier costs of maintaining troops
> on long front lines further removed from the main sources of trustworthy
> manpower and supplies.

14 Russett and Starr (1981: ch. 18).
15 Rasler and Thompson (1983) carefully recognize the particular private benefits, to the
    commercially extended hegemon, of providing defense and deterrence for others. This
    should be set against the more familiar argument that military expenditures become a
    private "bad" by inhibiting capital formation and growth in the hegemon. For evidence,
    see Rasler and Thompson (1988).
16 For the argument that free trade is not necessarily a collective good, see Conybeare (1984).
17 Arrighi (1982: 57).
18 In a brilliant article, Snidal (1985), notes that both Krasner (1975) and Gilpin (1981),
    fully recognize the degree to which the postwar regimes benefited the United States and
    that Gilpin particularly argues that the United States was significantly able to extract
    contributions as a quasi government.
19 Without tying it completely to Marxist analysis, this is akin to the concept of cultural
    penetration that I have employed in work with my colleagues. See Duvall *et al.* (1981),
    especially 320–321. I have long been concerned with the political impact of a great power's
    cultural penetration—see, e.g., Russett (1963:, chs. 6–8).
20 Persuading someone to do something he or she would not otherwise do; see Dahl (1984).
21 Cox and Jacobson (1982: 7):

> World hegemony is founded through a process of cultural and ideological
> development. This process is rooted mainly in the civil society of the founding
> country, though it has the support of the state in that country, and it extends to
> include groups from other countries.

See also Elias (1982):

> Just as it was not possible in the West itself, from a certain state of interdependence
> onwards, to rule people solely by force and physical threats, so it also became
> necessary, in maintaining an empire that went beyond mere plantation-land and
> plantation-labour, to rule people in part through themselves, through the
> moulding of their superegos. . . . The outsiders absorb the code of the established
> groups and thus undergo a process of assimilation. Their own affect-control, their
> own conduct, obeys the rules of the established groups. Partially they identify
> themselves with them, and even though the identification may show strong
> ambivalencies, still their own conscience, their whole superego apparatus, follows
> more or less the pattern of the established groups.

Neither of these statements is meant to deny some reciprocal role of elites in the periphery
in helping to shape the dominant world culture.

22 They form, e.g., a key element in Alker's conception of power. See Alker (1973).
23 For a good but now slightly dated survey, see Singer (1972: chs. 4–5). It is tempting for
    the cynical academic to bemoan the pervasiveness of American popular culture, from
    the presence of the *Today Show* by satellite in the wee hours of television programming
    in the Western Pacific to the Tokyo branch of Disneyland. But the influence of liberal
    American human rights policy must not be ignored. I was told that the Japanese
    government recently passed legislation for women's rights primarily out of a desire not
    to be embarrassed by ridicule from the US delegation to the Nairobi Conference
    concluding the United Nations Decade for Women.

24 British influence was heavily facilitated, and consciously promoted, by the rise of English as an international language and the popularity of English literature from Shakespeare to contemporary authors. It is the United States' good fortune, for its present influence, that its language is also English. Of other countries, France has had the most success in promoting its influence through the cultural medium of its language; one of the French motivations in trying to keep Britain out of the European Community was the hope that with Britain excluded the Germans could be made to learn French as the Community language. Japanese has not proved to be an exportable tongue. The West German government, through its Goethe Institute, has tried to promote fluency in German. But the primary German cultural product is probably music rather than literature; knowing the language is of little importance, and perhaps some artifacts (e.g., Wagnerian opera) are more attractive when one doesn't understand the words. Russian has proved not very exportable either, outside the regulated market of Eastern Europe. The classics of Russian literature (Dostoevsky, Tolstoy) are not favored by the Soviet government, Marx wrote in German, and socialist realism just is not very attractive.

25 Kennedy (1984a) similarly notes the role of Britain's cultural force in prolonging its influence abroad.

26 The theme of military expenditures coming at the expense of long-term economic viability is a common one, including in my own work. For some observations on the historical experience of great powers, see Kennedy (1984b) and Rasler and Thompson (1983). The contemporary Soviet example also suggests how the excessive pursuit of military power produces economic stagnation.

27 Keohane (1984a: ch. 9) gives some reasons for optimism.

28 Carr (1939: ch. 14) thought a "pax Americana imposed on a divided and weakened Europe would be an easier contingency to realize than a pax Anglo-Saxonica based on an equal partnership of English-speaking peoples."

29 Snidal (1985) is very good on this matter.

5

THE REAL DECLINE IN NUCLEAR HEGEMONY[1]

Some time ago I wrote a piece (Russett 1985) arguing that the decline in US hegemony of the international system had been greatly exaggerated. I contended that the US ability to influence outcomes, as derived from its economic strength, military capabilities, and global cultural and ideological penetration, remained at least as high as that of previous "hegemons" and not substantially below that which the United States itself wielded in the preceding decades. I still believe that characterization is essentially correct.[2] But the discussion of military instruments of power, especially the role of nuclear weapons, needs to be very carefully nuanced. Observers have been too quick to proclaim the decline of economic hegemony by the United States, and too slow to recognize the decline in nuclear hegemony generally.

In this chapter I contend that the primary purpose of superpower nuclear weapons—extended deterrence—has always been of somewhat doubtful utility, and that the doubts have grown substantially, and with good reason, over the past two decades. Concurrent with the military situation, international norms have evolved to reinforce the unusability of nuclear weapons. Their unusability has meant that the role of nuclear weapons in reinforcing hierarchies of centralized power (hegemony), whether globally, within alliances, or within states, has declined, with uncertain consequences for the world system.

What are nuclear weapons good for?

Nuclear weapons remain extremely effective instruments to achieve some military and political purposes; they have little utility—less than previously—for others. They are not necessarily very important for those purposes for which they seem useful.

Nuclear weapons remain most useful for the purpose for which they are least needed, and have always been least needed: deterrence of nuclear or conventional attack on the home territory of a superpower. Whatever Soviet leaders may have feared following World War II, it is clear that they did not need to fear a deliberate, unprovoked attack by the United States on their home territory, either in the form of conventional invasion or nuclear strike. Despite some talk on the fringes, "preventive war" never remotely approached acceptance as US policy; moral restraints, the vast challenge of subduing and occupying the Soviet Union, and the inability to prevent Soviet conventional devastation of Western Europe in the meantime were, in some mix, fully sufficient deterrents long before the Soviet military actually received operational nuclear weapons in 1952. Similarly, the United States deployed its nuclear weapons long before the Soviet Union had its, and has always been fully as immune from invasion.[3]

Now that both sides have vast numbers of nuclear weapons it is plausible that if either one undertook total nuclear disarmament while the other did not the side retaining nuclear weapons might be tempted to strike with them. That would present an opportunity to end the troublesome rivalry, and to eliminate the risk of subsequent nuclear rearmament by the adversary. But unilateral nuclear disarmament by either side is not very likely. So long as both sides maintain sophisticated, diverse systems of nuclear deterrence, the chance of deliberate, unprovoked nuclear attack is close to nil. This principle is well recognized by even the most cautious strategic analysts. Even the strongest proponents of the idea of a "window of vulnerability" worried about the risk of attack during the escalation of a severe crisis, not about an adventurous strike "out of the blue."

The fact is that nuclear weapons were originally built and deployed not to deter direct attack but for the purpose of extended deterrence or compellence; that is, to protect the security of allies and client states. As such, they were to be a pillar of American post-World War II hegemony. The first implicit threat to use nuclear weapons was by the United States to defend West Berlin and West Germany in 1948; subsequent ones were to try to roll back nascent Chinese entry into the Korean War, to coerce China to accept US terms to end that war, and to deter Chinese attack on the offshore islands of Quemoy and Matsu. In each case the target of the threat was a nonnuclear power. After the Korean War the US principle of "massive retaliation" with nuclear weapons in response to conventional attack by a Soviet "satellite" was made explicit policy. During the 1950s the British developed their own "independent" nuclear deterrent not because they feared being the object of a direct attack, but to cover threats to remaining imperial interests that might be too peripheral to engage US commitment. And the first Soviet nuclear threat was a rather transparent bluff to try to halt the British and French advance at Suez; Britain's nuclear weapons at that time posed little threat to the Soviet Union, and the French still had none. Extended deterrence and compellence formed the game.

The Soviet Union's achievement of an assured retaliatory capability sharply limited any use for US nuclear weapons in making compellent or extended deterrent threats. If one side's assured retaliatory capability were really in serious doubt, then it might be subject to compellent or deterrent threats. But the doubts would have to be very substantial, more than seems plausible with anything like current technology and the numbers of weapons on either side. Otherwise the risks of catastrophe would seem too high for any remotely rational decision-maker actually to carry out the threat.

Paradoxically, with a deliberate nuclear strike in full peacetime virtually out of the question, nuclear weapons as deterrents become the problem rather than the solution. A direct nuclear attack on a superpower's homeland would happen, if at all, only during an extended deterrence crisis. To the degree either power's retaliatory capability is in any doubt, the danger of preemption in the face of threat raises its head. (A few such threats have been made, but to no apparent effect, as we shall see below.) Perhaps if, and only if, a nuclear power were faced either with the imminent loss of a truly vital national interest, or with the perception that the other nuclear power was about to attack it in desperation, a nuclear strike might appear to be the least unattractive option available. In an interacting high-level alert, where *they* might preempt because they think *I* might preempt, and so on, the risks of *not* striking might be high. To wait might mean losing the capacity for any effective "damage limitation" or even retaliation. If it is no longer possible to win a nuclear war, it is possible to lose one, with degrees of losing on an absolute scale (rather than one merely relative to the condition of the adversary) ranging from very bad to dreadful. Under those conditions, and given vulnerability and counterforce capabilities, nuclear weapons create a very real problem of crisis stability. Thus nuclear weapons prevent what they are little needed to prevent (a direct attack "out of the blue") but become a lightning rod to draw fire during the storm of an extended deterrence crisis.

A brief history of nuclear threats

A review of the full history of nuclear threats will show their decreasing frequency and utility. Table 5.1 lists these threats, with the following characterizations: for their purpose, I distinguish between general deterrence, immediate deterrence, and compellence. General deterrence applies to an adversarial relationship with no particular overt challenge; immediate deterrence, by contrast, is "where at least one side is considering an attack while the other is mounting a threat of retaliation in order to prevent it" (Morgan 1983: ch. 1). Whereas a deterrent threat says "don't do it," a compellent threat says "stop doing it," or "do something else." Threats may be conveyed explicitly by verbal communication, overtly by the manipulation of military forces or only implicitly and ambiguously by words. Finally, a threat may succeed or fail in its purpose, or be irrelevant. If the adversary defies the threat, it has failed. If the adversary does as directed, it may be because the threat succeeded, or because action was taken for some reason other than the nuclear threat—because of some other influence, or because the act was intended anyway. If the latter, the nuclear threat is simply irrelevant.

There are often doubts and ambiguities attached to any of these judgments, and it is not possible to clear them all up or document all the judgments here. I indicate

TABLE 5.1 Nuclear threats since 1945

Year	Threatener	Recipient	Interest	General/ immediate/ coercive	Explicit/ overt/ implicit	Succeeded/ failed/ irrelevant
1948	US	USSR	W. Berlin	I	O?	S?
1950	US	China	Korea	C	E	F
1953	US	China	Korea	C	I	S?
1955		China	Quemoy and Matsu	I	E	S?
1956	USSR	UK and France	Suez	C	E	I
1958	US	USSR	Lebanon	G	O	I?
1958	US	China	Quemoy and Matsu	I?	E	I?
1958	USSR	US	W. Berlin	C	I	F
1959	US	USSR	W. Berlin	I?	I	I?
1961	US	USSR	W. Berlin	I?	I	I?
1962	US	USSR	Cuba	C	O and E	S
1969	USSR	China	Border	I?	I	I?
1969	US	N. Vietnam	S. Vietnam	C	E?	F
1973	US	USSR	Israel	I	O	I?
1975	US	N. Korea	S. Korea	G	E	I?
1980	US	USSR	Persian Gulf	G	I	I

Sources: Principally Betts (1987); also Ellsberg (1981), Bundy (1984), Halperin (1987).

the more serious cases of doubt with question marks, and I do not believe that a contrary judgment would severely compromise the conclusions to be drawn. Before trying to draw any conclusions from Table 5.1 it will be helpful to explain very briefly some of the question marks.

In the 1948 Berlin crisis the US threat constituted movement of B-29 bombers to bases in Britain. Whereas the B-29 was then the primary delivery instrument for US atomic bombs, those B-29s were not equipped to carry nuclear weapons and Soviet intelligence may well have known that. Hence the nature of the threat and its efficacy are questionable.

Coincident with its three threats to China between 1953 and 1958 the United States achieved its goals, but it is questionable what role the nuclear threats played in that achievement. Evidence that the Chinese intended to invade Quemoy and Matsu is weaker for 1958 than for 1955.

There is no indication that the Soviet Union had any intention of opposing the 1958 US landing in Lebanon or taking other military action.

Soviet intentions in the later Berlin crises are also in doubt. Arguably the Soviet Union achieved its primary goal by erecting the Berlin Wall.

Chinese intentions in 1969 are likewise unknown.

Halperin (1987: 41) declares that Nixon and Kissinger conveyed several explicit nuclear warnings in demanding that North Vietnam accept a negotiated settlement.

Documentary evidence to support Halperin is not publicly available. If the threats were made they certainly failed.

Betts (1987: 129) says of the 1973 alert, "More than in most cases, the circumstantial evidence for inferring efficacy in the US nuclear threat is weak, and much points in the direction of concluding that it was beside the point."

Halperin (1987: 44) includes Defense Secretary James Schlesinger's warning to North Korea, delivered in 1975 soon after the fall of South Vietnam, but there is no evidence that North Korea was seriously considering military action. The "threat" was directed more toward a South Vietnamese audience as part of American post-Vietnam reassurance.

Truman said that he made a nuclear threat when in 1946 he demanded that the Soviet Union leave northern Iran. The consensus of historians, however (see Bundy 1984: 45), is that all relevant documents are available and none show a nuclear threat; hence it is not listed in the table. The widespread belief that such a threat was made, and succeeded, may nevertheless have contributed to policymakers' faith in the efficacy of nuclear threats.

Table 5.1 shows why Bundy can characterize the record of nuclear diplomacy as "unimpressive." The most nearly unambiguous success was in the Cuban missile crisis of 1962. Weaker and less plausible, but not refutable, arguments can be made for two of the US threats to China in the 1950s and, still more weakly, for what was only an ambiguous threat in the first Berlin crisis. Other cases range from very weak indeed to clear evidence of the failure of nuclear threats. This corresponds to the results of several studies that have been made of the role of the *existence* of nuclear weapons (not necessarily a threat to use them) in extended deterrence crises. Systematic comparative analysis, including multivariate statistical examination of a fairly large number of cases of extended deterrence crises, concludes that nuclear weapons in the hands of the defender have not increased the probability that deterrence will succeed, at least since the 1950s. Rather, other elements of the balance of power—especially local military forces in the immediate region at stake—and interests, plus the bargaining behavior and reputation of the principals, make the difference. This conclusion is put forth with some tentativeness, but when stated carefully—there is little evidence that nuclear weapons systematically make a difference—it is important (see Blechman and Kaplan 1978; Kugler 1984; Huth 1990; Huth and Russett 1988; with a contrary conclusion by Weede 1983).

Save for the Cuban missile crisis, all the plausibly successful threats were made in the first decade of the nuclear era and against adversaries who did not themselves possess nuclear weapons. Even allowing for Soviet nuclear weaponry in the 1953 and 1955 US threats to China, this was undeniably a period of very great American nuclear superiority. Ten of the nuclear threats were made in the first sixteen years of the nuclear era, before the Cuban missile crisis. Only five have been made in the subsequent twenty-six years, even counting the doubtful 1969 Nixon threat to North Vietnam.

Reference to the Cuban missile crisis inevitably raises the question of how important strategic nuclear superiority has been in determining both whether nuclear threats were made and whether they would succeed. Participants and analysts disagree vehemently about whether US strategic nuclear superiority or US local conventional superiority in the Caribbean made the greater difference in persuading the Soviet Union to pull out its weapons. But the facts of US nuclear superiority, the threat to use nuclear weapons, and Soviet acquiescence are not in doubt.

Some participants in decision-making during the Cuban crisis emphasize their hesitancy, even given superiority, in light of Soviet retaliatory capabilities:

> They were finally forced out, but it was not through the threat of use of nuclear weapons. We never conceived of using nuclear weapons under those circumstances. It was our tremendous conventional power in the region which forced the Soviets to take those missiles out.
>
> (Robert S. McNamara, quoted in Charlton 1987: 23)

The crisis showed "not the significance but the insignificance of nuclear superiority in the face of survivable thermonuclear forces" (Bundy 1984: 55). Henry Kissinger, who was not there, says a bit differently, "Khrushchev withdrew from Cuba because we had local superiority. On top of it, what made it easy was that we also had strategic superiority" (quoted in Charlton 1987: 55). Revelations at a 1987 "reunion" of Cuban missile crisis participants made it clear how much of the received wisdom on that event (for example, Allison 1971) is misleading, and how difficult it is to reconstruct motives and decisions in national security crises.

Nuclear threats were more common in the years up through the Cuban missile crisis than afterward. If made by the United States, with its nuclear superiority, they were more likely then to have at least some semblance of success. Is this because US leaders believed that their nuclear superiority gave them near-immunity from Soviet retaliation? The most thorough review of the historical documentation concludes that was not the case. US leaders usually believed that a Soviet retaliatory strike would impose severe costs on the United States; they did not feel immune and perhaps felt more vulnerable than now-available information about the nuclear balance suggests they need have been:

> There may, conceivably, have been a golden age when US leaders could be confident in their ability to limit damage from Soviet nuclear retaliation to a remotely acceptable level—say, total blast and fallout fatalities under 10 percent of the population. But it was an age that comprised, at best, only two brief periods: the years before the mid-1950s and a few years in the early 1960s.
>
> (Betts 1987: 174)

Even in the possible "golden age," this is a very weak statement about immunity.

Betts's conclusion is carefully balanced: US escalation dominance perhaps "made nuclear superiority if not a rational comfort, a visceral one" (178). US decision-makers were not prepared deliberately to make nuclear war, but were willing to take some risks that matters might escalate to nuclear war. One may or may not judge that willingness to have been adventurism, but the circumstances that made it possible passed with the advent of nuclear parity and "essential equivalence."[4]

The five cases since the Cuban missile crisis deserve some attention. The Soviet nuclear threat to China was verbally somewhat ambiguous, but we know the Soviet leadership seriously considered using nuclear weapons—if with the assent of the United States. When the United States failed to reply favorably, the Soviets then did nothing. The Chinese moved to reduce military tensions in the border conflict, for reasons we cannot fully know. Relieved of the immediate danger and devoid of any US support for relief from their longer-run worries about China as a nuclear power, the Soviets stood down despite their overwhelming nuclear superiority over the Chinese. The alleged US threat to North Vietnam in 1969 may never have been made; if it was, it is clear the Nixon administration had no intention whatever of carrying it out. The 1973 nuclear alert and signaling was a pale shadow of the Cuban missile crisis. Neither Schlesinger's 1975 threat nor Carter's in 1980 was made at a time of international crisis or immediate threat of communist attack. Delivered under conditions of general deterrence the threats were not very provocative, and did not create problems of crisis alert and signaling; Schlesinger and Carter were not at immediate risk of having to put up or shut up. None demonstrated the credible willingness to initiate nuclear war that might have been inferred in some previous crises. There have been no nuclear threats since 1980. Whereas Betts points out that US leaders have been willing to make nuclear threats without possessing nuclear superiority, those few threats simply do not carry the same weight (note that Betts does not even include the 1969 and 1975 US threats in his list).

Crises without nuclear threats

Further clues to the infrequency and ineffectiveness of nuclear threats emerge when we look at the instances when nuclear threats might have been made and were not. Elsewhere a colleague and I have examined the universe of extended immediate deterrence crises over the past century (Huth 1988; Huth and Russett 1988). Omitting several crises that were included in Table 5.1 as nuclear threats, these fourteen involved nuclear powers as defenders. Table 5.2 presents them somewhat in the format of Table 5.1. The labels "defender" and "attacker" replace "threatener" and "recipient," however, precisely because no nuclear threat was made. For that same reason the second column for characterization of the threat is omitted, and the first such column is not needed because these are by definition all cases of immediate deterrence.

Several observations can be made. First, of these fourteen cases, three were instances when deterrence did not succeed, despite the fact in two of them only the defender, and not the attacker, had nuclear weapons. The mere existence of those weapons in a one-sided relationship was no guarantee of success. Nor in the third instance (1979) was clear Soviet nuclear superiority over China very helpful.

TABLE 5.2 Extended immediate deterrence crises with nuclear-armed defenders

Year	Defender	Attacker	Interest	Deterrence: succeeded or failed
1946	US	USSR	Iran	S
1946	US	USSR	Turkey	S
1950	US	China	Taiwan	S
1957	USSR	Turkey	Syria	S
1961	UK	Iraq	Kuwait	S
1961	US	N. Vietnam	Laos	S
1964	UK	Indonesia	Malaysia	F
1964	China	US	N. Vietnam	S
1964	US	N. Vietnam	S. Vietnam	F
1971	China	India	Pakistani Kashmir	S
1975	UK	Guatemala	Belize	S
1977	UK	Guatemala	Belize	S
1979	USSR	China	Vietnam	F
1983	France	Libya	Chad	S

Source: (with definitions and qualifications) Huth and Russett 1988.

Second, all of the failures occurred after 1964. Third, in one instance (China in 1964) deterrence succeeded against a thermonuclear superpower even though the defender's nuclear capability was but nominal (tested but not operational). Fourth, in many of the successes, especially recent ones, it is impossible to believe that the defender's possession of nuclear weapons played any role in the attacker's decision not to press forward. It is absurd to think of the United Kingdom "nuking" Guatemala, and whatever Gaddafi's provocations, it is not much more plausible to postulate a French nuclear strike against Libya. Full multivariate examination of the conditions for success or failure of deterrence is properly left elsewhere. But it is hard to see here any evidence that nuclear weapons have made much difference and, if they once did, that they have done so in the last fifteen years or so.[5]

The essential irrelevance of nuclear weapons even against nonnuclear adversaries emerges even more clearly in a case that did not make either of the above tables: the Falklands/Malvinas war between Britain and Argentina in 1982. It did not appear in the tables because the British never made any deterrent threat at all; they avoided doing so before the Argentine invasion in order not to be provocative. Some British ships in the South Atlantic had nuclear weapons aboard and the Vulcan aircraft used to bomb the occupied airstrips were originally built for carrying nuclear weapons. Nevertheless, even during the course of the war the British made no threat, explicit or implicit, to use those weapons. (Recall that the United States was quite ready to make such threats against China over an equally piddling set of islands in the 1950s.) At no time did the Argentine government, though powerless to retaliate in kind and not under the US nuclear umbrella, ever seriously fear that it would be hit by British nuclear weapons.

The evolution of norms

Nuclear weapons were understood to be normatively disproportionate in the Falklands/Malvinas war; perhaps licit in the defense of a homeland or some truly vital national interest, but not of a peripheral one even though British soldiers and sailors were dying in defense of that "peripheral" interest. There has emerged in the global community a recognition that nuclear weapons are unusable across much of the range of traditional military and political interests; that recognition has been strengthened by actions as diverse as the Reagan administration's repeated statements that it does not target Soviet population centers per se, the US Catholic Bishops' Pastoral Letter (USCC 1983), and Soviet pledges—however reliable—to take a no-first-use posture.

First use, as a doctrine of deliberate action in a policy of extended deterrence, is in disrepute around the world. In 1982, McGeorge Bundy, George Kennan, Robert McNamara, and Gerard Smith became the first members of the national security establishment to issue a public call for a no-first-use policy. McNamara (1983: 79, his emphasis) subsequently declared, "*Nuclear weapons serve no military purpose whatsoever. They are totally useless—except only to deter one's opponent from using them,*" and said that at least the leaders he served seemed quietly to agree: "In long private conversations with successive Presidents—Kennedy and Johnson—I recommended, without qualification, that they never initiate, under any circumstances, the use of nuclear weapons. I believe they accepted my recommendation." A survey of generals and admirals in 1984 found 61 percent saying they could not justify a nuclear first strike against the Soviet Union (Kohut and Horrock 1984). (Technically, of course, abjuring a first strike does not necessarily mean abjuring first *use* in the face of conventional attack.)

The people of Western Europe (as distinct from their governments) have for three decades expressed themselves in favor of a no-first-use policy. By 1981 fewer than 20 percent of the population in any of the big Western European countries (Britain, France, West Germany, and Italy) thought that NATO should use nuclear weapons to defend itself even "if a Soviet attack by conventional forces threatened to overwhelm NATO forces," and sentiment has not changed significantly since then (Russett and DeLuca 1983; Adler 1986). Americans were somewhat slower to reach this conclusion, but by the late 1960s a majority were opposed to using nuclear weapons to defend their European allies, and by 1982 it was a two-thirds majority. In 1984, three-quarters said they favored a policy of no-first-use in general (Kramer *et al.* 1983; Yankelovich and Doble 1984; Graham 1987). In this respect popular sentiment has run ahead of elite attitudes.

The disillusionment with first use is of course not just a result of normative developments, and certainly norms themselves are hardly fully independent variables. The numbers and destructive power of the weapons, plus the achievement of a secure second strike capability by the superpowers and probably the secondary nuclear powers (Britain, France, and China) are almost surely the major factors. But fear of retaliation does not account for many of the instances when nuclear weapons were useless to deter nonnuclear states, especially those states like Argentina, which lacked any plausible nuclear defender. No one wants to be the first since 1945 to use a nuclear weapon in war. "Self-deterrence" of the use of nuclear weapons began in the Truman administration (Gaddis 1987: ch. 5); the experience of forty-two years has more firmly established a de facto norm of nonuse.[6]

Betts is inclined not to credit US post 1962 restraint too much to the Soviet achievement of nuclear parity. He rightly points out that US leaders made nuclear threats on two subsequent occasions (1973 and 1980), and Halperin somewhat tenuously adds two more (1969 and 1975). Nuclear superiority is not a necessary condition to making such threats, and lack of it did not prevent the Soviets from making nuclear threats (ineffective ones) in 1956 and 1958. Some decision-makers may be sufficiently risk-prone, or see such vital interests engaged, that they will do so from positions of parity or even inferiority. But they are less likely to do so, especially in real crises where the escalation dynamic of alert and counter-alert might become engaged. General deterrence threats, as against North Korea in 1975 or regarding the Persian Gulf in 1980, are much safer—and therefore less impressive.

Reasons for restraint

Betts also rightly points out that superpower conflicts since 1962 have occurred exclusively at the periphery of superpower interests (that is, not in Europe). Two explanations come to mind. One is that the superpowers have grown more cautious in Europe, with its vital interests to both, and have perhaps done so because of their mutual fears of nuclear weapons use. That is almost surely true. But it is not because the deliberate use of nuclear weapons in Europe is more credible. The deliberate use of those weapons has rather become less credible. That threat has been replaced with what Schelling (1966: 99) called "the threat that leaves something to chance." The threat is that nuclear weapons may be used without the intention or authorization of the central command authorities. In normal peacetime the weapons are under tight control; in a high-level crisis they would likely be widely dispersed, with the capabilities to fire them delegated to low-level military commanders. In wartime those commanders could readily find themselves in situations of "use them or lose them," and of losing their troops, if they hesitated to fire their nuclear weapons. Moreover, commanders of the opposing forces would be aware of those pressures, and consequently be under great temptation to preempt (Bracken 1983; Charles 1987). All these pressures are made worse by the use of dual-capable aircraft and missiles and by the close integration of nuclear and conventional weapons in the field.

These are not the threats of the archetypal rational nuclear deterrent theorist, but threats of losing "rational" centralized control. They illustrate a certain continued utility for nuclear weapons, ironically a perhaps greater utility than against a nonnuclear state. But it is hardly what was envisaged for a dominant nuclear power. The risk is that the political events that give rise to crises may be no more controllable than are military events in the "fog of war." The reluctance of the superpowers to challenge each other in Europe is therefore hardly an indication of their confidence in nuclear weapons as deliberate, manageable instruments of deterrence or war. Such a potentially unstable equilibrium in crisis is hardly what most of the classical nuclear theorists thought they were buying. In the best-informed study of these problems with strategic weapons, Blair (1985) considers the risks of crisis instability to be so serious that he recommends adopting a posture of no immediate *second* strike, allowing time for an informed decision and reducing the pressures on an adversary to preempt. Doing so would, by eliminating the threat that leaves something to chance, mark the end of extended nuclear deterrence as a viable strategy.

A second reason for the credibility of deterrence in Europe has everything to do with the network of economic and political interests, cultural and institutional ties, and past commitments that exist between each superpower and its group of European allies. The superpowers stand ready to fight in Europe not because they think they would benefit by some tilt in the nuclear balance, but because they cannot afford to lose their varied investments (Quester 1987). That fear makes them willing to accept the risks inherent in the threat that leaves something to chance. To counter any possible adventurism on either side there is also, and perhaps as important, the fear of conventional war. Europeans (including Russians) have lived with the experience of full-scale conventional war in their homelands. Nuclear war is an extra and still more horrible threat, but the prospective levels of casualties and property damage from conventional war alone provide an enormously powerful deterrent.

Conventional war among rich industrial states is particularly horror-inducing. They are rich and industrial and could sustain the production of great quantities of war material; they could be self-sufficient enough to fight long and hard enough to level the continent. Being rich already, they have all the more to lose by the large-scale devastation of war, and virtually nothing worth gaining. If the deterrent effect of memories of World War II has faded slightly, the entrenchment of interest in preserving postwar prosperity can balance it. Prosperity also is embedded nontrivially in East–West ties of economic interdependence.[7] Even without taking nuclear weapons into account, Europeans in effect are operating at points on the marginal cost and benefit curves where those curves become very flat, and the pattern of incentives is already heavily against war. As Mueller (1988a) nicely put it, "A jump from a 50th floor window is probably a bit more horrible to think about than a jump from a 5th floor one, but anyone who finds life even minimally satisfying is extremely unlikely to do either."

A more general reason for the recent infrequency of nuclear threats worldwide is the irrelevance of the dangers they are best designed to deter: loss of territory or the extinction of national sovereignty. By historical standards, national borders have been extraordinarily stable since the end of World War II. Boundaries have been unchanged in Europe. Even in Africa, with so many ethnically arbitrary colonial boundaries, there have been almost no postindependence changes.[8] Cases of loss of sovereignty have been even rarer: only the peaceful union of Tanganyika and

Zanzibar into Tanzania, and the hardly peaceful reunification of North and South Vietnam. The essence of nuclear threats is, "Don't cross the boundaries."

Nuclear weapons may have made a contribution to the stability of borders and statehood in Europe. Many observers think so, and think that the effect has on balance been desirable.[9] But it is hard to maintain that they have much to do with the experience in, for example, Africa. Furthermore, whereas nuclear weapons help to deter change in the formal boundaries in Europe, they can do little to deter the kinds of changes that are much more probable—for example, the shift toward market economies in Eastern Europe, or maybe toward greater political pluralism there. These, not boundaries, are what matters for the quality of life in that part of the world. Outside of Europe, US nuclear superiority could not prevent the Soviet Union from aiding armed insurgencies against pro-Western governments; now Soviet nuclear parity does nothing to keep the United States from aiding guerrillas in Afghanistan, Angola, Ethiopia, Kampuchea, or Nicaragua.

The nonusability of nuclear weapons has little to do with the fine points of the strategic nuclear balance. Henry Kissinger's exclamation, "What in the name of God is strategic superiority? . . . What do you do with it?" is well known. True, he later stepped back, saying, "If we opt out of the race unilaterally, we will probably be faced eventually with a younger group of Soviet leaders who will figure out what can be done with strategic superiority" (Betts 1987: 212). Yet even the later qualification means only that we must not, by opting out of the race, permit our adversary to achieve superiority; it does not mean that either side can achieve a politically or militarily significant imbalance so long as the other follows the rules of normal prudence.

It may not even be extreme to say that a no-first-use of nuclear weapons regime has grown up, de facto, despite efforts of the nuclear powers (especially the United States) to prevent it. Certainly there are major common norms, expectations, and decision-making procedures for crisis behavior and hence crisis stabilization. The hotline, crisis management centers, and a series of arms control agreements such as for managing contacts between warships at sea and monitoring troop movements in Europe all are intended to stabilize crises. That in turn must mean an ability to assure the other side that one is not intending to use nuclear weapons, or if a few are used inadvertently to establish the inadvertence.

Arenas of nuclear hegemony

Nuclear hegemony has operated in two senses. First is the hegemony of the nuclear powers in the international system. Initially it was US hegemony, and then the bipolar nuclear hegemony of both the United States and the Soviet Union within their own blocs. The superpowers talked about nuclear disarmament, but studiously avoided doing it. The late Alva Myrdal characterized their activities as "the game of disarmament." "Behind their outwardly often fierce disagreements . . . there has always been a secret and undeclared collusion between the superpowers. Neither of them has wanted to be restrained by effective disarmament measures." For her the reason was rooted in international politics: "Military competition results in an ever increasing superiority—militarily and technologically—of the already over strong superpowers, thus sharpening the discrimination against all lesser powers" (Myrdal 1976). They kept an enormous lead over the other nuclear powers (about ten thousand warheads apiece for the United States and the Soviet Union as compared with only a few hundred for any of the others), and sponsored the Nonproliferation Treaty to prevent the rise of any other nuclear powers.

Indeed, the nonproliferation arena has consistently marked the high point of Soviet-US cooperation on arms control. The form of that cooperation has become a matter of bitterness among many of the nonnuclear states. The bargain for "horizontal" nonproliferation was supposed to be that the superpowers would reduce their "vertical" nuclear proliferation, which they have not done. A major hurdle to any truly substantial reduction of the US and Soviet nuclear armories remains their worry about significantly reducing the gap between themselves and secondary nuclear powers. A European nuclear deterrent—perhaps of substantial capability— is a real possibility in the long run.

Nevertheless, whether or not they fully realize it their position of dominance is beginning to erode. Britain, France, and China all are engaged in programs to expand and modernize their nuclear retaliatory forces. When these programs are completed, each will then have something like a secure second-strike capability— not remotely enough to permit them to engage in extended nuclear deterrence of conventional attack on their own allies, but enough pretty reliably to deter direct attack on themselves. Many knowledgeable observers fear that the nonproliferation regime is about to break down. Even allowing for frequent cries of wolf in the past, the situation is worrisome. Israel has an unannounced but significant de facto nuclear capability; South Africa may well also have joined the club, and efforts to control the situation in South Asia (India and Pakistan) are clearly faltering. It is worth noting that all of these new or candidate nuclear powers are among the minority of states with serious problems about where their boundaries should lie.

The Strategic Defense Initiative (SDI) can be seen as a desperate effort by the United States to either restore its own unilateral nuclear hegemony, as the Soviets apparently fear, or to reestablish on a firm basis the conditions of Soviet-US nuclear co-hegemony. Modernization of the British, French, and Chinese forces will give them an assured retaliatory capability only so long as the superpowers do not have a decent SDI. A good SDI for either superpower—however unlikely it may seem —would give that superpower nuclear hegemony. A good or even pretty good SDI for both superpowers would give them joint hegemony against ICBMs in their game of duopoly, because that SDI would be much more effective against the smaller retaliatory force of a secondary or nth nuclear power than against the other superpower. Notice the terms of the Reagan administration's characterization of SDI: something that would include America's allies as contractors and protégés and something for which—if one believes in the tooth fairy—the technology could be shared with the *Russians*.

The other last-gasp means of restoring US nuclear hegemony or co-hegemony is represented by the effort to create feasible and credible "limited nuclear options." An ability to fight limited nuclear war, and to keep it limited, would revitalize the principle of extended deterrence as a rational act for a superpower. The effort has proceeded at both the strategic and tactical levels. Kissinger, looking back at his 1956 advocacy of tactical nuclear weapons for the European theater, said, "Sooner or later (I thought it would come sooner than it did) strategic nuclear weapons would tend towards a kind of parity that would make absolute war impossible, and I called for alternatives" (Charlton 1987: 33). Some Americans may like the idea because it implies a "limited" nuclear war could be kept limited to, say, Europe. For the same reason, neither European governments nor their people like the idea.

Ironically, a variety of small accurate weapons, theoretically usable, now exist. More lacking than ever is a sane scenario for limited nuclear war. I have already indicated some of the reasons why the effort to make the deliberate initiation of limited nuclear war credible is unlikely to succeed. The matter cannot be settled to everyone's satisfaction, but there is an impressive array of opinion, from academics to national security professionals to senior military officers that the effort must fail (Ball 1981; Steinbruner 1981–1982; Bundy et al. 1982; Collins 1982; Bracken 1983). To these, as well as to most members of the mass public, limited nuclear war is an oxymoron advocated by morons. (Limited nuclear options are essential if the goal is quick war termination, and I agree [most recently in Russett 1988] that such planning for very limited "counter combatant" use is, with great caution, appropriate. Plans for protracted war-fighting, escalation dominance, and war-winning are not.)

If nuclear weapons represent an instrument of centralizing power in the hands of a hegemon or alliance leader, they must secondly be recognized as an instrument for retaining societal hegemony by the leadership of the central government. Governments are regarded as the "legitimate wielders of the instruments of violence." "Terrorists" often are defined as nongovernmental wielders of collective violence, ignoring what others would characterize as state terrorism. Nuclear weapons are the instruments of violence par excellence—the instruments of state terrorism if you will. Only a large modern central government can gather the resources to build, deploy, and control nuclear weapons. Even it can do so only under perceptions of great national danger. The need to limit access to nuclear weapons, and the knowledge of how to build them, becomes the basis for legitimizing state control over a wide range of information. Local governments are not permitted to play with those instruments; small national governments and private individuals can afford to do so with only the greatest of difficulty. States around the world would applaud the extermination of any nonstate actors who tried to use nuclear weapons. Nuclear proliferation into the hands of nonstate actors would erode the basis for state hegemony over national societies.

In his book, John Ruggie (1988) maintains that the global system of rule is becoming transformed, that the assumptions of territoriality and differentiation among states are becoming ever more invalid. One can argue about whether that is true, and if true whether it will be a "good thing" for humanity. One can also argue about whether the ability of nuclear weapons to reinforce hegemony and territoriality is in fact declining, and whether, if so, that is a good thing. I have no doubts that nuclear weapons have served that function, and am at least inclined to believe that their utility in that function is diminishing. That diminution carries great dangers as well as opportunities. The result may be decentralization of power and reduction of hegemonies in the global system into a form of "patterned chaos," the chaos of war of each against all, or the imposition of a new hegemony in the form of a global state. Whether any of those would prove to be a good thing must be the subject for another occasion.

Notes

1   I thank William Foltz, Joshua Goldstein, Paul Huth, Peter Katzenstein, Robert Keohane, Joel Rosenthal, and Dieter Senghaas for comments on an earlier draft.
2   One exception: the emergence since then of the enormous US trade deficit and net foreign indebtedness, which endangers the economic foundations of hegemony.
3   A stimulating and unorthodox argument for the existence of mutual superpower security without nuclear weapons is Shepherd (1986).
4   Halperin (1987: ch. 2) dismisses the efficacy of nuclear threats virtually throughout the era, and so underplays the significance of this trend.
5   The situation is reminiscent of that in the sixteenth century, when the weapons and tactics of war among the great powers proved of little use in the periphery. See Braudel (1984: 58). Remember also that the context here is immediate deterrence—whether nuclear weapons make a difference once a crisis has arisen—not general deterrence preventing a crisis even from occurring.
6   This argument has been elaborated, in a formulation that to be sure is not legally binding, by a group of international lawyers in the statement by Lawyers' Committee on Nuclear Policy (1981, 1984).
7   West Europeans are of course richer than Russians and other East Europeans, but the easterners still are far better off than in their past and hardly about to jeopardize those hard-won gains. On Soviet motivations, see MccGwire (1987). The argument that modern war (not merely nuclear war) rarely has any utility for rational purpose has a long tradition, from Sir Norman Angell before World War I, to a provocative statement by Deutsch and Senghaas (1971).
8   The important exception would be the border between Chad and Libya. There have been only two others: negotiated minor adjustments between Mali and Mauritania and between Mali and Burkina Faso. South Africa has wanted to make several changes in its area, but despite its status as regional hegemon has been unable to do so.
9   Weede (1983, and in Chapter 12 here) is one who holds that they have helped the hegemons to keep the peace within their alliance systems as well as between them. He sees the Falklands/Malvinas war and the Soviet failure to deter China in 1979 as dangerous portents of decline in this ability. In my opinion (for example, Russett and Starr 1989: ch. 14) there are other, much more persuasive, explanations for the achievement of peace, at least among the Western industrialized states.

6

THE FUTURE AS ARBITER OF THEORETICAL CONTROVERSIES

Predictions, explanations, and the end of the cold war[1]

James Lee Ray and Bruce Russett

Some analysts assert that a failure by the discipline of international relations to predict the end of the cold war reinforces their conviction that predominant theories as well as systematic empirical analyses of international politics have proved fruitless. Accurate predictions are an important product of useful theory, partly because predictions cannot be modified in order to accommodate the events upon which they focus, since the outcomes to be accounted for are unknown. But predictions are contingent statements about the future, not unconditional assertions, which might more accurately be labelled prophecies.

Three related streams of work—a political forecasting model that relies on rational choice theory, insights and information provided by traditional area specialists, and democratic peace theory—together constitute an emerging basis for making accurate predictions about the political future, and deserve attention in any evaluation of the utility of systematic empirical analyses of politics. Moreover, the systematic empirical approach is not entirely bereft of potential to provide a better understanding of the end of the cold war. The democratic peace proposition suggests that if the autocratic protagonist in a confrontation becomes more democratic, tensions should be significantly reduced. This implication of democratic peace did not go unnoticed in the years before the cold war ended.

"The role of theory," according to John Lewis Gaddis, "has always been not just to account for the past or to explain the present but to provide at least a preview of what is to come" (Gaddis 1992/93: 10).

Having reviewed the recent performance of international relations theorists, Gaddis also points out, correctly, that the vast majority of those theorists failed to predict the end of the cold war. But then he argues further that star-gazers, readers of entrails and other "pre-scientific" methods were as effective in providing foreknowledge of the fundamental transformations that took place from 1989 to 1991 as allegedly "scientific" methods were (Gaddis 1992/93: 18.[2] His critique ultimately becomes an indictment not only of the inadequacies of predominant theories of international relations, but of "scientific" methods for predicting international affairs in general. We disagree with that indictment.

Gaddis's opinions on these matters are hardly unique, nor based solely on the absence of accurate predictions regarding the end of the cold war. Yosef Lapid referred over five years ago to the "demise of the empiricist–positivist promise for a cumulative behavioral science," and to the "ruins of the positivist project" (Lapid 1989: 236). In 1990, *International Studies Quarterly* devoted a special issue to "Dissidence in International Studies" containing several examples of postmodern, deconstructionist, discourse analyses (Ashley and Walker 1990). Donald Puchala, in an essay entitled "Woe to the Orphans of the Scientific Revolution," defended the thesis implicit in that picturesque title by declaring that international relations theory "does not, because it cannot in the absence of laws . . . invite us to deduce, and *it does not permit us to predict*" (Puchala 1991: 79, emphasis added).[3]

Yet the scientific (or quantitative, or systematic empirical) approach to political science or the subfield of international politics survived—and even flourished through—earlier celebrations of its demise. David Easton, for example, praised the "post-behavioral revolution" in political science long ago (Easton 1969).

Our central claim here is that current reports of the death of the scientific study of international politics are also exaggerated. In support of that claim, we will discuss several issues regarding the use of predictions in the evaluation of different, competing approaches to international politics. We then evaluate the ability of the scientific approach to international politics to produce accurate predictions about political events in general, and about the end of the cold war in particular. We conclude that the thesis regarding the demise of the systematic empirical study of international politics advanced by Gaddis and others ignores a substantial body of work that we believe justifies a more positive judgement.

Predictions, explanations, and useful theory

Gaddis asserts that theories should highlight patterns from the past in a way that makes them useful guides to the future (Gaddis 1992/93: 6). Hans Morgenthau argued that "realism" would allow analysts not only to foresee but to influence the future (Morgenthau 1948: 4–5). No less an authority on science than Stephen Hawking declares that "a good theory . . . must make definitive predictions about the results of future observations" (Hawking 1988: 9).[4] Similarly, Robert Keohane in his essay on "Theory of World Politics" emphasizes that foreknowledge is one of the most important products of good theory (Keohane 1983).

But J. David Singer, a founder of the quantitative approach to international politics, argues that prediction demands less of a theory than does explanation, or even description. He points out, for example, that it is relatively simple to predict that pressure on the accelerator of a car will increase its speed. Explaining why that is the case is a more demanding task, in his view (Singer 1961). Joining Singer in this skeptical attitude about the utility of accurate predictions as an "acid test" of the validity and quality of theories are rather strange bedfellows: an array of "anti-" or "post-positivists," and more currently of postmodernists who disagree with the idea that hypotheses can be tested by comparing their implications with experience. In the postpositivist view, there is no way of describing or observing the "real world" in a way that is independent of the theory that produced the hypothesis. This means that no one can "objectively" observe the correspondence between theory-based predictions and happenings in the "real world." "There are no 'brute' facts—no facts prior to interpretation . . . *Facts are always theory-dependent*" (Hollis and Smith 1990: 54–56, emphasis added).[5] Postmodernists "consider both [causality and prediction] uninteresting . . . They argue [that] the requirements of temporal priority and independent, external reality assumed by these concepts are dubious" (Rosenau 1992: 212).

Some postmodernists also feel that any correspondence between theory-based predictions and "real world" events will be doubly misleading, not only because the perceived correspondence will be produced spuriously by theory-driven perceptions of the "facts" in question, but also because any correspondence that is perceived will also be in part the result of a self-fulfilling prophecy. That is, being aware of the theory, people will behave in the way it predicts because they believe in its validity, or because they think that the common expectations produced by it in the culture in which they operate make it "rational" to behave as the theory predicts (Vasquez 1994).[6] Related to this idea is the postmodernist belief that theoretical predictions constitute a form of political oppression. In this view, communities of people ought to be allowed to supply their own meaning and truth for themselves. Any attempt to generalize across communities involves the destruction of differences. Such generalizations are in effect "hegemonic power plays" (Vasquez 1994: 4). In the opinion of Richard Ashley, "Any knowledgeable practice that participates in the inscription of sovereign voice and the narrative structure of history—and the conduct of social theory is certainly one such practice—is an arbitrary practice of power" (Ashley 1989: 280).

Evaluating theories: the case for predictive accuracy as a criterion

In contrast, A.F.K. Organski and Samuel Eldersveld, for example, find "troubling" the persistent view that the capacity to predict is of little consequence because explanation is the real commitment of the social sciences (Organski and Eldersveld 1994).[7] One of the origins of such discomfort is the influential argument of Carl Hempel that "the logical structure of a scientific prediction is the same as that of a scientific explanation" (Hempel 1965: 234). This argument implies that explanations and predictions should both be defined as contingent statements, and contrasted with "prophecies," or assertions about the future prefaced by no conditions or contingencies (Dessler 1994).[8] It is true, as Singer has argued, that "any informed layman" can predict that if pressure is applied to an accelerator of a car, it will increase its speed (Singer 1961: 79–80). But the prediction will be wrong if the car has run out of fuel. The contingency "if the tank contains gasoline," or any other contingency that would improve the explanation might also usefully be considered part of a more complete or accurate prediction.

This is not to say that we accept unconditionally Hempel's argument that explanations are identical in structure to predictions, nor are we advocating what some would term a "naive falsificationist" view that scientists are analogous to bookkeepers who can mechanically tally up the extent to which the predictions based on a theory are supported by events in the real world. We acknowledge, for example, that scientists can be and often are influenced by predominant "paradigms" or "research programmes" in ways that make them quite different from accountants adding and subtracting columns of numbers (Kuhn 1962; Lakatos 1970). We are also aware of, and in partial agreement with, scientific "realists" who contend: that explanations focus on causal mechanisms and processes; that many intuitive notions about explanations and causality do not fit into Hempel's arguments regarding the symmetry between explanations and predictions; that many successful explanatory schemes do not necessarily provide a basis for accurate predictions; and that in general explanations cannot be equated with predictions, or vice versa.[9] But the Hempelian and the "realist" conceptions of explanation (and prediction) are not in irreconcilable competition with each other. "The two explanatory modes are complementary; a full science will recognize both" (Dessler 1991: 346).[10]

While we acknowledge, then, that explanation may be in general a more demanding or important task for theory (and theoreticians) than prediction, we are also inclined to argue that in one important respect, at least, predictive accuracy is a more stringent criterion. Explanations may be—but predictions cannot be— modified, consciously or subconsciously, in order to accommodate the events upon which they focus, since the outcomes to be accounted for by predictions are unknown. This makes the future an important, even irreplaceable, arbiter between contrasting claims based on competing theoretical or epistemological approaches. In other words, we have no quarrel with those who insist that "understanding," not prediction is the main purpose of science. But "prediction can be a purpose too . . . It is the *test* of a theory, whatever the purpose" (Quine 1992: 2).[11]

We adopt such an argument even though we agree with postpositivists, post-modernists, and hermeneutically inclined analysts that there are no "facts" out there in the real world to be observed independently of theoretically derived expecta-tions and inclinations. Since human beings cannot be totally objective, even the most seemingly innocuous descriptive observations about international politics are "theory-laden." Consider the assertion that "Germany initiated the Second World War in 1939 by attacking Poland." It involves anthropomorphizing the states in question ("Germany" and "Poland") in a way that is not only theoretic-ally based, but objectionable to some scholars of international politics. The phrase "Second World War" is ethnocentric. It might, more objectively, be referred to as the second phase of a European Civil War.[12] To designate the point in time as "1939" is equally ethnocentric, accepting the Gregorian calendar as opposed to the Chinese or Hebraic methods of assigning numbers to the passing years. Potentially even more substantial issues raised by this statement include whether Germany really was responsible for initiating the Second World War, or when it really began.

But to go from a valid assertion that observations of facts about the "real world" are inevitably theory-laden to the conclusion that one cannot usefully compare derivations from theories to the results of empirical observations is to press a valid point to an extreme which is unnecessary. "Difficult cases make bad law." Analogously, it is a mistake to conclude from the impossibility of making "neutral" or "objective" observations of the real world that it will be impossible to achieve any meaningful degree of consensus about whether predictions derived from a theory are accurate or valid. In short, we acknowledge that observations are inevitably theory-*laden*; they are not, however, theory-*determined* to the degree that comparing observations to theoretical expectations is a pointless exercise.[13]

Admittedly, it is possible that a majority of observers will form a theoretically based consensus around ideas that only *appear* to be validated, because the social actors being observed are infused with the same theoretical notions and behave accordingly. But especially if one considers the number of null findings that never see the light of published day, then the proportion of empirical analyses that fail to support the hypothesis in question suggests that most of them are not self-fulfilling prophecies. In addition, many analyses address the past, sometimes more than two millennia ago. Since the theories in most cases did not exist during the times on which such analyses focus, there is no danger that they will be confirmed in a self-fulfilling way. Similarly, the geographic scope addressed by predictions in the field of international politics, at least, militates against the self-fulfilling prophecy. Such points are even more compelling in the light of the significant number of competing, diametrically opposed propositions in the field of international politics, even though their adherents share epistemological commitments to systematic empiricism.

In response to the fear that accurate predictions (or the theories on which they are based) constitute a form of oppression, we would not deny that those who attempt to predict political events typically have an interest in having an impact on them. In fact, scientifically oriented analysts will often proclaim proudly that their work is "policy-relevant." Nor is it possible to deny that the knowledge producing accurate forecasts of political processes or events can fall into the hands of people who will use it for nefarious purposes. But to eschew the pursuit of scientific knowledge because of its potential for exploitation for undesirable ends is a step towards ensuring that fate for such knowledge. In other words, if "good" people (by definition) avoid the generation of scientific knowledge on the grounds that it can serve undesirable ends, then only "bad" people will produce such knowledge. "Although science may or may not require prediction, we do. It is a large part of what we look to science for. It is what we need to ameliorate the human condition or at any rate to prevent further deterioration" (Rosenberg 1992: 51).

Fortunately, too, science as a human endeavour is opposed in principle to the imposition of ideas by *authority*, or by the power inherent in formal authoritative roles. An essential character of scientific evidence is that it be reproducible—that anybody, but *especially* critics or opponents of ideas espoused by scientists, should be able to reproduce the results or evidence in support of those ideas on her or his own, independently. Admittedly this is an ideal often not attained in the "real world." But even approximations of the idea provide some protection against the use of scientific knowledge for oppressive purposes.

Predicting the political future

The assertion by John Gaddis that the field of international politics has failed to provide a basis for making accurate predictions about political events (such as the end of the cold war) is based on a thorough review of theoretical and empirical work in the field. But he does not mention a set of related streams of research and theory that justifies, we believe, a more optimistic evaluation of the field's ability to deliver accurate predictions.[14] The streams of research to which we refer are, specifically: a rational choice approach to political forecasting; the wisdom and insights of traditionally trained country and regional specialists upon which that approach relies; and the developing body of work devoted to an elaboration and evaluation of the democratic peace proposition.

The origins of the political forecasting model based on rational choice theory can be traced to *The War Trap* by Bruce Bueno de Mesquita (Bueno de Mesquita 1981). The theory introduced there was refined in 1985 (Bueno de Mesquita 1985) and served in turn as the basis for a model designed to produce forecasts of policy decisions and political outcomes in a wide variety of political settings. "The expanded domain of the theory required no modification of the formal mathematical structure of the model, although it did require additional definitions to make it useable outside the international context" (Bueno de Mesquita 1993).

The original forecasting model[15] has been updated in a way which is closely linked to the international interactions model presented in *War and Reason* (Bueno de Mesquita and Lalman 1992) and described in detail in a recent edited volume on the European Union.[16]

This "expected utility" forecasting model has now been tried and tested extensively. It has been utilized to make predictions regarding over 2,000 policy decisions and outcomes of political interactions taking place in over sixty different countries (Bueno de Mesquita 1993).[17] For example, a recently declassified Central Intelligence Agency (CIA) publication reveals that in May 1983 a forecast based on the model asserted that after the People's Republic of China claimed the China seat at the Asian Development Bank, Beijing would modify its position to permit some Taiwanese participation in the bank. As this publication acknowledges, "At the time, even PRC [People's Republic of China] statements that hinted at a 'two Chinas' attitude were considered impossible" (Feder 1995). The rise to power of Hasheimi Rafsanjani in Iran was predicted in an article published in 1984 at a time when Rafsanjani was widely viewed as an unimportant figure, and the Ayatollah Khomeini had officially designated Ayatollah Montezeri as his successor

(Bueno de Mesquita 1984). In October 1988, the model was used to generate an accurate prediction that Daniel Ortega and the Sandinista government would be defeated in the election of 1990 (Bueno de Mesquita and lusi-Scarborough 1988). In February 1989, an analysis based on the same model "predicted that China was facing a period of severe political instability in which relative hard-liners were likely to slow or stop economic and political reforms and in which students and other reform-minded interests would face severe repression" (Bueno de Mesquita 1993). In June 1989 that severe repression occurred in Tiananmen Square. Also, in the late 1980s, a study based on this model suggested critical elements of a strategy that led to successful elections in Cambodia. That study is now declassified and an executive summary completed in 1989 predicted the essential elements of a peace agreement signed in November 1991. An article published in 1991 accurately predicted the admission of two Koreas into the United Nations (Bueno de Mesquita and Kim 1991).[18] And a report completed on August 19, 1991 predicted that the coup in the Soviet Union would soon fail.[19]

The "expected utility" model has also been utilized successfully in a wide variety of private sector settings. A nonprofit organization in Washington, DC, for example, relies on it in its efforts to lobby the US Congress when it makes decisions regarding the funding for family planning programs; the organization reports that it has provided precise and ultimately accurate projections about the amount of funds that will be provided by Congress for family planning. It has also been utilized by a large, international consulting firm in its work involving General Agreement on Tariffs and Trade (GATT) negotiations. This firm is provided with projections regarding which negotiating strategies are most likely to result in desired outcomes. Another consulting firm has utilized the model to develop forecasts about the impact of various international bargaining processes, such as those which occur within the Organization of Petroleum Exporting Countries (OPEC), on the price of oil. Price projections based on the model are reportedly "unbelievably accurate."[20]

We recognize the shortcomings of this evidence. Many (but not all) of the forecasts were not publicly available before the predicted events occurred. Most of the predictions have either been classified, or provided for exclusive use by private-sector clients. The secrecy surrounding many of the predictions and forecasts based on this model has, understandably, generated suspicions about it. But we also would argue that the evidence in the form of testimonials from government and private-sector clients is not *entirely* useless. Clearly, it is not systematic scientific evidence. However, even in this article in which we defend the utility of a scientific approach to the study of international politics, we would not insist that scientifically generated evidence is the *only* kind worthy of serious consideration. So that when Stanley Feder, an analyst in the Office of Research and Development in the CIA, asserts that this model "has been gaining increased acceptance at the agency and has resulted in accurate predictions in 90 percent of the situations in which it has been utilized" (Ray 1995a: 147), his assertion might be thought of as roughly analogous to interviews (confidential in some cases) with decision-makers involved in crucial policy-making processes regarding their insights, thoughts, motives, etc., as a basis for achieving a better understanding of those processes. (Feder is less anonymous than the "informed sources" often cited by journalistic accounts of international political events, another type of evidence which cannot be ignored entirely, in our opinion.)

Furthermore, the structure of the expected utility model and an increasing number of predictions based on it have been, and are, publicly accessible. The structure has been described at length in several published sources.[21] A substantial number of predictions based on this model have either been available ahead of time, or at least sent in for publication or presented at a conference before the predicted outcomes actually occurred.[22] Even predictions published after the event in question would be difficult to fiddle with for the sake of making them come out right, because of the necessity of adhering to the procedures publicly available and consistently adhered to in literally thousands of cases. This suggests that predictions published after the fact deserve *some* credence, and several important examples of such predictions are also available for scrutiny.[23] In short, the amount of publicly available information and evidence regarding this model and the accuracy of its forecasts is sufficiently substantial, it seems to us, to make it deserving of serious consideration as a "scientific" enterprise.

Admittedly, rational choice approaches in general have provoked substantial criticism and suspicion recently because of their ostensible shortcomings in political science (Green and Shapiro 1994) as well as economics.[24] But the rational choice approach discussed here is different from rational choice approaches in general in ways that may be crucial to its success and potential.[25] For example, rational choice approaches in international politics are often criticized for their reliance on the unitary actor assumption, especially when it is applied to states. One of the key characteristics of the approach under consideration here, however, is that it rests on a general bargaining model that can treat states as unitary actors[26] or analyze bargaining among subnational actors, even individual leaders.[27]

In addition, this particular rational choice approach combines the parsimony characteristic of its breed with a comprehensive, detailed look at the interactions involved in the negotiating processes upon which it focuses. Each pair of players involved in those processes is analyzed individually, and from the separate points of view of each player in every pair, in precise, consistent and comprehensive ways that are practical only with the aid of computers. Psychological factors ignored or glossed over by other approaches are emphasized in this expected utility model; for example, estimates are made from the basic data about each player's attitude towards risk, and the impact these attitudes have on each player's perceptions of the others.[28]

This expected utility approach also benefits from the virtues of computer simulations. Once the original data have been processed and analyzed, "what if" questions can be addressed systematically. One of the more important questions of this sort is, "What if the data are faulty?" In such a context, the original data can be modified to see how sensitive the bargaining, negotiation, or competitive process is to the estimated values of various data points. In this sense, this expected utility model also shares important similarities with the "artificial life" approach to the study of complex systems—where unit-level behavior that is assumed to be a function of a few simple rules is analyzed through multiple iteration simulations (Waldrop 1992; Horgan 1995; Suplee 1995).

Rational choice approaches in political science and economics have come under much criticism recently (and rightly so, in our opinion) because of their protagonists' apparent reluctance to confront their mathematical creations with empirical data.[29] But the rational choice forecasting approach in question here is virtually *always* confronted with data about the "real world"; its major purpose is to produce predictions, as well as strategic advice, which are then evaluated in the light of precisely defined empirical outcomes.

Rational choice approaches have also generated much hostility in the subfield of comparative politics, especially among area specialists. David Laitin recently acknowledged, "a specter is haunting comparative politics; it is the specter of pure theory." By pure theory, he meant rational choice theory (Laitin 1994).[30] Asian specialists Chalmers Johnson and E.B. Keehn have recently worried that when applied to other cultures rational choice theory is not merely often wrong but it also tells us surprisingly little about the subjects it purports to study. Its simplification of human behavior, inability to conceive of institutions as anything more than rules that are extensions of behaviorism, and its total lack of interest in culture and social meaning suggest that political scientists have adopted some of the worst tendencies of economists (Johnson and Keehn 1994: 18).

But area studies specialists and "experts" on individual countries are crucial to the expected utility approach described here. The model relies on information regarding the players, their power, their preferences, and their priorities within the political context or situation being analyzed. These data are based on the impressions of area specialists or experts on individual countries, regions, political leaders, or relevant political systems. The experts themselves translate their impressions into numerical estimates of the kind exemplified in the Appendix to the version of this chapter as originally published in the *British Journal of Political Science*. That Appendix contains an analysis of the prospects for the passage of the North America Free Trade Agreement (NAFTA) in the US Congress.[31] In short, area experts and country specialists provide wisdom and insights that enhance the potential of the expected utility forecasting model to generate accurate predictions about the political future.

This approach to political forecasting is not, however, totally dependent on area expertise for its success. It is not akin to the Delphi method, nor is it simply an atheoretical computational algorithm for aggregating the opinions of experts. (In fact, quite often only one expert is consulted.) The experts are in fact virtually never asked what they believe will happen with regard to the political events and interactions being analyzed. They often disagree with the projections based on the information they provide. Stanley Feder asserts that "a number of predictions [by Policon] have contradicted those made by the intelligence community, nearly always represented by the analysts who provided the input data. In every case, the Policon forecasts proved to be correct."[32]

The evidence regarding the validity of the expected utility approach to fore-casting political events is not definitive. There is a lot of room for increased confidence in it if and when it is utilized by larger numbers of people less closely associated with its originators, and if it proves possible to arrange more systematic (and unclassified) comparisons of its performance with that of potential competitors. However, we would argue in a Lakatosian fashion that in terms of the range of issues and political settings to which it has been applied, and the body of available evidence regarding its utility and validity, it may be superior to any alternative approaches designed to offer specific predictions and projections regarding political events, and that it should not be rejected until and unless something better comes along. Moreover, in the light of that evidence, assertions that current international relations theory or systematic empirical approaches offer no better guide to the future than "star-gazers" or "readers of entrails" or that "international relations theory . . . does not allow us to predict" need to be modified.[33]

Predicting the end of the cold war in particular

It is true, as John Gaddis points out, that few scholars of international relations specifically forecast the end of the cold war in the years before its demise.[34] Gaddis absolves international relations theorists of the need to produce deterministic predictions or even contingent predictions, asking that they offer "only a prob-abilistic forecast," with a "specification in advance" of one of several outcomes as "*likely*."[35] We concur in his assumption that probabilistic statements rather than deterministic laws or point predictions are the proper goal of social science, but we would also insist that it is necessary to embed those probabilistic statements within a specific set of contingencies. We will argue here that in fact international relations theory was not entirely bereft, as Gaddis charges, of probabilistic state-ments with appropriately specified contingencies which amounted to an accurate prediction regarding the end of the cold war.

Realism and neorealism have come in for severe criticism regarding their record for forecasting the end of the cold war. Admittedly, "the competing pre-dictions of realist theories make realism difficult to falsify. Almost any outcome can be made consistent with some variant of realist theory."[36]

Retrospectively, a realist story can be told to explain the end of the cold war in some partial manner. William Wohlforth provides a particularly persuasive exam-ple, but with a weakness that stems from its flexibility. By emphasizing *perceptions* of power, and its "significant nonmaterial elements," as well as the wide range of options available or suggested to policy-makers by those perceptions of power, Wohlforth does construct a plausible realist account of the end of the cold war.[37] Our doubts about its utility involve questions about its falsifiability well expressed by Wohlforth himself:

> Realist theories can be made more determinant, but only in *ex post* explanation rather than *ex ante* prediction. Realist theories are terribly weak.

They are too easy to confirm and too hard to falsify. They do not come close to the ideal of scientific theory.

(Wohlforth 1994/95: 93)[38]

These doubts are similar to those posed perennially about Morgenthau's emphasis on the actions of nations based on the national interest defined in terms of power.

Even a realist like Wohlforth acknowledges that neorealism or structural realism (as opposed to realism) is hard-pressed to account for the changes that marked the years from 1989 to 1991. In the terminal stages of the cold war, Gorbachev's actions went beyond what one would have expected from a neorealist perspective. He "confounded neorealist expectations when he discarded the Brezhnev Doctrine, allowed revolutions overthrowing Eastern European communist regimes, and accepted the demise of the Warsaw Pact. Even less can one account for American behavior within a neorealist framework" (Koslowski and Kratochwil 1995: 129).

> According to neorealist assumptions, the United States should have taken advantage of Soviet weakness with an aggressive foreign policy and efforts to compound Soviet difficulties so as to make the Soviet Union as weak as possible. Instead, the United States extended to the Soviet Union . . . large-scale financial aid . . . and even supported Gorbachev's efforts to hold the Soviet Union together.
>
> (Koslowski and Kratochwil 1995: 131–132)[39]

Neorealism posits the distribution of power in the international system as the fundamental driving force behind whatever changes might occur in international relationships. Yet changes in the distribution of power within the international system were substantially a *result rather than a cause of the end of the cold war*. Both the general Soviet-American military balance and the nuclear balance in particular—the essential features of the bipolar system—remained in place while the most dramatic changes in Soviet policy and in the US-Soviet relationship occurred. "Until 1989 [Gorbachev] made no major cuts in defense spending. Between 1985 and 1989, defense consumed about the same percentage of gross national product as it had under Brezhnev. After 1989 it consumed more."[40] In other words, the dramatic changes in Soviet-American relations took place even though the distribution of power in the system remained quite stable.

So the criticisms by Gaddis and others about the inability of predominant international relations theories to cope with or account for the end of the cold war apply quite persuasively to realism or neorealism.[41] Some other theories—realist and nonrealist—lend themselves to stories that have some plausibility, but only after the fact, applying selective versions of theoretical traditions as they might have predicted the end of the cold war. Hardly any, however, were told before the events in question, actually making the prediction.[42] Those few that did were of the "sooner or later" variety with little specification of time frame or contingency.

At best, events can be said to "confirm" such propositions only with a *post hoc propter hoc* account. A forecast with such vague content as to time or contingency can never be falsified; the prophet can always claim "not yet, but keep waiting."[43]

There is, however, a burgeoning sector of international relations theory less vulnerable to such criticism, namely that which focuses on the democratic peace proposition, or the idea that democratic states have not and are not likely to initiate international wars against each other. The arguments and evidence for the democratic peace proposition are impressively diverse; they are epistemological (Rummel 1975), philosophical (Doyle 1986b), historical (Ray 1993; Owen 1994; Weart 1994), experimental (Mintz and Geva 1993), anthropological (Ember *et al.* 1992; Crawford 1994), and statistical in nature.[44] The proposition receives empirical support not just in the nineteenth- and twentieth-century international system where it first became evident, but in some earlier eras and in ethnographic material on pre-industrial societies.[45] As a research program, it has spun off hypotheses, and evidence, that democracies will be more likely to ally with one another; that the legal systems of democratic states will recognize and enforce each other's law in their own systems; that in disputes between democratic states the parties will be more accommodative, and more likely to accept third-party intervention for conflict management or binding third-party settlement; that states with competitive elections generally have lower military expenditures, which in relations with other democracies promote cooperation; and that as the politically relevant international environment of democracies becomes composed of more demo-cratic and internally stable states, democracies tend to reduce their military allocations and conflict involvement (Bercovitch 1991; Siverson and Emmons 1991; Slaughter 1992; Brecher 1993; Dixon 1994; Garfinkel 1994; Raymond 1994; Maoz 1996).

The democratic peace proposition is also supported by theoretical analyses, some of them formal in nature.[46] Moreover, in a work with important theoretical ties to the political forecasting model we have discussed, there is a formal argument developed by Bruce Bueno de Mesquita and David Lalman (1992: 156–157):

> Whenever democracies confront one another, it is common knowledge that each has unusually high confidence that the other is likely to be con-strained to be averse to the use of force. And that common knowledge about the magnitude of the prior belief encourages states under all but the most unusual circumstances to negotiate with one another or to accept the status quo.

Advocates of the democratic peace proposition did not anticipate with any precision the timing of changes in Soviet policy that marked the last days of the cold war. Like neorealism, democratic peace theory does not attempt to explain or predict transitions in domestic political regimes, and neoliberalism did no better in forecasting the initial Soviet domestic changes. All assume that such transi-tions are matters to be dealt with by specialists on the domestic politics of states in the international system, i.e., comparative politics specialists, or in this case, Sovietologists. Hardly anyone predicted far in advance that the key contingency for a democratic peace—a more democratic Soviet Union—might transpire.

We summarize our interpretation of the actual *events* marking the end of the cold war as follows. In 1986, Mikhail Gorbachev set in motion a process of domestic liberalization and the reduction of international tension, both of which gathered force in subsequent years. Not later than November 1989 the bipolar cold war system can be termed defunct, with the fall of the Berlin Wall and the peaceful acceptance by the Soviet leadership of the collapse of its political and military control over Eastern Europe. By this interpretation, the dissolution of the Soviet Union at the end of 1991 was merely the "ratification" of the end of the cold war. The internal character of the Soviet system moved importantly towards democracy during the 1986–1989 period, though some of the greatest changes occurred only in 1991.

Establishing the validity of a neoliberal story regarding the end of the cold war would require at a minimum persuasive evidence that the Soviet Union in fact did become more democratic during these crucial years. A detailed historical analysis of political developments in the Soviet Union is clearly beyond the scope of this effort. However, we can point out that both the Polity III codings and the annual Freedom House ratings judged that substantial movement in the direction of democracy in the Soviet Union (and ultimately Russia) did take place between 1986 and 1991.[47] A remarkable feature is thus, that when the Soviet Union did break up, a reasonably *democratic* Russian government permitted it to happen, *peacefully*. (Most observers would concur that Russia has become less democratic since 1991.)

Indeed, any understanding of the change in the Soviet Union's international behavior *before its dissolution*, and reciprocated by the West, demands attention to the three legs on which the liberal Kantian vision of *Perpetual Peace* stands: (1) movement toward democracy in the Soviet Union, with consequent changes in free expression and the treatment of dissidents at home, in the East European satellites, and in behavior toward Western Europe and the United States; (2) the desire for economic interdependence with the West, impelled by the impending collapse of the Soviet economy and the consequent perceived need for access to Western markets, goods, technology and capital, which in turn required a change in Soviet military and diplomatic policy; (3) the influence of international law and organizations, as manifested in the Conference on Security and Cooperation in Europe (CSCE) and the human rights basket of the Helsinki accords and their legitimation and support of political dissent in the communist states.

In the light of this experience, it seems to us that acceptable standards of social science prediction (not prophecy) would require a prior set of statements somewhat along the line of the following: certain contingencies, such as economic stagnation or decline, or rising ethnic and national tensions within the Soviet Union, are likely (not certain) to occur. Such a contingency would in turn be likely (not certain) to force the leaders of a still-intact Soviet Union to seek (and obtain) a very substantial reduction in East–West conflict that we could appropriately term a peaceful "end of the cold war." Whereas a strong causal relationship from democratization to the end of East–West conflict might be difficult to establish, a further condition for a "democratic peace" prediction would be that the end of conflict should closely follow or coincide with some significant democratization. The end of the conflict should not come first. Such a prediction would not necessarily first require a full collapse of the previous system.

By these—possibly high—standards, hardly anyone did very well. Predictions that economic stagnation or rising ethnic conflict might occur were common, and also that they would likely force some sort of change in the Soviet economic and/or political system. But few predicted substantial liberalization of the system. Zbigniew Brzezinski edited an early book addressing the likelihood of major change in the Soviet political system. The great majority of the twenty contributors to the symposium either made no clear-cut prediction at all, or came down as considering conservative adaptation, degeneration or collapse as most likely at some time in the future. Only three—Jayantanuja Bandyopadhyaya (a scholar from India), Joseph Clark, and Arrigo Levi (an American and an Italian journalist respectively)— considered "renovative transformation" (substantial liberalization) as a serious possibility.[48] Later, some creators and supporters of Reagan administration policies in the early 1980s anticipated that pressures of an intensified arms race on the Soviet economy could ultimately force the Soviet Union to behave more co-operatively— but few specified how that might happen, or under what type of political regime.

Some theories (and theorists) did predict the demise of the Soviet Union as such. Helene d'Encausse published *Decline of an Empire: The Soviet Socialist Republics in Revolt* in 1979. Randall Collins delivered a paper in 1980 with a "geopolitical theory" based on five main principles, each of which "pointed in the same way: collapse of the Russian empire."[49] But by the criteria above these works fail on at least two counts. First, the cold war came to an end before the Soviet Union collapsed. Second, theories of this type generally anticipated a violent end to the cold war. Collins acknowledges, for example, that his geopolitical theory predicted that "ultimately the world simplifies down to two rival empires which engage in a 'showdown' war . . . carried out with unprecedented ferociousness and cost" (Collins and Waller 1992: 33). Wohlforth acknowledges that "realists of all types tended to associate large-scale international changes with war. In particular, those who did contemplate Soviet decline in the context of the cold war tended to assume that Moscow would not face decline gracefully" (Wohlforth 1994/95: 102–103).

An alternative basis for anticipating the end of the cold war emphasizes the impact of internal regime changes on relationships among states. Its contemporary origins can be traced to Karl Deutsch's work on pluralistic security communities, now being recognized as perhaps the principal alternative paradigm to realism (Deutsch *et al.* 1957; Adler and Barnet 1994; Wendt 1994). This work was an important precursor to the democratic peace proposition, with its emphasis on peaceful relationships, especially among democratic states. Harvey Starr points out the connections between Deutsch's work and the international interaction model developed by Bueno de Mesquita and Lalman (Starr 1992: 211). And as Bueno de Mesquita and Lalman (1992: 248–249) themselves declare in defense of that model:

> The predominant realist or neorealist viewpoint suggests that broad international structural characteristics . . . not the individual qualities of decision makers or particular domestic political institutions of states, [are] the essential explanatory factor in international affairs . . . Recent Soviet developments make more sense if understood from a domestic viewpoint than from a realist viewpoint, which interprets demands and foreign policy actions strictly in their international context. Internal imperatives, rather than external constraints, seem to have shaped the revolution in Soviet foreign policy.

In other words, neorealism and democratic peace theory (or neoliberalism) are affected quite differently by arguments and evidence that the cold war relationship between the United States and the Soviet Union was changed dramatically by reforms internal to the Soviet regime. The democratic peace proposition clearly implies that if major regime transitions do occur they can fundamentally alter the pattern of relationships between states.

Typically, if physical scientists offer propositions about the future of the "real world," they must be specifically qualified. Their ability to predict in an unconditional way is limited. For example, physical scientists cannot predict with consistent accuracy where and when the next large earthquake will occur (or when the Big One will hit southern California), nor exactly when and where, next year, a hurricane will strike North America. Yet it would clearly be unjustified to conclude that the inability to predict in this fashion demonstrates that geologists or meteorologists have no real understanding of phenomena such as earthquakes or hurricanes, or that their theories regarding them are "bankrupt."

Similarly, we would argue, it is unfair to argue that the absence of predictions about the end of the cold war by advocates of the democratic peace proposition demonstrates their (or their theory's) inadequacies. It is more important that democratic peace theory could generate probabilistic forecasts about the cold war, contingent upon regime transitions. Specifically, it leads us to expect that *if* the autocratic half of an antagonistic pair of states becomes more democratic, then the relationship between those states will improve. Thus one could readily derive the proposition that if the Soviet Union becomes more democratic, the cold war will probably end.[50]

Finally, a prediction (that is, a contingent statement about the future, as opposed to either a prophecy or a *post hoc* explanation) specifically regarding the end of the cold war is not merely a logical possibility existing only in the abstract. Writing in 1980, one of us ended his discussion of the democratic peace proposition by asking whether the

> experience of OECD countries gives us any basis for hope that 'stable peace,' based on something more just than dominance or more stable than mutual

deterrence, can be achieved in other parts of the world or by the OECD countries with other states.

Addressing the question of whether "relations with the Soviet Union could ever be like those within a security community," he concluded that "stable peace could be possible only if the government of the Soviet Union were to evolve into something more democratic than the current 'state socialism'." Nonetheless, he shared with other analysts the error of treating that key contingency of liberalization as unlikely—and particularly because of the potential for ethnic conflict.[51]

Other than the perceived unlikelihood of the contingency, why was such a prediction not shouted from the housetops, or taken up by other advocates of the democratic peace proposition? After all, the basic idea had been around for two decades or more (not counting Immanuel Kant and Woodrow Wilson). The problem was that only quite lately did enough people—including many of its advocates—conclude that the evidence for the democratic peace proposition was in fact correct. It took time for the necessary scientific process of specifying the theory and gathering empirical evidence. The theory had to be tested for the influence of confounding variables like wealth and alliance ties, and the underlying logic of the process had to be spelled out. For this very reason many social scientists who are now believers in the democratic peace were initially agnostic or even atheist.[52] And well they might have been. The twentieth century has seen quite enough instances of going from "imaginatively generalizing" (Puchala 1991: 57) to strong policy recommendations without getting the facts and logic right. Who wants to wind up in the dustbin with Lenin, having done incalculable harm to humanity?

Conclusion: scientific prediction is possible

The scarcity of accurate predictions by scholars of international politics regarding the end of the cold war has apparently reinforced skepticism in some circles regarding the utility of the "scientific" or systematic empirical approach to the field. That skepticism is, in part, on firm ground, since an ability to provide foreknowledge is one important attribute of useful theories, and advocates of systematic empiricism have had several decades now to help develop such theories. This is not to say that accurate predictions are the sole aim of "science," or even the most important or stringent criterion by which theories can be evaluated. But the future can serve as an important arbiter between competing theoretical (and epistemological) approaches to the study of international politics, because predictions, unlike explanations, cannot be modified in order to make them conform to the (unknown) outcomes they address.

John Lewis Gaddis, among others, has seized upon the nearly complete absence of accurate predictions regarding the demise of the cold war as evidence of the bankruptcy of predominant theoretical approaches in the field, as well as of scientific or systematic empirical analyses. Our thesis here accepts predictive accuracy as an important criterion by which to evaluate theories and systematic empiricism, and argues that there are three related streams of research in the field that justify a more optimistic evaluation of theory in the field of international relations, as well as systematic empirical methods of developing and evaluating theory. In short, we believe that a rational choice approach to political forecasting, the inputs relied upon by that approach from country and regional specialists, and the expanding body of work focusing upon the democratic peace proposition have collectively demonstrated an ability to produce accurate forecasts about political events in general, and even to provide a basis for anticipating the end of the cold war.

Many criticisms of rational choice approaches in economics and political science are justified. However, the approach to political forecasting discussed here differs from rational approaches in general in several ways that contribute to its apparent success as a forecasting tool. It can and does treat states as unitary rational actors, but it also can be utilized to analyze interactions between subnational groups, or even individuals. Some rational choice models suffer from excessive simplicity. The rational choice approach to forecasting discussed here is based on parsimonious assumptions and rules, but it takes advantage of the information-processing capabilities of computers to analyze bargaining, negotiating, and competitive processes in considerable detail, analyzing (for example) such processes from the points of view of each pair of actors involved. Rational choice approaches tend to overlook psychological factors, but this expected utility approach integrates attitudes towards risk, and the impact of these attitudes on perceptions with the more purely logical calculations that constitute the heart of the model. Computer simulation techniques allow this approach more flexibility than many models based on mathematical calculations. The original, as well as the processed, data can be modified in order to run "experiments," or to address counterfactual questions. Finally, this rational choice approach takes into account political context through its reliance on traditionally trained area and country experts to supply the original data on which its forecasts are based. These strategies and characteristics have allowed this approach to political forecasting to produce a substantial history of success. Some of that history is not publicly available for scrutiny, but the number of predictions and forecasts that are accessible, combined with the substantial information about the model's structure in published sources, make it worthy, we believe, of serious consideration as a "scientific" enterprise.

Since social science is necessarily a probabilistic rather than a deterministic exercise, the failure to produce an accurate forecast about one particular event is not sufficient to discredit any theory in any field, and the absence of predictions by realists and neorealists about the end of the cold war should not be considered definitive contrary evidence. Nevertheless, that absence, and the tendency of realism and neorealism to create expectations of a violent end to the cold war, can fairly be considered evidence tending to weaken confidence in such theoretical approaches to international politics. The theoretical approach producing the democratic peace proposition, in contrast, leads to an expectation of the peaceful demise of the cold war if the autocratic antagonist in that confrontation becomes more democratic. The Soviet Union did become more democratic in the years from 1985 to 1991, and the emphasis on the impact of domestic political regimes on foreign policies as well as international interactions that is a fundamental attribute of the democratic peace proposition seems well-founded in the light of the way the cold war came to an end. Even in advance of the dramatic events of 1989 to 1991, at least one advocate of the democratic peace proposition pointed out the implications for the course of the cold war of substantial changes in the domestic political system of the Soviet Union.[53]

That ultimately justified prediction (defined as a statement about the future based on specified contingencies) is one reason for rejecting a blanket condemnation of theoretical approaches in the field of international politics. Systematic empirical evidence in support of the democratic peace proposition provides an important basis for hope regarding the utility of scientific analyses in that field. The evidence regarding the potential of a political forecasting approach based on a rational choice model that relies extensively on the wisdom and insights of traditionally trained social scientists and historians suggests that political events in general are on the way to becoming more predictable. In short, the scientific, or systematic empirical approach to international politics is not dead, and evidence regarding its ability to produce accurate predictions about the political future is one of its more encouraging signs of life.

Notes

1 We thank Janice Bially, John Lewis Gaddis, John Mueller, William Odom, R.J. Rummel, Steve Smith, Harvey Starr, John Vasquez, and Alexander Wendt for comments, Ram Krishnan for research assistance, the United States Institute of Peace for support of the first author, and the John D. and Catherine T. MacArthur Foundation for support of the second author.

2 Gaddis's sharpest criticisms are directed at North Americans pursuing a social scientific research agenda; we therefore respond primarily by reference to that literature.

3 Puchala here, like Gaddis, condemns not just contemporary theories in the field of international politics, but also, as the title clearly implies, "scientific" approaches to that subject matter.

4 Gaddis (1992/93) cites both Hawking and Morgenthau in support of this view.

5 Hollis and Smith (1990: 54–56) here are reporting the view of Quine (1961).

6 Some of the works cited by Vasquez (1994) are: Berger and Luckman (1966); Foucault (1972); Lyotard (1992).

7 Such a view has been expressed recently, for example, by Singer (1994a); Rosenau (1994).

8 "World War III will begin at 2 p.m. on 11 October 1997" would be an example of a prophecy as opposed to a prediction.

9 Ian Shapiro and Alexander Wendt, for example, cite an article by Philip Kitcher as an authoritative source on "the incoherence of explanatory-predictive symmetry." See Shapiro and Wendt (1992: 222); Kitcher (1989). But in that same volume Merrilee Salmon (1989: 408), having reviewed the controversy regarding Hempel's views on "nomological" explanations (and predictions of the same structure) concludes:

> Despite protests of the critics of causal and nomological explanation in the social sciences, the best approximations to a satisfactory philosophical theory of explanation seem to embrace successful explanations in the social sciences as well as successful explanations in the physical sciences. None of the critics, I believe,

has demonstrated that the admitted differences between our social environment and our physical environment compel us to seek entirely different methods of understanding each.

On this controversy, see also Keat and Urry (1982); Wendt (1987: 335–368); Bhaskar (1978).

10 Shapiro and Wendt (1992: 212) assert that "realists are not hostile to logical empiricists' reliance on predictions of empirical regularities as evidence for the validity of claims," while Alexander Rosenberg observes in a similar vein that "among philosophers of science in recent years at any rate, the most central debate, between realism and antirealism, is about whether prediction of observations is merely necessary for knowledge, as realists hold, or all we need from science, as antirealists hold." See Rosenberg (1992: 51). For a more extended and somewhat less conciliatory discussion of this issue, see Ray (1995b: ch. 4).

11 Quine also notes that "A sentence's claim to scientific status rests on what it contributes to a theory whose checkpoints are in prediction" (20).

12 "It makes more and more sense, the farther in time we are from them, to view World Wars I and II as a single European civil war . . ." See Gaddis (1992a: 5).

13 "Observation, however, is not *determined* by theory or discourse; unlike some 'strong' interpretivists, realists contend that well-established theories do refer to, and are constrained by, external reality" (Shapiro and Wendt 1992: 211).

14 In their otherwise excellent review of many of the same epistemological issues that serve as our focus here, Hollis and Smith (1990) also fail to cite most of the sources to which we are about to turn our attention.

15 Described in Bueno de Mesquita (1984: 226–236) and in Bueno de Mesquita (1985).

16 See in particular Bueno de Mesquita (1994).

17 Most of the forecasts have been produced by a corporation called Decision Insights, established by Bueno de Mesquita, Jacek Kugler and A.F.K. Organski in 1981 under the name of Policon.

18 This article appeared after the vote in the United Nations, but the editor notes on the first page that it had been submitted and accepted before the vote.

19 "Outcome of the Soviet Coup and its Political Aftermath" (Decision Insights Incorporated Assessment, August 19, 1991).

20 This statement was made in a telephone conversation with the chairman of the consulting organization in question. In the preceding eighteen months, Decision Insights had provided political forecasting and strategic planning services to more than thirty-seven private-sector clients.

21 Bueno de Mesquita (1984; 1990: 317–340; 1993; 1994). Manuel Oroszco, currently a graduate student at the University of Texas, replicated the software that produced analyses reported in Bueno de Mesquita et al. (1985). Bueno de Mesquita offers his own exposition of the record of success achieved by his approach in Bueno de Mesquita (1996).

22 For example, Bueno de Mesquita (1984, 1990); Bueno de Mesquita et al. (1985); Bueno de Mesquita and Lusi-Scarborough (1988); Bueno de Mesquita and Kim (1991); Bueno de Mesquita and Organski (1992: 81–100); James (1992); Kugler (1987: 115–144); Morrow et al. (1993: 311–331); Newman and Bridges (1994: 61–80); Organski and Bueno de Mesquita (1993); Wu and Bueno de Mesquita (1994: 379–403).

23 See especially several chapters in Bueno de Mesquita and Stokman (1994: 113–148).

24 Rosenberg (1992). According to J. David Singer, "'Rational choice' explanations for the behavior of political elites in general, and statesmen in particular . . .[are] not only redolent of failed models that litter the landscape of modern economics, but dramatically at odds with the more solid findings in psychology" (Singer 1994b: 28).

25 The discussion that follows owes much to the recent critiques of rational choice approaches by Green and Shapiro (1994) as well as that by Rosenberg (1992), which, in general, we might add, have much to recommend them. It probably should be pointed out here that the focus of *Pathologies of Rational Choice* is on American politics (so it does

not address Bueno de Mesquita's rational choice approach explicitly), and that Rosenberg's volume is dedicated to (among others) Bruce Bueno de Mesquita.

26 See Bueno de Mesquita (1981, 1985); Bueno de Mesquita and Lalman (1992).

27 For example, Bueno de Mesquita et al. (1985); Bueno de Mesquita and lusi-Scarborough (1988); Feder (1995).

28 Bueno de Mesquita (1994) and Kim and Bueno de Mesquita (1995: 51–65).

29 "A theory of politics has no payoff if its hypotheses do not survive empirical scrutiny. In this light, it is surprising that both defenders and critics of rational choice theory have paid so little attention to empirical testing" (Green and Shapiro 1994: 32).

> Over a ten year period the proportion of papers in the *American Economic Review* that elaborated mathematical models without bringing the models into contact with data exceeded 50 percent and . . . a further 22 percent involved indirect statistical inference from data previously published.
>
> (Rosenberg 1992: 66)

Another 15 percent of articles in the *American Economic Review* during this period, according to Rosenberg, involved neither mathematical formulation nor data.

30 Laitin goes on to observe that "having a specialist for every piece of international real estate may soon seem as arcane as having a specialist for every planet in the astronomy department" (4).

31 "Through the judicious use of modelling and area expertise, it is possible to derive issue-specific analyses that are more reliable and more informative than can be achieved through modelling alone or through area expertise by itself" (Bueno de Mesquita 1990: 340).

32 Feder (1995). Policon is the name of the original corporation founded by Bueno de Mesquita and his associates (see fn. 16). Kugler, Snider and Longwell (1994).

33 Gaddis (1992/93: 18); Puchala (1991: 79). Even John Lewis Gaddis might now agree with our statement. Gaddis and Bruce Bueno de Mesquita have discussed in some detail what amounts to a simulation of the history of the cold war based on Bueno de Mesquita's model, in a paper with a working title of "The End of the Cold War as an Emergent Property: Complexity in International Affairs." These conversations have led Gaddis to conclude (in an email message to Bueno de Mesquita on February 8, 1995) that

> as I understand it, what you've done is to confirm Axelrod's 'evolution of cooperation' model in iterated prisoners' dilemma games, and then extend it beyond where he went to show how what looks like a robust system over time (a 'long peace'?) can suddenly break down. You've shown that this can happen not through war or mutual convergence, which always seemed to be the only choices while the Cold War was going on, but by one side's suddenly shifting to the other's point of view. That strikes me as an important advance over earlier approaches to predictive modelling because it takes into account the emergent properties of complex adaptive systems. It's getting closer to how historians think.

This is from a copy of this email correspondence (sent via email) to James Ray by John Gaddis, in which Gaddis also acknowledges that "there has been a sort of BdM-JLG convergence" (February 8, 1995).

34 Decision Insights, however, did produce forecasts of the break-up of the Soviet Union shortly after the coup attempt of August 1991. John Mueller also asserted in 1986 that

> we may be coming to the end of the world as we know it. The predominant characteristic of international affairs over the last 40 years has been competition and confrontation between the United States and the Soviet Union, and there is a great deal in the present situation to suggest that this condition could be on the verge of terminal improvement; the incentives for the Soviet Union to reduce its commitment to worldwide revolution are considerable. This could eventually result in the end of the cold war.
>
> (Mueller 1986: 1)

This paper is informed by international relations theory to some extent, particularly in its conclusion about the low probability of an international war between the United States and the Soviet Union. It might be fair to say, however, that its impressive prescience regarding the demise of the cold war is based more on wisdom, intuition and a pragmatic logic of cost-benefit analysis than a well-developed explicit theory of international politics.

35 Gaddis (1992/93: 18, emphasis in the original).

36 Lebow (1995: 24). In the same volume, Oye (1995: 58) states, "Because realism is underidentified, it cannot be tested with reference to the end of the Cold War or any other sequence of events."

37 In defense of the idea that this account is consistent with realism it might be pointed out that David Sanders provides an account based on realism of the withdrawal of Great Britain from its colonies in the late 1940s and the 1950s with some similarities to Wohlforth's realistic account of the withdrawal of the Soviet Union from Eastern Europe (see Sanders 1990, esp. 265–269). However, unlike Wohlforth, Sanders emphasizes that realism calls for ensuring that the evacuated areas are left in the hands of the "firmest and most trustworthy ally" (267), something the Soviets did not accomplish. And like Wohlforth, Sanders provides this realistic account of a withdrawal from imperial holdings only well after the fact.

38 It is only fair to point out that Wohlforth goes on to argue that the strength of realist theories is only evident "when they are compared to the alternatives, which suffer from similar or worse indeterminacy but do not possess comparable explanatory power" (93). We intend to compare realism not only to some ideal standard, but also to a specific alternative.

39 Similarly, Gaddis asserts that "the second most 'powerful' state on the face of the earth did voluntarily give up power, despite the insistence of international relations theory that this could never happen." See Gaddis (1992b: A44). And Lebow (1995: 41) argues that

> the most fundamental tenet of realism is that states act to preserve their territorial integrity. Gorbachev's decision to abandon Eastern Europe's communist regimes wittingly called the integrity of the Soviet empire into question. It triggered demands for independence from the Baltics to Central Asia that led to the demise of the Soviet state.

Thinking about whether Gorbachev's behavior was both pivotal and not to be expected from other possible Soviet leaders constitutes a useful counterfactual exercise to help sort out the role of systemic forces in constraining leaders. On such exercises, see Tetlock and Belkin (1996).

40 Lebow (1995: 39). Also Chernoff (1991).

41 John Mueller of the University of Rochester expressed the following in a September 1994 personal communication to us:

> Insofar as anyone can figure out what realism in its various forms (neo, structural, quasi, crypto, semi, defensive, last-ditch, kinky, etc.) actually was, therefore, it seems to me it was (I like the past tense here) not only flawed in that it was incapable of predicting the end of the Cold War, but that it had a negative, even blinding or at least blinkering, effect in that it caused people for decades to focus on the wrong dynamic and to be incapable of seeing what was going on. It ignored domestic issues willfully and to its ultimate peril.

42 Various examples are reviewed by contributors to Allan and Goldmann (1992). In his chapter, "The Events in Eastern Europe and the Crisis in the Discipline of International Relations," Philip Evarts does a particularly devastating job of compiling forecasts that turned out very wrong.

43 This is the characterization by Kjell Goldman, "Bargaining, Power, Domestic Politics, and Security Dilemmas: Soviet 'New Thinking' as Evidence," and Isabelle Grunberg

and Thomas Risse-Kappen, "A Time of Reckoning? Theories of International Relations and the End of the Cold War," in Allan and Goldman (1992). This is certainly not to imply that such a forecast should, by contrast, have taken the form of a point prediction.

44 Bremer (1992); Maoz and Russett (1993). These and additional sources in each of these categories are reviewed in Russett (1993), and Ray (1995b). Also see Oneal *et al.* (1996).

45 Cohen (1994), Layne (1994), and Spiro (1994) argue that the democratic peace proposition fails on conceptual, historical, or statistical grounds. We believe we refute these arguments in Russett and Ray (1995) and Russett (1995). In his reply in the same issue of *International Security*, Layne (1995) makes the novel charge that Russett is guilty of practising postmodernism.

46 Bueno de Mesquita *et al.* (1992); Lake (1992); Fearon (1994); Schultz and Weingast (1994); Bueno de Mesquita and Siverson (1995). One implication of these works considered together is that democratic states might avoid war against each other because they are formidable opponents in war, and because democratic states are particularly vulnerable to a loss of power in the wake of a lost war. See Ray (1995b: ch. 1).

47 In Polity III, the Soviet Union received a score of 0 on the institutionalized democracy index (on a scale from 0 to 10) in 1986, a score of 5 in 1989, and 7 in 1991. On the institutionalized autocracy index (also a 0 to 10 scale), it had a score of 7 in 1986, 1 in 1989, and 0 in 1991. On the Freedom House indicators, the Soviet Union received the worst (least democratic) possible scores on political rights and on civil liberties (that is, 7s) in 1986, and moved to scores of 6 and 5 by 1988; at the end of 1990 it was coded as 3 on both scales. Gastil (1989); McColm (1992); Jaggers and Gurr (1995).

48 Brzezinsky (1969). Summary characterizations of each contributor's position appear on 157.

49 d'Encausse (1979). Collins's paper is cited in Collins and Waller (1992): 34.

50 Ray (1995c: 350). Interesting testimony regarding the logic of such a derivation from democratic peace theory can be found in a passage (first published in a 1987 article) by John Lewis Gaddis:

> Michael Doyle has recently pointed out [that] there is a historical basis for arguing that liberal democracies tend not to go to war with one another. This raises the question: could the extension of democracy—especially within the superpower that has not, until now, had much of it—bring an end to the Cold War? Stranger things have happened.
>
> (Gaddis 1992a: 140)

51   The prospects for liberalization in the Soviet Union are complicated, because it is not just the matter of political control by the current leaders that is at issue— or even just the maintenance of Socialism vs. some restoration of capitalist institutions. The very unity of the USSR itself is at stake. A major barrier to liberalization of the Soviet government is the suppressed desire of ethnic groups or 'nationalities' for self-determination. Liberalization could revive these potential separatist movements, bringing the potential fissioning of the world's last great colonial empire.

Both this passage and the one above are from Russett (1982: 191). Both repeat verbatim material that appeared in the more widely available book by Russett and Starr (1981: 442). Writing in mid-1988, he treated the key contingency as more plausible:

> As Soviet ideology and practice begins to shift, the distinction between ruling elites and their people loses some of its force. If both sides see each other as in some sense truly reflecting the consent of the governed, the transformation of international relations begins.
>
> (Russett 1989: 259)

52 We believe this accurately characterizes many scholars cited here as ultimately contributing to the theory and evidence for the democratic peace, including Bremer,

Bueno de Mesquita, Dixon, Maoz, and Ray himself. Policy-makers also were appropriately cautious both in taking up the democratic peace proposition and in applying it to the Soviet Union. Nevertheless, by April 1989 US Secretary of State James Baker was saying, "And a kind of democratization—something, I think that's far from democracy, but, nevertheless, a kind of democratization, has begun," and GIST, an unauthored State Department publication which generally follows the tone and observations of high-ranking officials, said a month later that should moves towards internal democratization "continue and become irreversible fact, the basic nature of the US-Soviet relationship could be altered profoundly, but we are not there yet" (US Department of State, Bureau of Public Affairs, S 1.128: Un 5/2/1989). Both quotations are from Mason (1998). By early 1992 Baker had thoroughly bought into the idea of a democratic peace with Russia (see Russett 1993: 128–129). The late Deputy Assistant Secretary of Defense for European and NATO Affairs recently observed:

> One of the most powerful [propositions] to come out of international relations research in decades is the notion that democracies do not go to war with each other. This proposition has had a substantial impact on public policy . . . There are very few propositions in international relations that can be articulated this cleanly and simply, but when you have one, you can really cut through the clutter of the bureaucratic process and make an impact.
>
> (Kruzel 1994: 180)

53 One anonymous reviewer of this article argues that "Wohlforth's realist account—that if a state perceives its power is radically declining it may retrench without resorting to conflict—the authors reject. Their own claim they call 'conditional prediction.' Wohlforth's assertion they call 'ex post facto' explanation. What's the difference?" We feel there are three important differences. The first is that the predominant thrust of realism, as Wohlforth admits, leads to an expectation that the cold war would end violently, even if, or perhaps especially if, the power or capability of one of the protagonists should change dramatically. The second is that Wohlforth's realist account depends on a change in the distribution of power between the United States and the Soviet Union which arguably occurred only after the end of the cold war. It seems to us that political changes within the Soviet Union more clearly preceded a change in the cold war relationship than did the change in the military–industrial capabilities of the Soviet Union. The final difference is that Wohlforth's explanation was offered after the end of the cold war, while Russett's admittedly contingent assertion occurred well before the events of 1989 to 1991. That is a distinction of some importance. It might also be prudent to acknowledge that political changes in Russia in the autocratic direction, which some current accounts suggest are already under way, would have negative effects on its relationship with the United States. (See Stanley 1995.)

7

COURTING DISASTER

NATO vs. Russia and China[1]

Bruce Russett and Allan C. Stam

The process of NATO expansion is on track. For a combination of bad reasons—domestic politics, organizational inertia, sloppy strategic analysis—NATO expansion up to but not beyond the boundaries of the former Soviet Union is a done deal.[2] But in its current limited incarnation it is a bad deal, an ill-considered and potentially regressive move. By limiting NATO expansion to small Eastern European states, NATO leaders preclude the alliance from developing the capabilities it will need to confront the coming security challenges of the twenty-first century.

Current plans for limited NATO expansion ignore the biggest future security problem for the West, which is not Russia itself, but the long-run possibility of a global power transition with China sometime in the next century. In this geo-strategic scenario, Russia matters because of the potential power of a Russian-Chinese alliance. The need to prevent any such alignment should be central to all thinking about the future of NATO. In the short run, the problem of securing Russian respect for the boundaries of its neighbors in Eastern Europe is best managed within the context of NATO's proven capacity for reducing and resolving conflicts among its members, of whom Russia should be one.

We will not review the standard objections to limited NATO expansion without Russia. They were, for example, well laid out by the forty-eight senior analysts in their June 26, 1997 statement,[3] and in any event are now largely moot. For small gain, limited expansion poses great risks. Whatever Westerners may say, that kind of expansion is directed against at least a hypothetical danger from Russia. It has no compelling purpose otherwise. But if it is too late to stop the first round of NATO expansion, it is not too late to consider including Russia in the next. Many Russians see an extended NATO as a direct threat against them. This threat risks reviving old Russian fears of the West, strengthening Russian militarists and nationalists, and inducing greater instability in Russian domestic politics and foreign policy.

For the near future, the risks may appear tolerable. Right now, Russia can do little more than complain.[4] Over time, likely results include intransigence on arms control issues, an increase in the resources Russia devotes to rebuilding its military capabilities, and a turn of its diplomatic orientation in a hostile direction.[5] Expanding NATO as currently planned may ultimately create from Russia a threat that is now absent.[6] The best-case future includes a hostile and isolated Russia. More plausible is a much worse outcome—an emergent alliance of Russia and China.[7] Such an alliance would look very attractive to two big powers that saw themselves as excluded from a hegemonic Western community. If Russia remains reasonably democratic, no further NATO expansion should be undertaken without it, tying Russia securely to the West.

From a cost-benefit perspective, it is not only about what the Russians might bring to NATO, but what NATO brings to the Russians, and what the Russians then *do not* bring to the Chinese. A future round of NATO expansion that fully incorporated Russia into NATO—not just in a second-class NATO-Russia Joint Council—would eliminate Russian concern about western encirclement and address the long-term problem of growing Chinese power. It would allow Russia to become a normal democratic state within the Euro-Atlantic community.[8] That would firmly bind Russia's future to Western Europe's and ensure substantial global peace for the next century.

Russia's options

From a geostrategic perspective, expanding NATO without Russia runs the risk of creating a severe security dilemma for both the East and the West.[9] What are the choices available to a state faced with an alliance far stronger than it is or can hope to be? One possible reaction is bandwagoning.[10] A state may try to join in cooperation with those who might threaten it. This is, in essence, the policy that Mikhail Gorbachev began and is the policy that led to the end of the cold war. To date, Boris Yeltsin and other Russian democrats have largely followed Gorbachev's precedent. Russian integration into NATO would be a giant step in that direction.

Russia's second option is to hide or to withdraw into heavily armed isolation, greatly dependent on its nuclear weapons and rooted in a perception of being surrounded by potential enemies (Western, Islamic, Asian). A Russian xenophobia based in some degree on reality (many paranoids do have enemies), an economy once again autarkic and burdened by militarization, and the revival of autocratic government are surely not in Western interests. Nor are Russians likely to see it as a viable option for the long run.

If NATO will not take Russia in, Russia's third choice, therefore, will be more attractive: to look eastward for a partner with whom to balance against the perceived growing threat from the West. Expanding NATO without Russia will likely lead to a Russo-Sino rapprochement and even a formal military alliance.

True, there is a long history of trouble in Russian-Chinese relations (Repko 1966), and such an alliance would experience real friction; but it would not be a type of alliance without precedent. To protect their interests, states will find allies where they can and must. Russian leaders have never liked to face adversaries on two fronts (Ching 1996). It is naive to think they would not eventually (probably sooner) turn to China. Imagine Russia allied with a hugely populous partner for whom Russian military technology represents the high end of what is available to the new partnership. A Russo-Sino alliance would vitiate the single and most effective foreign policy initiative of the cold war: Richard Nixon's opening to China, a move that then deprived the Soviet Union of any hope of recovering its most powerful potential ally. Limited NATO expansion risks recreating the world of bipolarity that Nixon deftly managed to shatter.

Is such an alliance so implausible that the West can safely ignore its possibility? It would have big benefits for each side. For Russia, China's expanding economy and 1.2 billion people would prove a weighty counterbalance to NATO. For China, a Russian partner with 150 million people, great natural resources, and a GNP perhaps a third of China's would be a big catch. Russia's military technology, while now largely inferior to that of the West, remains the most modern part of the Russian economy and has the potential to serve as a catalyst for future military development. In virtually every category, Russia's capabilities are far superior to China's. From submarines to communications, to missiles and aircraft, to nuclear weapons, the Russians have much to offer a large and increasingly wealthy state. Easy access to Russian technology would hasten Chinese military modernization at reduced cost. It would also reduce incentives for the continued contraction of Russia's military-industrial-complex.

Evidence for improved Chinese–Russian relations can already be found in arms sales and diplomatic efforts alike (*Current Digest of the Post-Soviet Press* 1997; Holloway 1997). China recently agreed to buy seventy-two advanced SU-27 fighter planes from Russia[11] and build a production line in Shenyang to make more.[12] A similar agreement on the SU-30 may be next, and Moscow recently announced a new sale of two advanced cruise missile warships (Holloway and Bickers 1997). Even more unsettling is evidence pointing to renewed missile sales between the two countries.[13] On the diplomatic front, Russia has been flirting with Beijing. In December 1996, President Yeltsin and Chinese Foreign Minister Li Peng announced a package of large troop cuts on their borders, trade agreements, and further arms deals. The April 1997 meeting in Moscow between Yeltsin and Chinese President Jiang Zemin called for a "multipolar" world in contrast to a unipolar one where, in Yeltsin's terms, "someone else is going to dictate conditions."[14] While disavowing any causal linkage from NATO expansion, Russian Defense Minister Igor Rodionov recently affirmed the development of neighborly relations with China, which "even bind Russia to strengthen relations of partnership also in the military sphere." A Russia–China partnership would place the destiny of much of the Eurasian landmass and the western Pacific in the hands of an antidemocratic alliance.[15] This alliance would operate outside the structure of international law and the norms of universal human rights associated with Western democracies for the past two centuries.

How to avoid the dangers of a Russia–China alliance

China, not Russia, presents the only remaining long-term credible potential threat to Western and global peace and security. This is not said to impute particular intentions or malice to China's people or to its current leaders. Nor does it imply that the Chinese government's intentions are fundamentally more than defensive, to secure a territorial integrity that includes but does not exceed historic Chinese regional claims. Rather, it is stated simply to recognize what diplomats and scholars have long understood. The period of transition from one great power system leader to another is marked by tremendous potential for instability and cataclysmic conflict, as a challenger catches up and ultimately surpasses the power base of the previously dominant state. If the rising power is dissatisfied with its place in the international system, war between the system leader and the challenger may well result.[16] Germany's ambitions earlier in this century illustrate but by no means exhaust the list of challenges. Moreover, the dangers exist even when the challenger is not particularly aggressive or expansionist. The fears, uncertainties, and potential miscalculations of each other's intentions and capabilities provide danger enough. The approaching dangers of Western–Sino military and economic parity pose in power terms a Realist problem. Two complementary strategies—one Realist, one Liberal—are available to manage the problem.

The Realist's way is to prevent the rising state from being able to approach the dominant state's power. A preponderance of power concentrated in the hands of the system leader will often deter the initiation of the overt conflict. Deterrence can work in the short run, so long as the capabilities of the dominant alliance continue to exceed the rising state's by a considerable margin. But a pure deterrence strategy, emphasizing counter-threat and military containment, can intensify conflicts and increase the challenger's commitment eventually to achieve its own dominance.[17] Deterrence—especially nuclear—should not be relied on indefinitely, and so long as it is practiced, it can become a self-defeating strategy. It can, however, buy valuable time, during which other means of ensuring the peace can be brought to bear.

The Liberal's way is to ensure that the rising power and the dominant power have few quarrels over the nature of the international order and the distribution of goods therein. This kind of transition occurred when the United States passed Great Britain as a world power. America did not fundamentally oppose the system that Britain had put in place. In turn, Britain was not willing to fight to oppose the marginal changes to the international system that resulted from subsequent US leadership. Both states shared many common interests and values, and both British and American leaders made a deliberate decision to strengthen Anglo-American ties (Perkins 1968; Campbell 1974; Rock 1989: ch. 2). Integrating Russia into NATO provides time and means to guard against the rising power of China in the short run. In the longer run, it creates a mechanism and a model by which China can over time become fully integrated into the international system, allowing the future rising power to be accommodated without cataclysmic conflict.

The one factor that most constrains a state's potential power is its population (Organski and Organski 1961). With but 150 million people, Russia is a fragment of its former self. Even a reconstituted Soviet Union, developing economically once again, could pose no fundamental danger to NATO's roughly 700 million people. Russia is not today, nor could it be in the future, a threat to the demographic and economic preponderance of the West. China is another matter. An economically growing China, with 1.2 billion citizens, is the single state that could pose a threat to the future security and prosperity of the NATO countries.

Expanding NATO to include the Visegrad countries and Russia would produce a population base of more than 900 million people. More important, the combined wealth and technological superiority of the alliance would postpone the day of reckoning with China's overtaking of the West. China can only achieve geostrategic parity by growing its economy to the point at which its income approaches that of the West, a development that is simply impossible in the near term. Even in the longer future, if the Chinese economy were to grow at 8 percent a year, while the expanded NATO's grew at only 2 percent per year, it would take nearly until the year 2030 to reach parity with the West.[18] There is no historical precedent—Japan included—for a long-sustained growth rate as high as 8 percent.[19] Nor is there much chance that China could maintain that rate with growing environmental problems[20] and, as its technological gap with the West narrowed, with less room for catching up simply by copying Western goods and services. Given an expanded NATO's power preponderance, a growing mercantilist China[21] would find it very hard to develop the military or economic capabilities needed to challenge America and NATO for system leadership by force or beggar-thy-neighbor policies.

As for potential Chinese fears, the Chinese have their deterrents against Russian or Western aggression. An invasion and occupation of China's vast territory and population is unimaginable, particularly by a NATO limited to a defense orientation. China also possesses the world's third-largest nuclear deterrent force. In this scenario, both sides would have ample time to develop a long-term solution to the parity problem, which will require a convergence of both preferences and interests.

Why not bring Russia in?

There are some standard objections to admitting Russia to NATO, which we list and then rebut. Carefully considered, the logic behind the argument to admit Russia is compelling, and far outweighs the concerns.

Objections

First, the Russian military establishment is too degraded to meet NATO countries' high standards. Thus, the costs of bringing Russia's military up to NATO's level are too high and the potential benefits too low. Russia's population and GNP more closely resemble Brazil's than that of a nation that could threaten or substantially contribute to one of the most powerful, stable, and enduring alliances in history.[22]

Second, even if the Russians were allowed into the alliance, we could not trust them to behave as loyal members. NATO members must be able to depend on each other to meet their commitments during potential crises. NATO cannot rely on the Russians, because their only real interest lies in blocking NATO's expansion, not in actually joining an alliance that would compromise their sovereignty and military secrecy.[23]

Third, Russia's economy is insufficiently market oriented and too corrupt to provide a match with the West. Nor is Russia's political system sufficiently democratic, stable, or even governable to provide any meaningful contribution to NATO's overall security.

Rebuttals

Cost and benefits

Yes, today the Russian military is in bad shape. The Red Army's poor performance in Chechnya does not presage a serious Russian threat to NATO now or in the reasonable future. Nor does it provide a basis for confidence that Russia will be able to meet the high military standards necessary for incorporation into NATO. Nevertheless, in the history of admissions to NATO (Greece, Turkey, Spain) the yardstick correctly applied was not the standard of a state's existing military capability. Rather, it was the potential of that state once integrated into the alliance for a range of political as well as military contributions. On the ground of potential, Russia rates highly.

Russia—our greatest former threat—over time can contribute greatly to the overall security of NATO. The equation of Russia with Brazil misses one big point. Russia possesses something quite significant that Brazil does not: its own high-technology military industrial complex with associated research and development potential waiting for the opportunity to be exploited again as it was during the cold war.

Estimates of the costs of integrating the new Eastern European members vary wildly, for political as well as technical reasons. The RAND Corporation study put the price at approximately $42 billion over ten years. This is the cost for upgrading their forces and readying NATO for rapid deployment to their territory in a crisis, but without stationing NATO troops there otherwise.[24] The Defense Department's (DOD) estimate for the most comparable upgrading is a little lower: $35 billion over twelve years, whereas the Congressional Budget Office's (CBO) closest option comes in much higher at $61 billion. For the sake of an illustration, let us take the DOD figure. Suppose that for Russia, with two-and-half times as many people, the cost of upgrading Russian systems to bring them into line with NATO standards were as much as $100 billion. (This is probably too high, since increased costs for NATO rapid deployment would not be proportional.) While that is a significant sum, in the context of Reagan's historic $4 trillion arms build-up it would represent a tremendous bargain, far more than the return from bringing in just the East Europeans. Those states have no indigenous aircraft industry, no submarine manufacturing industry, no nuclear weapons, no ability to make a self-sustainable contribution to their defense and security obligations. Moreover, since the Russian military needs a retrofit anyway, the Russians will pay part of the cost.

Although the costs cannot be ignored, the potential gains from Russian integration should not be ignored either. A major benefit would be the reduced burden of acquiring information through covert means. How much have we paid in the past and are we planning to pay in the future to get information covertly on Russian intentions and capabilities? To be able to integrate Russian nuclear weapons into NATO's command and control system would alone be worth the price. One of the greatest fears about Russia concerns the loss of control of its nuclear weapons. Admitting it to NATO provides the means to control its fissile materials more directly than by buying up excess warheads or trusting the Russians to convert surplus plutonium to reactor fuel. By contrast, leaving Russia out encourages its continued reliance on nuclear deterrence, maintaining thousands of warheads on alert and immensely complicating all high-priority arms control efforts to reduce nuclear weaponry (Turner 1997).

Trust and murky motives

Why was France brought into the Quintuple Alliance in 1818 (Schroeder 1994)? Did we trust the Germans forty years ago? One of the principal reasons for bringing West Germany into NATO in 1955 was fear of revived and unconstrained German nationalism. In Lord Ismay's phrase, Germany belonged to NATO to "keep the Germans down" as well as to "keep the Russians out." The allies recognized that the best way to contain German expansionism was to include the Germans in security structures, not to exclude them.[25] Similar concerns brought West Germany into the whole range of European institutions, led to Gorbachev's acceptance of a United Germany in NATO (Zelikow and Rice 1995; Maier 1997: chs. 5–6) and continue to motivate French and German policy today. These same motivations should hold toward Russia. We should bring the Russians in precisely because we do not fully trust their intentions. Integrating Russian and NATO military forces will require a convergence of doctrine, command, training, and equipment. For example, NATO aircraft have IFF—identify friend or foe—devices to prevent them from firing on one another. This integration of standards and equipment will require and create a level of openness impossible to obtain otherwise. Openness exposes secrets, creating conditions in which no hidden preparations, as those of Nazi Germany for Barbarosa in 1941, are possible. A large-scale German surprise attack on any current NATO member is simply inconceivable today. Much of the explanation lies in changed German intentions. But in no small part, our dismissal of such a scenario stems from the openness that NATO provides, and in the institutional binding of Germany to Europe and the United States, including the unified NATO command. Military integration into NATO will become a guarantee of effective civilian control of the Russian military.[26]

Will Russia simply obstruct NATO's now relatively smooth operations and sow seeds of dissent among the alliance members? There are real conflicts of interest within the alliance, but NATO has a decent record of accomplishment in handling them. Consider the seemingly intractable dispute between Greece and Turkey. Although NATO has not been able to resolve all their problems, NATO's conflict-resolution techniques—a combination of mediation (as by US Secretary of State Cyrus Vance and NATO Secretary-General Manlio Brosio in 1967) and deterrence —have kept them from going to war (Ehrlich 1974; Markides 1977; Mandell 1992). Without NATO, they probably would have done so by now. Fears of conflict within NATO should not preclude the expansion of one of the few organizations that truly can make a difference in solving the thorniest security dilemma the major powers will face in the coming century.

Do the Russians really want to come in? Although in 1991 Boris Yeltsin repeatedly requested NATO admission,[27] maybe Russia would not be serious. Joining NATO imposes significant constraints on a state's ability to exercise privacy rights and sovereignty. While the loss of autonomy for NATO members does not match that embodied in the European Union (EU), Russian entry into NATO would bring a substantial loss of control. Indeed, that would be part of NATO's motivation in inviting the Russians.

Russia could decline the invitation just as it declined Marshall Plan aid following World War II. However, if it does refuse a sincere offer, it will be by its own choice, not by way of NATO exclusion.[28] This should defuse many Russian objections and hence reduce the political backlash in Russia to limited expansion of NATO. A refusal to accept an offer of NATO membership would be a useful early indicator of the future direction of Russian foreign policy, making limited NATO expansion more justifiable.

Alternatively, Russia could accept the offer but not in good faith. What happens if NATO lets the Russians in and the expanded partnership does not work as hoped for? Or what if the gulf between the two cultures cannot be bridged by intrusive NATO institutions? Certainly, the Russians would have learned a lot about Western military doctrine and weapons. Nevertheless, the West will have learned a great deal about the Russians' command postures and intentions as well.

Or Russia might join, even intending to stay, but then throw sand in NATO's gears, with the alliance losing much of its capacity for joint action in situations such as in Bosnia. In this scenario, the Russians could effectively veto NATO actions or otherwise obstruct NATO's already limited capacity for out-of-area operations.

Even in this admittedly dismal situation, Russia would not and could not pose a credible threat to NATO's security. It would chiefly limit NATO proactive offensive capacity, a risk worth taking by an alliance whose principal purpose is providing for the common defense of its members. Nor would a continuation of a security frontier in Europe—like the cold war's, only farther east—exist to feed irrational fears and resentments within Russia's borders.

Ultimately none of these objections carries much weight. If the Russians do prove obstructive, NATO would simply become a defense-only alliance, albeit one still serving to protect its members from attacks both from the outside and from each other. Ironically, this scenario produces a new NATO, which is in the end what it has claimed to be from the outset. NATO efforts at proactive out-of-area cooperation are already tenuous. More than ever, NATO will have evolved into a transparent defense alliance with little offensive capacity, a collection of states that pose no aggressive threat to anyone. It will, however, have evolved into a structure that can both inwardly and outwardly guarantee the borders of its members. Indeed, it should include a general guarantee of borders in Eastern Europe, avoiding the mistake of the Locarno treaties of 1925 (Keylor 1996: ch. 3). By creating a division of labor, pushing states to pursue technical specialization and military comparative advantage, NATO hampers its members (other than the United States) from acting alone. NATO provides powerful restraints on adventurism by its members.

Furthermore, cooperation of the sort NATO demands of its members has already begun to grow in many nonmilitary areas between Russia and current NATO members.[29] The United States is risking the lives of its astronauts in cooperative aerospace projects. Russian rockets will launch critical components of the planned space station. NATO expansion would merely extend the type of cooperation already under way between the Russian space agency and NASA. Civilian firms also are cooperating in joint ventures that require exchange of technology and human resources.[30] Boeing technology and equipment will be used on Russian and Ukrainian rockets to launch communications satellites.[31] Allied Signal has established two joint ventures, to design and manufacture avionics and landing systems for Russian-built aircraft and a software development center in Zhukovsky.[32] Additional partnerships are in progress for cooperative development of environmental controls, auxiliary power, fluid systems, and engines.

Political and economic institutions

Fears of political instability in Russia are not unfounded, but limited NATO expansion will exacerbate the conditions that generate those fears. Rather than increase the risks of political instability, rising ultranationalism, and the general decline of democratic institutions, including Russia in NATO as a full partner would tend to defuse the aura of external threat that strengthens the hands of the radical conservatives in Russia. It would also eliminate the greatest external threat the Russian military can point to in the internal battles for budgetary and political influence.

Concerns about Russia's political instability should not preclude consideration of her suitability as an alliance partner. Although most NATO members have been free-market democracies, Portugal joined under the Salazar dictatorship, and neither Greece nor Turkey was expelled during its periods of military rule.[33] NATO does not maintain the very high admission standard for democracy and free markets that we associate with the European Union. Russian democracy and free-market economics are surely as well developed as those of Romania, where hopes for inclusion in the next round of NATO expansion are being fanned. If we expect the Russians to continue to develop open political and economic institutions, we must address their security fears. In the long run, the best way to promote sustainable democracy is to integrate Russia into some Western institutions, NATO in particular, with the prospect of further integration when its democracy becomes firmly established. Including Russia follows directly from Secretary Madeleine Albright's characterization of more limited expansion, when she declared, "The purpose of NATO enlargement is to do for Europe's east what NATO did 50 years ago for Europe's west: to integrate new democracies, defeat old hatreds, provide confidence in economic recovery and deter conflict."[34]

Russian entry into NATO will not and cannot happen immediately. It will take years of preparation, as did European integration.[35] The point is to start that process now, with a firm commitment and a credible timetable. If the United States wishes to remain the leader of NATO, this is the issue on which to exercise leadership and persuade reluctant Europeans. Bringing Russia into NATO would finally complete what Tsar Peter the Great and other Westernizers aimed to do from the eighteenth century onward: integrate Russia with the West, to their mutual benefit. It would bring security and enhanced stability at a lower cost than would bringing Russia into the EU, and it more directly addresses concern over the rising power of the military within Russia.

The Chinese reaction?

Both the United States and the Soviet Union exacerbated the cold war conflict by being insensitive to the fears of the other. Would our proposal simply create a replay of the old cold war with a potentially more powerful adversary?[36] It should not, and need not. Any coming confrontation with China will be fundamentally different from the old ideological conflict between NATO and the Warsaw Pact. During the cold war, US–Soviet ideological differences made conflict virtually inevitable, as the two systems not only differed in their domestic and world-views but also were fundamentally opposed to the continued existence of the opposition. Leninist doctrine, which provided the theoretical underpinnings of the Soviet system, was based on a revolutionary world ideology—despite its rejection of Leon Trotsky's overt call for world revolution (Gaddis 1997). The endgame in the Leninist framework was to be world revolution driven by inevitable class struggle among a growing urban proletariat. The communist system would win out in the end in part because Lenin and his followers argued that the Soviet state had the superior economic system.

The ideological foundations of the Chinese system do not carry those ambitions. Mao Zedong's ideological goals were fundamentally local, driven not by an ever-expanding worldwide urban revolution that could spread from one city to another like wildfire before a strong wind, but by his vision of a rural revolution. Moreover, today's Chinese leaders have largely abandoned Marxist economics, and in an attempt to modernize rapidly, they vigorously embrace capitalism and more open markets. In China we are left not with an expansionist regime driven by an ideology fundamentally opposed to the continued existence of the West, but rather confront a growing power governed by what is essentially a variant of Asian authoritarianism. The Asian authoritarian model does pose an ideological challenge to Western liberalism, and to some provides an attractive organizing principle for the relationship between economics and politics (Mahbubani 1993). It does not, however, carry a fundamentally subversive and mutually exclusive ideological appeal, as did the old Marxism/Leninism.[37]

Consider how states gauge or measure success in the international arena. For the Soviet Union, success was a new communist country. Not so for contemporary China, where Mao's communist ideology is no longer at its core. Today, the Chinese gauge success by making money and increasing their influence abroad. Of course, we should not discount the antagonism of a hegemonic democratic ideology and an expanding authoritarian ideology (Monk 1996). Democracies prefer to be surrounded by other democracies in an inherently peaceful relationship (Russett 1993). The Western democracies should continue to engage China on human rights and democracy, not abandon their many advocates within China. Those advocates will in time gain influence. Nevertheless, democracies also are accustomed to surviving in relationships with nonaggressive autocracies. Economic insularity today is much more difficult for both democracies and autocracies to sustain.

Confronted with a growing NATO, China will have the same three basic options as Russia does. China could try balancing. Fear of Russian balancing behavior drives our willingness to have Russia join NATO. For those in China who wish to balance against the Western alliance, if NATO follows our prescriptions it will have taken China's obvious partner, Russia.[38] China might conceivably attempt to balance by striking an accord with India or Japan. These developments are largely unthreatening in the former case and implausible in both cases. India has long been China's greatest regional rival. A Sino-Indian alliance would totally reverse those countries' traditional geopolitical strategy without bringing China the advanced industrial and technological support it needs.[39] While a Russia outside of NATO can threaten to balance by allying with a stronger state, China has no such options, save possibly for a deal with Japan. Moreover, it is difficult to see Japan, ever more integrated economically and institutionally with the West, throwing its weight to the Chinese side. If Japan is to line up with anyone, Chinese economic and military growth could eventually bring the Japanese into a closer arrangement with NATO.[40] Chinese balancing against an expanding NATO is very unlikely to work.

Some Chinese efforts to expand regionally against weaker neighbors are likely regardless of whether Russia joins NATO. Threats to nearby Pacific islands, including Taiwan, are to be expected.[41] For these, deterrence based on a stable overall military balance, coupled with the carrots of engagement with the West and respect for China's ability to defend its existing territorial integrity, are the proper counters. The original NATO members would not be much involved; nor do they possess the capacity or physical proximity needed to have much influence over Pacific Rim affairs. Russia, however, could be an invaluable NATO member in this regard, given its geographic proximity, naval and military bases in the Far East, and potentially respectable military capabilities.[42] Denying these potentially valuable strategic assets to China will help restrain it.[43] The inclusion of Russia would make NATO the first truly global alliance. Both northern oceans would have a NATO state on each side, with a stable Europe as the keystone. Articles 5 and 6 of the NATO treaty exclude Asia from those regions in which an armed attack against any member "shall be considered an attack against them all." While this could be amended, an amendment could be seen as a provocation to China. It is already understood that common action may occur elsewhere, outside the narrow boundaries of the North Atlantic Ocean, if unanimously approved as a Combined Joint Task Force operation.

Beijing's next possible response could be hiding, or pursuing an isolationist policy. A Chinese foreign policy stance of armed political, if not economic, isolationism would pose some difficulties for the United States and NATO. Moreover, in the short run this may be the most likely policy reaction to a broad expansion of NATO. Yet this would not necessarily lead to very bad results. To the contrary, it solves the thorniest dilemmas of the coming global power transition. An isolationist China would confront an intractable political predicament. The new leaders in China face a series of political challenges and trade-offs that they will be forced to confront in the near future. These choices will be impelled by the high and competing costs associated with military modernization, the economic and technical difficulties associated with rapid economic modernization, and the problems of maintaining an autarchic regime in the face of a growing middle class. In the emerging global economy with its constant competitive pressures, the challenge of attempting to develop the Chinese economy while simultaneously expanding its immediate military base may prove intractable. Unlike the current Russian leaders, who have so far survived a near-stagnant economy, the legitimacy of the Chinese rulers depends almost entirely on their continued ability to deliver rapid growth.

If China aspired to match the Western alliance in military power and economic capacity, armed isolation would be very costly. Chinese leaders would have to devote proportionally more resources to the military than do the United States and NATO. While the data are imprecise at best, the following numbers are reasonable within a rough magnitude. China's military expenditures in 1995 amounted to 2.3 percent of its GNP; its per capita expenditure was a paltry $53. In the same year the United States spent 3.8 percent of its GNP on the military.[44] The US GNP alone is more than two-and-half times China's. China would have to spend

10 percent of its GNP on defense to match the American level and nearly 18 percent to keep pace with the combined capabilities of all of NATO with Russia and the other new members. Although the Chinese army is potentially huge, the Gulf War in 1991 demonstrated that sheer numbers no longer carry the same weight in conventional war that they did during the Korean War, which was the last large-scale direct conflict between China and the West.[45] China's military is now in far worse shape than the Soviet Union's was before its collapse. To try to match the West's overwhelming capability, China would be forced into either of two courses of action.

If the Chinese decided to be isolationist and to rely principally on domestic investment, they would likely have to choose between the military and domestic consumption or investment.[46] Given the growing strains on China's internal stability, diverting significant resources to the military is not a viable alternative if the Chinese truly hope to achieve strategic parity with the West. The Soviet Union's history suggests what would happen to a China that tried simultaneously to catch up militarily, satisfy growing civilian consumer expectations, and sustain the economic growth rate needed to bring itself up to par with a far richer Western alliance.

Alternatively, China might turn to outside sources of direct investment, as is its current policy. Doing so could free domestic capital to be invested in the military, but this policy also serves Western interests. An economy sufficiently robust to be able to support high levels of military investment clearly would be dependent on Western investment. China already receives more than a third of all foreign investment in manufacturing in developing countries. From the perspective of NATO—an alliance seeking both global stability and the maintenance of the global territorial status quo—that would be a good thing. All else being equal, economically interdependent states are more likely than others to live in peace with each other.[47]

Would Western investment keep flowing to a hostile China?[48] Karl Marx long ago claimed that the capitalists would end up making the rope with which to hang themselves. Of late, European firms have demonstrated great willingness to invest in potentially unstable areas of the world. However, they do so at a price to the investment recipient. Bellicose states and political adversaries pay a high cost for the foreign capital they import. Investors put a higher discount on politically risky investments, with demands for higher interest rates and expected profits. Such penalties will raise the costs to China to develop its military or develop economy at a pace sufficient to allow it to catch up with the West. Therefore, the Chinese become bound by strong incentives to maintain stability and to keep sending reassuring signals to Western investors.

The Chinese dilemma is this: if they do not want to be dependent on Western investment, then they cannot afford the military needed to confront the West. If they do rely on Western investment to be able to divert domestic capital to support the military, then they become over time interdependent with the West. Already China's dependence on foreign trade and investment, and its eagerness to participate in multilateral international organizations like the World Trade Organization (WTO), put it on a path of cooperative relationships that will be strongly resistant to reversal. Such growing interdependence reduces the likelihood that China will choose a confrontational military and foreign policy.

China's final alternative would be to bandwagon, or to join the growing alliance and bind its security interests with those of former adversaries. The Chinese have bandwagoned in the past. They turned west with the Nixon initiatives, although the United States at the time anchored the dominant pole in the international system. In doing so, the Chinese did not simply balance power nor strictly balance against an immediate military threat (Qingshan 1992). They could have interpreted western outposts around China—South Korea, South Vietnam, Taiwan, SEATO—as being fully as threatening as their Soviet neighbor was. Instead, they saw improved relations with the United States as the key to building their economic and long-term military security. China bandwagoned west in a way that presaged the Soviet bandwagoning that ended the cold war.

If Russia is to be kept out of NATO for fear of antagonizing China, much the same logic should have stopped NATO expansion into Eastern Europe for fear of antagonizing Russia. Rather, the first round of NATO expansion should be the first step toward one last big cycle of bandwagoning. NATO would then expand to include a democratizing Russia. Until China is also ready to join, it is important that NATO not gratuitously threaten Chinese security. The Chinese leaders should be encouraged to see their security vested in a policy of increasing political and economic openness.[49] China should be engaged in an ever-deepening network of international organizations and economic interdependence.[50] Ultimately, a great security management system might come to include all but the rogue states. In a sense, that would be the end of international political history. Perhaps Francis Fukuyama called it one move too soon, with not quite enough attention to geo-strategic matters (Fukuyama 1992). Such an alliance would constitute a triumph both of Western ideology and of Western power and organization.

A new future for NATO

NATO exists to provide for the security of its members. For that purpose, con-siderable benefits would accrue from extending an offer of membership to Russia. Such an offer would integrate a potentially threatening state into NATO and increase the overall power base of the alliance. For Russia, the new NATO would provide security assurances on its western front and deterrent power vis-à-vis its eastern front. Membership criteria should be on both political and economic grounds similar to those required for membership in the EU. But rather than raise the bar to such heights as to preclude marginal states from joining the new NATO, the membership hurdle should be set just a notch lower than the stringent conditions for the EU.

It is far easier for states to reform their economies and polities in the absence of security concerns than when faced with powerful and potentially bellicose neigh-bors. Integration into the NATO alliance provides stability for a state's domestic political regime and external security that allows it to focus on the tough job of political and economic development. Any defensive alliance serves two purposes.

The first is to prevent an external power from trying to alter the international territorial status quo. The second is to prevent any of the member states from wishing to do the same. NATO supplies greater physical security for all its members by integrating them into the full NATO system. Key is the integration of command, doctrine, training, and equipment. The NATO system is much more than just a traditional alliance: it creates common expectations and notions of defense versus offense and common beliefs in the stability of the interstate system. That means integration and interdependence in the broadest possible sense—ideological, institutional, and economic.

The bigger the alliance becomes, the less is the burden on any single state and the greater the security provided.[51] If smaller states cheat on defense expenditures—as some did and do in NATO past and present[52]—those states will then become even less able to mount any serious threat on their own. This potential demilitarization would provide a downward spiral of the security fears of neighboring states. Why should not other states, such as Japan, Korea, and ultimately China be attracted to this and be welcome?

Wider NATO expansion will and must proceed slowly. Japan is clearly a potential member, an outcome to be encouraged. Nevertheless, Japanese domestic politics are not ready; and for now, Japan's ties to the other industrial countries are strong enough to allow NATO membership to remain a low priority.[53] Rapid global NATO expansion would only feed historically well-founded Chinese fears of encirclement and Western imperialism. The challenge of managing the peaceful power transition that China may present is a long-term one that does not require a current policy of containing China. American and Japanese engagement with China is much to be preferred.

The potential gains from limited expansion—with or without a second round extending to Romania or the Baltic states—include stabilizing the new members domestically and protecting them from a real or imagined Russian threat. But it damages the prospects for Russian democrats. Most likely, we would wind up with some gain from Eastern Europe being integrated into the rest of Europe at the real risk of a nationalist Russia turning to China. In the global geostrategic net, this is the worst possible outcome. The United States and its current NATO partners constitute a status quo alliance with every incentive to avoid great losses. Their goal should be to preserve their dominant global position as long as possible. They should not choose a policy that runs the very real and very large risk of creating a powerful opposing coalition.

Expansion with Russia also risks some losses as well as gains. The downside risk is that Russia would hamstring NATO in many respects. Even so, Russia would still be in a security system for moderating conflicts within the NATO alliance. With Russia no longer a potential ally of China, large net gains accrue to the West. Western ideological and institutional principles will lie at the core of world organization, even more than now. In effect, a continually expanding NATO provides an essential supplement to the United Nations, one with military teeth and an organizational structure to support them. It is a multilateral structure in which

American leadership is strong but tempered by common perceptions and the experience of negotiated cooperation.

If NATO chooses to include Russia, the very enemy it was created to guard against, what is the potential limit to NATO's expansion? NATO should in time welcome all states that meet certain criteria of economic and political stability. Potential members should be well into the democratization process, avoiding instability and any consequent tendency toward external disputation.[54] Democratic states have less internal violence and civil war than do other states (Krain 1997; Rummel 1997); once established, democratic regimes become permanent if the democracies are also reasonably wealthy (Przeworski and Limongi 1997). New NATO recruits would have to do what Germany, Japan, and now Eastern Europe did to enter the Western alliance: grow their economies and reform their politics. This is the kind of post-cold war security system worth striving for. NATO should expand to include anyone who meets the criteria, most certainly Asians, and especially the Chinese.

Notes

1 The authorship of this chapter is equal. We thank Charles Hill, Paul Kennedy, Mark Lawrence, James Lindsay, William Odom, Jack Snyder, Celeste Wallander, H. Bradford Westerfield, and William Wohlforth for comments.
2 Goldgeier (1998: 85–102) reports on the evolution of views in the Clinton administration. For a discussion of Russian views of the inevitability of limited NATO expansion, see Kondrashov (1997). Also, Doherty (1997).
3 One of the more persuasive presentations of the opposition is Mandelbaum (1995a). A comprehensive review is Kugler (1996). Other discussions of flaws in the expansion argument include Brown (1995); *Arms Control Today* (1997); Dean (1997); MccGwire (1997).
4 Complaints include Pushkov (1997: 58–62); and Fischer and Potter (1996).
5 A relatively early argument to this effect was Harries (1993).
6 The following review many of the current views about the possible evolution of Russian views towards the United States and NATO: Arbatov (1996); Kitfield (1997); Pushkov (1997); Yanov (1997).
7 Recent proclamations along these lines include Baoxiang (1997) and Holloway and Bickers (1997). For a more traditional grand strategy view, see Brzezinski (1996).
8 Goodby (1998). Leaders of the Democratic Choice of Party in the Duma have formed a deputies group called "For the Atlantic Union," *Ria Novosti*, May 28, 1997.
9 See Snyder (1990); and Christensen and Snyder (1990). Snyder (1994) discusses emerging trends in Russia and their consequences for European security. Walt (1987) is a standard citation on alliance politics.
10 Schweller (1994) addresses strategies for manipulating balancing versus bandwagoning behavior.
11 Tyler (1996) writes of a supposedly secret deal to modernize the Chinese Air Force with SU-27 fighter planes.
12 Koretsky (1996) points this out; and Fulghum (1996) addresses the issue of production rights for SU-27 fighters. Russia, for the first time since the 1960s, is ready to export military high technologies to China. This assumes great significance since the SU-27 is a transcontinental fighter and Moscow could come within its firing range.
13 Ukraine or Russia may sell SS-18s to China according to Erlanger (1996). This development is particularly dangerous given Chinese statements about developing

regional deterrent strategies based on nuclear weapons systems they do not currently possess. See Johnston (1995). For a more optimistic view see Garrett and Glaser (1995).

14 From *Beijing Review* (1996). See also Shinkarenko and Malkina (1996).

15 Discussed by Zhilin (1996).

16 For the earliest discussions of this idea, see Organski (1958). More recent treatments include Organski and Kugler (1980); Gilpin (1981). Tests of the underlying propositions include Houweling and Siccama (1988); Kim and Morrow (1992). Further empirical studies and literature review can be found in Kugler and Lemke (1996) and (1998).

17 For a discussion of what works and what does not in deterrence situations, see Huth and Russett (1993).

18 These estimates are at purchasing power parity: calculations based on exchange rates would put the Chinese economy much smaller.

19 Paus (1994) presents a skeptical view of the notion that economic liberalism can provide for long-term high-speed expansion.

20 See especially Esty (1997). Smil (1997), lays out China's current and coming environmental woes. Saywell (1997) addresses the problem of dwindling food stocks. As fleets compete for catches, the region may be heading into an era of fish wars. Niu and Harris (1996) also address China's coming environmental constraints.

21 Engardio (1996) discusses China's mercantilist tendencies.

22 For views that discuss the dilapidated core of the Russian army, see Loshak (1997); and Yurong (1995).

23 For specific and more general arguments that expansion increases demands more than the off-setting gains, see Kitfield (1996).

24 Kelley (1995); Asmus *et al.* (1996). On the DOD estimates, see Mann (1997). A comparison of the three estimates is Erlanger (1997). The chief author of the CBO study termed a recent estimate putting the cost at a mere $1.5 billion "ludicrous" (Shenon 1998).

25 Helpful reviews of the initial phases of NATO development include Artner (1985). A nice review of the social changes in Germany at the relevant time is Park (1986). Also see Baylis (1992); and Kirchner and Sperling (1992).

26 Posen (1984) provides a helpful exposition of the importance of civil control of military organizations. For a discussion of how the Soviets viewed US policies, see Lockwood (1983).

27 Yeltsin insisted it was inevitable that East and Western Europe be more unified and predicted that NATO will evolve into a single armed force for one free Europe. See Karpychev (1992); Persada (1992).

28 Many in the United States viewed this as a clear signal of future Soviet intentions. See Gaddis (1997). As we know from the debate about the origins of the cold war, intentions are very important but extremely difficult to divine.

29 For a discussion of US and Russian space issues and in particular the financial issues involving the Mir space station, see Covault (1996); Lawler (1996); Reichhardt (1996).

30 On cooperation between Lockheed and the Russian firm, NPO, see Asher (1997). See also Scott (1997). Scott notes that this particular project is coming in on time and under budget, unlike many of the governmental programs such as the European space station and the Mir project.

31 Covault (1997) addresses some of the lingering concerns over this type of cooperation.

32 On the joint agreement with Russian Institute to supply electronic systems for aircraft, see *New York Times* (1992); *Aviation Week & Space Technology* (1993).

33 On Portugal's role in NATO, see Bosgra (1969); and for a review of Greece and Turkey's entry and subsequent crises, Hart (1990).

34 Secretary Albright's comments reflect her Senate testimony on 23 April 1997 and her House comments 5 March 1997. See Albright and Obey (1997).

35 A volume that addresses some of the early integration issues in the context of German reunification and Russian democratization is Baranovsky and Spanger (1992).

36 The two contrasting policies for managing relations with China are known as containment and engagement, represented loosely by Bernstein and Munro (1996); and Nathan and Ross (1997). Most recently, see Nye (1997–98).

37 For a pessimistic view, see Huntington (1996); and a more optimistic one, Fukuyama (1992).

38 Alexandr Chudodeyev, Pavel Felgengauer, and Vladimir Abarinov, Russian political analysts, debate the possibility of an alliance between China and Russia since the Chinese political climate has changed considerably following the death of Deng Xiaoping in Chudodeyev et al. (1996).

39 Hunter (1996) addresses this somewhat outrageous possibility.

40 US government estimates put China's military spending as exceeding Japan's for more than a decade. US ACDA (1997). In an interview, Chen Jian, spokesman for the Chinese Foreign Ministry, highlighted the tension between Japan and China by noting that Japan decided to stop aid to China for the rest of the 1995 fiscal year, because it opposed Chinese nuclear testing programs. Cited in *Beijing Review* (1995).

41 A novel view of future security concerns in Asia is Simon (1996). For a more traditional perspective, see Mandelbaum (1995b). Roy (1994) reviews growing fears of increasing Chinese power in East Asia. See also Dreyer (1996).

42 Cronin and Cronin (1996) argue that multilateral containment and engagement will be the only way to manage relations with China in the future. Their key point is that not only the United States but other states as well will have to cooperate in order to prevent future East Asian regional spats from flaring into potentially global crises.

43 Recent problems controlling technology transfers to China highlight the difficulties that the United States will face if it tries to forge ahead alone in its containment policy towards China. For discussion of these problems see Holloway (1996). China bought hi-tech American machine tools, ostensibly for civilian use. Instead, it sent them to a weapons factory—exposing US export controls as ineffective.

44 US ACDA (1997). These estimates are at purchasing power parity rather than at current exchange rates, which would put the Chinese economy much smaller. Other economic and demographic data come from the 1997 *CIA World Fact Book* available online at: www.odci.gov/cia/publications/factbook/index.html.

45 Biddle (1996) argues that a powerful interaction between a major skill imbalance and new technology caused the radical difference between the rate of casualties of Iraqi and coalition forces in the Gulf War. He points out that technology alone is not sufficient to guarantee victory, but that the combination of technological superiority and high skill levels will likely create stunning defeats for unprepared states.

46 The idea that there is a trade-off between goods for domestic consumption and military security is frequently referred to simplistically as the guns versus butter choice. In actuality, the consequences are often complex, indirect, and vary over time and country. Nevertheless, "The price of national vigilance will have to be paid somehow. It may be paid by foregoing current consumption, by depleting past savings, or by mortgaging future economic growth" (Ward et al. 1993: 547). More generally, see Chan (1995); Ward et al. (1995).

47 Oneal and Russett (1997); Russett et al. (1998). World War I is commonly identified as a counter-example on economic interdependence. Even if the interdependence point is correct, the cited articles indicate that the likelihood of war between two states rises with geographic contiguity, a deterrence situation of power balance rather than dominance, a conflict of alliance ties, autocratic governments in one or both states, and a thin or absent network of international organizations. All these other influences were present in 1914, leaving trade alone as a conflict-mitigating force.

48 Nolan (1996) argues that China cannot have it all—economic gains, political autocracy, and a huge army.

49 Brzezinski (1996) argues that China should be treated with the same great power respect that the Soviet Union was accorded during the cold war. On the potential reaction to various US policies directed toward China, see Shambaugh (1996).

50 An argument for just this sort of engagement policy is Segal (1996).
51 The common starting point in this literature is Olson (1971). For more recent treatments of collective action in NATO, see Oneal (1990); and Sandler (1993).
52 Conybeare (1994). See also Murdoch and Sandler (1991); and Oneal and Diehl (1994).
53 In an interview, Japanese Prime Minister Morihiro Hosokawa argued that there is no present need for a NATO-like security organization in north Asia (Chanda 1993).
54 Whether democratization raises the likelihood of interstate war is hotly disputed. The positive case is by Mansfield and Snyder (1995). Challenges, rebuttals, and counter-rebuttals include the correspondence in *International Security* 20(Spring 1996): 176–207; the exchange between Mansfield and Snyder (1997) and Thompson and Tucker (1997a; 1997b); Maoz (1998); Ward and Gleditsch (1998).

8

A NEO-KANTIAN PERSPECTIVE

Democracy, interdependence, and international organizations in building security communities[1]

In this chapter I explore elements of a partial but arguably nascent global security community. To think about such a global scope requires treating the concept of security community somewhat loosely, and surely it applies unevenly, to some regions more strongly than to others. At one end of the spectrum, some "hot spots" manifest no security community whatsoever; other parts of the global system have plausibly reached the stage of ascendant (South America) and even mature (Europe) security communities. Overall, true interstate conflicts have become rare with the end of the cold war, just as intrastate conflicts have multiplied.[2] So what we must do here is to consider elements—partial and potential as well as actual—of a global security community. In doing so we take the hard case, focusing on global processes and institutions and thereby push the envelope of this discussion on security communities. What seems to be transpiring, at the very least, is a blurring and extension of the boundaries of regional security communities, as they exist or as they are emerging.

By focusing on the global parts, particularly the United Nations, I do not imply that everything about these organizations works as intended. Rather, I am trying to capture the essential vision of many of the founders of the UN, previous commentators, and recent contributions to the discourse on reforming the UN.[3]

A Kantian framework

As a way of introducing some of these elements in a Kantian framework, we begin with a puzzle about the end of the cold war. For this purpose the question is not simply why did the cold war end, but rather: why did it end before the drastic change in the bipolar distribution of power, and why did it end peacefully? Neither of these questions is well answered within the framework of a neorealist analysis. In November 1988 Margaret Thatcher proclaimed, as did other Europeans, that "the cold war is over." By spring 1989 the US State Department stopped making official reference to the Soviet Union as the enemy (Mason 1998). The fundamental patterns of East–West behavior had shifted toward those of a nascent security community, beginning even before the circumvention of the Berlin Wall and then by its destruction in November 1989. All of this precedes the unification of Germany (October 1990) and the dissolution of the Warsaw Pact (July 1991). Even after those events, the military power of the Soviet Union itself remained intact until the dissolution of the USSR at the end of December 1991.[4] None of these events was resisted militarily. Indeed, by fall 1990 the United States and the Soviet Union were cooperating closely against Iraq, formerly a Soviet ally.

Any understanding of the change in the Soviet Union's international behavior, before its political fragmentation, and in time reciprocated by the West, demands attention to the three legs on which the liberal vision of Immanuel Kant's *Perpetual Peace* stands:

1. Substantial political liberalization and movement toward democracy in the Soviet Union, with consequent changes in free expression and the treatment of dissidents at home, in the East European satellites, and in behavior toward Western Europe and the United States.[5]
2. The desire for economic interdependence with the West, impelled by the impending collapse of the Soviet economy and the consequent perceived need for access to Western markets, goods, technology, and capital. Obtaining that access would require a change in Soviet military and diplomatic policy, and would constrain that policy subsequently.
3. The influence of international law and organizations, as manifested in the Conference on Security and Cooperation in Europe (CSCE) and the human rights basket of the Helsinki accords and their legitimation and support of political dissent in the communist states. Whereas the UN itself was not important in this process of penetrating domestic politics, the CSCE as an inter-governmental organization, and the various human rights INGOs, most certainly were (Adler 1998; see also Mastny 1992; and Frye 1993).

These same three pieces—consolidation of democracy, economic interdependence, and transnational institutions—constituted the basis whereby Jean Monnet, Konrad Adenauer, and other founders of the European Community sought to foreclose the possibility of yet another great war in Europe. Peace among representative democracies, economic interdependence, and international law clearly emerge in a free translation and late-twentieth century reading of Kant's 1795 work.[6] It is also a view consistent with a definition of human security recently espoused as the protection of states, and their populations, from mortal danger.[7] It is a view subversive of authoritarian and autarchic concepts of state sovereignty, in the interest of popular sovereignty in control of states (liberal internal systems) operating with substantial autonomy but embedded in, and therefore supporting and actively promoting, the production of liberal states in an interdependent international system.

It is a view ultimately of a global authority structure, weak but with enough teeth to defend itself against illiberal challengers. In this it is a dynamic view of sovereignty.[8]

Ever since the Treaty of Westphalia, state juridical sovereignty has been the fundamental legal and ideological principle (and also myth) undergirding the world system. The United Nations, as an organization comprising sovereign states, is neither a world government nor an assembly of peoples. Yet states' practical sovereignty has in many areas been eroded. Some of these erosions have happened consciously and voluntarily—most strikingly in the case of the European Union, in other instances by a variety of treaty commitments binding states to common legal norms and procedures. Others have been involuntary, as when extreme violation of human rights or humanitarian distress becomes the basis for international intervention in what would normally be the domestic affairs of a state (e.g., Iraq, Haiti). Sometimes the collapse of civil authority (e.g., Somalia) may mean that there is no government capable of exercising the practical rights of sovereignty to which the country is nominally entitled. A normative fracture exists between Article 2(7) of the Charter, forbidding the UN "to intervene in matters which are essentially within the domestic jurisdiction of any state," and the broadened scope of authority under Article 39 "to maintain or restore international peace and security."

Conceptually, a Kantian view fits nicely with the thesis of the former UN Secretary-General Boutros-Ghali that democracy, economic development and interdependence, and peace are inextricably linked, in something of a triangle of positive feedbacks, with the United Nations and other international organizations able to make direct contributions to each. Boutros-Ghali makes this thesis explicit in his *Agenda* reports, first on peace, then on development, and finally on democratization (Boutros-Ghali 1992; 1995; 1996). Figure 8.1 illustrates this system.

It does not matter what item one places at any particular corner of the triangle, but for the sake of this discussion peace belongs at the center. The triangular image serves as a description and prescription for an ordered, just, and peaceful society at the domestic or international levels, with wide and equal political participation yet protection of minority rights, equality of opportunity with sharp limits on rents that are derived from control of a market by powerful political or economic actors, and institutions to facilitate and promote cooperation with some—but minimal—elements of coercion.

The basic perspective holds that each of these is interacting and mutually supportive, internationally and domestically as well, in a dynamic mutually reinforcing system. For example, each of the other elements is, or can be, supported and encouraged by international organizations; in turn, a world where international organizations can flourish must be one where peace, development, and democracy also flourish in most of the constituent states. Hence all the arrows go in both directions, to emphasize the mutual feedbacks. Again, this is a conceptual and theoretical schema. The empirical evidence for each of the links is in some instances weak and contradictory, and in any case I could not possibly review it in detail here. Nor would I deny that there can also be some contradictions and negative feedbacks.

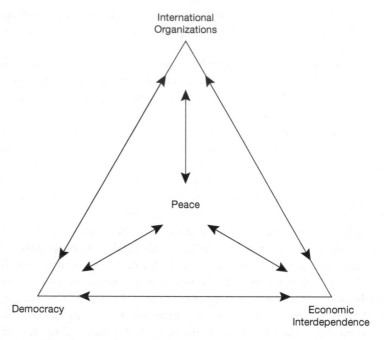

FIGURE 8.1 A Kantian security community

But there is enough evidence for most of the links to allow us to take "the whole ball of wax" seriously, if still somewhat speculatively. We begin with the linkages in the lower half of the figure, among democracy, economic development and interdependence, and peace, proceeding only later to the linkages to and from international organizations.

Democracy and peace

At the international level, the causal arrow from democracy (and perhaps human rights more generally) to peace is arguably the most solidly established generalization of the lot. It is not uncontested, but in my view the critics have yet to seriously dent the "democratic peace" proposition. To this point in time, no one to my knowledge has seriously argued the opposite (that democracies are *more* likely to fight each other than are other states); at most a few articles have held that, especially for particular times and places, the positive association does not appear, or if so is not statistically significant. I have responded to some of these critiques elsewhere, and refer the reader to that response. The response depends less on refuting a few particular critiques than on the now voluminous theoretical elaboration and empirical evidence (statistical and historical) which support not just the basic "democracies rarely fight each other" proposition, but, in the style of a progressive research program, move to elaborations of the program to such topics as alliance behavior, winning wars, military expenditures, and signaling. I characterize the state of the evidence as akin to that about the causal effect of smoking on lung cancer: autarchies are not the sole cause of war (nor is smoking the sole cause of lung cancer); not every autocracy or smoker experiences war or cancer; the micro-causal mechanism is still in some dispute; and some folks still haven't got the message. But the evidence is stronger than most of what we use as the basis for public policy (Russett 1996).[9]

For the security community perspective, it is important to note that the "democracies rarely fight each other" effect is specific to democracies. It depends on particular normative perspectives on the rightness of fighting others who share a commitment to peaceful conflict resolution, and on the absence of need to fight those who have political institutions that support peaceful conflict resolution internationally. It may apply to a degree to states which, though not especially democratic, nevertheless share some of the normative perspectives and institutional restraints typical of democracies. But little evidence suggests it is generalizable to other broad categories of political and cultural similarity (e.g., Islamic states, military governments, communist states). Whereas there surely are specific examples of similar "we feelings" that inhibit war-making, applying that expectation broadly risks frequent refutations unless one makes it virtually tautological. (If we don't fight them, despite some opportunity and perhaps cause to do so, it must be because we share mutual identity and we-feeling.) Deutsch's emphasis on compatibility of values rather than similarity seems sounder. I doubt, therefore, that it is necessary to make expectations of a global security community—however distant that may seem—dependent upon widespread acceptance of ideas of global citizenship or adoption of a common global culture. Globally, as well as within states, the need is to create institutions reflecting democratic principles which can protect cultural diversity while preserving a wider sense of common identity.

Within countries the evidence about peace and democracy may be less well developed, but it is still strong. Whereas civil wars do occur within democracies, they are relatively rare. The extreme cases of governments slaughtering their own citizens and otherwise engaging in massive violations of human rights are over-whelmingly concentrated in authoritarian and totalitarian states. Stable democracies, with guarantees of minority rights against majority tyranny, offer means of peaceful conflict resolution and are less likely to experience severe ethnic conflict (Sen 1981; Gurr 1993; Rummel 1994, 1997).

The return arrow plausibly also operates at both the international and national levels. Since democracies usually—80 percent of the time—win their wars against authoritarian states, and leaders of states who lose wars are more likely to be overthrown, an evolutionary mechanism may operate from democracy to peace (Bueno de Mesquita *et al.* 1992; Lake 1992; Stam 1996). Wars are nonetheless dangerous to democracy. In Charles Tilly's famous aphorism, "the state makes war, and war makes the state." A common criticism of the cold war, sometimes in terms of Harold Lasswell's prescient "garrison state" concept, was that it strengthened authoritarian political forces on both sides. International threats, real or perceived, enhance the forces of secrecy and repression in domestic politics. Relaxation of international threats to security reduces the need, and the excuse, for repression of democratic dissent (Lasswell 1941; Gurr 1988; Tilly 1990).[10] Similarly, domestic insurgencies frequently lead to the suspension of democratic liberties by the threatened central authorities.

Peace and economic interdependence

As for the effect of economic interdependence on peace, a long tradition—partly Deutschian and constructivist, partly straight-out rational and nineteenth-century liberal—argues in favor of the proposition. The nineteenth-century liberal version derives primarily from a viewpoint of rational economic interest: it is hardly in my interest to fight you if in fact my markets, my sources of supplies, raw materials, and other imports are in your country. If my investments are located in your country, bombing your industry means, in effect, bombing my own factories. The Deutschian argument is that economic exchange becomes a medium for communicating perspectives, interests, and desires on a broad range of matters not the subject of the economic exchange, and that these communications form an important channel for conflict management. Both these versions probably operate empirically. In these ways dense linkages of economic interdependence are part of a wider variety of international transactions that help build a sense of shared identity among peoples.[11]

It is true that there is a competing proposition, that in many circumstances economic ties, especially in the form of asymmetrical dependence rather than true interdependence, do not promote peaceful relations. The final judgment is not yet in. The preponderance of systematic evidence for at least the post-World War II era, however, suggests that mutual economic interdependence, measured as the share of dyadic trade to GNP in the country where that trade is proportionately smaller, is strongly associated with peaceful relations in subsequent years. This is so even after the now-customary controls—distance, alliance, relative power, democracy, and wealth or economic growth rates—are included in the equation and prove also to have positive independent effects (Kim 1988; Oneal and Russett 1997).[12] To this should be added the possibility of an interaction between democracy and interdependence with a stronger effect than just the additive one. For example, Lisa Martin argues within the context of the principal-agent framework that in order to reach credible agreements with other states, democratic executives have to persuade, and accommodate themselves to the perspectives of, their legislatures. In doing so, they make it more likely that they will be able to keep their commitments, that the commitments won't become unglued in quick or arbitrary fashion. She applies this, appropriately, both to security issues and issues of trade and economic interdependence. From it one can plausibly impute not just the direct arrow from democracy to peace, but one running from democracy to interdependence and then to peace. Another kind of interaction may be seen in some "two-level games," whereby interdependence brings extra-state actors into the domestic political process to a degree facilitated by a pluralistic political system (Martin 2000).[13]

The possibility of reciprocal effects—states do not allow themselves to become too economically dependent on states with whom they are in military conflict or anticipate such a possibility—is of course also plausible and likely; a full sorting-out of these relationships is in progress.

Democracy and interdependence

The final set of relationships concerns the base of the triangle, between democracy and economic interdependence. At the international level, it may be that economic interdependence supports democracy; at least the European Union seems to operate on this principle, requiring all applicants for admission to the common market to demonstrate their commitment to stable democratic rule and human rights. In the other direction, democratic states presumably feel their security less threatened by other democratic states, and hence can enter into relationships of economic interdependence for absolute gain without worrying as much about the relative gains that so centrally impact the realist model of relationships. One would there-fore expect more trade between democracies than between democracies and non-democracies, or between two nondemocracies, holding constant other relevant cultural and economic influences.[14] Economic interdependence typically is greater between states with competitive markets (somewhat more common in democracies) than operating under state or private monopolies.

Purely at the domestic level, the relation between economics and democracy requires a conceptual shift away from simply economic interdependence to a broader focus on income levels and distribution, and to a focus on peaceful means of con flict resolution and the maintenance of stable democracy. These relationships are somewhat problematic and in dispute. Most scholars readily agree that there is an association between democracy and per capita income, and that economic development facilitates democratization. But they do not agree on whether any significant causality operates from democracy to development, nor fully on the causal relationship between economics and domestic political stability and peaceful conflict resolution. The role of free markets is also part of the discussion. Arguably, a key component of economic development is the determination of peaceful pro-cesses of economic interdependence more by market considerations than by state fiat or ethnic preference. As this debate is both voluminous and also not central to the focus of this chapter I will simply summarize my understanding of the results.[15] Nevertheless, these relationships are important to the triangular perspective of the Secretary General:

- Economic development and democracy are strongly correlated; the causal arrow seems to be from development to democracy, rather than the other way. There are nonetheless a fair number of exceptions, with successful democracy in poor countries like India, and strong resistance to democratization in Singapore (as rich as France). But once a democracy reaches an income level of $6,000 per capita in 1985 dollars, it is "impregnable and can be expected to live forever" (Przeworski *et al.* 1996: 41).

- Democracy does not in any systematic way inhibit economic growth, nor does autocracy promote it. For every authoritarian government that represses political opposition while promoting growth, several dictatorial kleptocracies steal billions of dollars from their people (e.g., Zaire). The generalization that political opposition must be repressed in the interest of development is a lie.
- Great inequality of incomes severely reduces the likelihood of establishing or preserving stable democracy. Inequality damages the sense of common identity in a community.
- Gross economic inequality is more likely to damage economic growth than to promote it.

International organizations and peace

Let us now turn to the role of international organizations—potential as well as actual. The same kind of statistical analysis that has established a relation between democracy and peace, and at least since 1950 between economic interdependence and peace, has recently found an additional, independent relationship between peace and dense networks of intergovernmental organization membership (Russett *et al.* 1998).[16] Here I focus primarily on the UN and its associated bodies—in promoting peace, democracy, and development and interdependence. We can treat the different parts of the United Nations, and other intergovernmental organizations and international nongovernmental organizations (INGOs), as instances of institutions capable of carrying on some of various processes of international transformation:

1. Coercing norm-breakers.
2. Mediating among conflicting parties.
3. Reducing uncertainty by conveying information.
4. Expanding material self-interest to be more inclusive and longer term.
5. Shaping norms.
6. Generating the narratives of mutual identification.

These possibilities range from standard liberal understandings of institutions as facilitating the rational pursuit of self-interest in ways that also serve existing mutual interests, to "teaching" a set of norms and appropriate political organization that may sharply revise actors' preferences and sense of their self-interest (Finnemore 1993). To illustrate them I draw on a perspective on the United Nations which I characterize as "the three UNs." Although the UN is not neatly and formally divisible into three separate sets of functional agencies, it can be helpful to group its activities under these three headings and purposes.

The direct relationship of international organizations to peace is straightforward, and largely derivable from realist theories of international relations rather than liberal ones. Realist theory does not attribute great importance to international organization, but allows it a possible role. The "first UN" is the UN concerned directly with security from threats or actuality of violent conflict. It chiefly comprises the Security Council, and to some degree the office of the Secretary General. The realist founders of the UN recognized the difficulties these institutions would have if the great powers were in serious conflict, but nonetheless saw these units as having the potential to make a contribution under the right circumstances.

The Security Council was designed as an agent of collective security and enforcement, in principle to be carried out by forces of the UN itself directed by the Military Staff Committee, as provided for in Chapter VII. Of course the Military Staff Committee was fossilized at the outset of the cold war, and ideas of a standing UN military force or even of national military and air forces on call from member states by the UN (Articles 43 and 45), were totally still-born. The Security Council has been able to agree on major collective security/enforcement operations twice during its history (the outset of the Korean War, while the Soviet Union boycotted the Council, and in the Gulf War of 1990). It has embarked on "peace enforcement" actions (as ultimately developed in the newly independent Belgian Congo, and later in Somalia and ultimately Bosnia) with mixed and controversial results. The Security Council has also repeatedly authorized not direct military action, but the enforcement of economic sanctions on actors judged a threat to the peace. The widespread opinion that economic sanctions generally have little effect is exaggerated. They seem to have been important in bringing Serbia to the peace table, and at great civilian cost in preventing Iraq from rebuilding its biological, chemical, and nuclear arsenal.

The concept of peacekeeping, however (by impartial forces, to monitor a cease-fire already agreed by the parties, lightly armed and authorized only to use lethal force in self-defense), developed outside the explicit authorization of the Charter, and has overall been more successful. In recent years the UN has increasingly been drawn more into largely internal conflicts of states than into interstate conflicts as its founders anticipated. A further innovation has been the development of post-conflict peacebuilding activities (e.g., Cambodia, Mozambique, Namibia) that has been only partially military, devoted more to creating or strengthening the political and economic institutions deemed essential to achievement of stable peace following civil wars. Because these are not primarily military, and impact more on other corners of the triangle than principally on peace directly, I will discuss them below.

If the Security Council constitutes the most visible realist part of the UN, and the "teeth" to defend whatever liberal world order exists, other parts are devoted to constructing institutions and practices which may directly moderate or mediate conflicts. Such international organization functions generally compatible with modest realist expectations include confidence building (as part of an arms control agreement, or a peacekeeping or peacebuilding operation perhaps), preventive diplomacy, mediation, arbitration, and abjudication. During the cold war opportunities to exercise these functions were not frequent, but less uncommon outside the arena of East–West military confrontation. Here are a few examples: Secretary-General Javier Pérez de Cuéllar made a major preventive diplomacy effort, coming rather close to success, to avert the Argentine/British war over the Malvinas/ Falklands. (For such purposes it is essential as a general principle that the Secretary General always retain a position of impartiality, "out of the loop" of, and above, enforcement actions that inevitably cast him as a partisan.) One of the great achievements of his tenure was to mediate an end to the Iran/Iraq war in 1988. Former US President Jimmy Carter is virtually a one-man INGO devoted to such good works. Another relevant INGO is the Papacy increasingly trusted, especially by predominantly Catholic states, since it has been shorn of its secular power. Argentina and Chile trusted John Paul II to arbitrate their dispute over the Beagle Islands.

The International Court of Justice rarely gets the chance to adjudicate major security disputes, but this does happen. The ICJ arbitration of fishing rights in the Georges Bank off Canada and the United States illustrates the established generalization that democratic states are more likely to accept third-party settlement efforts, even up to formal arbitration (Bercovitch 1991; Brecher 1993; Dixon 1994; Raymond 1994, 1996);[17] when Chad and Libya accepted its decision on allocation of the Ouazou Strip between them it illustrated that such willingness is not limited to democracies. On the theme of interactions between democracy and international law and organization note also the finding that interdependent democracies are more likely to recognize and enforce each other's law in their own states than are other types of regimes (Slaughter 1992, 1995).

International organizations and interdependence

A "second UN" is that attempting to build the economic and institutional foundations on which the liberal vision of peace rests. Established alongside the realist institutions, it owes its origin to elements of the tradition of Kant, Richard Cobden, and Woodrow Wilson. It is perhaps in symbiosis with the realist parts of the UN, able to operate only where realist considerations initially inhibit the outbreak of violent conflict, yet where these foundations deepen they increasingly make realist calculations tangential or irrelevant. Conditions of "dependable expectations of peaceful change" diminish the fear of losing out in relative terms, and hence facilitate the pursuit of absolute gains through commerce (Powell 1991). The importance of interdependence is variously implied in Deutsch et al.'s (1957) specification of several other conditions for integration: superior economic growth, expectation of economic gains, strong economic ties.

Major institutions here include the United Nations Development Programme (UNDP), the Bretton Woods institutions (World Bank and IMF), the World Trade Organization, as well as regional trade and development institutions. These institutions are devoted to the economic development of poor countries, financial stability, and the freer flow of international capital and goods. Their activities apply both to establishing norms and rules for international exchange, and, increasingly with the emphasis on "good government" and "transparency" (near-synonyms for democracy) as well as market economics, to constitutive norms within states. Initially, and again recently, they have taken a major role in providing the resources to reconstruct war-shattered societies.[18] Such a role means both building institutions and teaching the relevant norms.

The record of these organizations is mixed and controversial to be sure, diluted not just because of politics in the UN and between its member states, but from the conflicting recommendations of economics professionals. Nonetheless, their achievements—especially in the realm of freeing world trade and capital markets —are often impressive. Recognition of their achievements need not obscure important critiques that they have been too attuned to the interests of international capital, and too inattentive to the needs of the poor and of environmental preservation (Rich 1994; Hurrell and Woods 1995). But the record of the chief ideological alternative—state ownership and the command economy—is surely not superior. If the prospect, and the experience, of human betterment is necessary to human security, and so too is some expectation of greater economic equality between rich and desperately poor peoples, then the practice of these international organizations needs appreciation as well scrutiny for the faults of their practice or their ideological underpinnings. It too is appropriate to mention the environmental organizations, some of them engaged in serious monitoring and facilitation of norm-development, and the agencies devoted to public health aspects of human security. UNICEF and the World Health Organization deserve the credit for the global eradication of smallpox. A similar operation against malaria was making great progress until member states decided, disastrously, that it was no longer a major concern.

International organizations and democracy

Finally, we come to the "third" UN of democracy and human rights. One can begin with the UN High Commissioner for Refugees, performing massive services for 30 million refugees worldwide. In addition one should include the fragmented, cumbersome, and weak apparatus directly assigned to monitor and promote human rights: among its parts are the UN High Commissioner for Human Rights, the Center and the Committee for Human Rights, and various functional units. Their record is controversial, primarily because of the unwillingness of many member states to permit these organizations the "teeth" to intrude effectively into "sovereign" areas of domestic law and political practice. Nevertheless, they do matter.

Various NGOs and INGOs (Amnesty International and the International League for Human Rights, for example) make governments accept some transparency, and press them to observe standards of human rights explicitly labeled, despite some vigorous resistance, as "universal." The widely ratified (if also widely violated) 1948 Universal Declaration of Human Rights, and many subsequent Conventions (for instance, on the rights of women, and civil and political rights), protocols, and other agreements establish norms which give nongovernmental organizations a basis for comparing the performance of states. Increasingly these international agreements have become embedded in the domestic law of states. Important too are the various UN-sponsored Conferences: talk shops, yes; but talk shops with an ability to develop a common narrative and promote constitutive norms by which governments can in some degree be held accountable. They may give rise to customary international law constraining even states which dissent (Charney 1993).

A little-appreciated part of the United Nations system is the Division of Electoral Assistance, in the Secretariat. Since its establishment about ten years ago it has assisted and monitored democratic national elections in more than seventy states, typically easing the transition from authoritarian rule or to independence. Success stories for the election process include such widely recognized cases as El Salvador, Nicaragua, Cambodia, Ethiopia, Mozambique, and Namibia. Its services (and those of many NGOs) include far more than just observing elections, such as advice on building political parties, constitutions, electoral laws, and press freedom.[19] Democratically elected governments do not always stay democratic, but free and competitive elections are the prerequisite for democracy. It would have been unthinkable for the UN to have taken on this task a decade ago, but with the recent shift toward democratic practice and democratic ideology it is an accepted function. The governments of many autocratic member states resist the norm-setting elements of this effort, but former Secretary-General Boutros-Ghali determinedly (and bravely) pushed it as a normative constituent of what it means to be a "modern" civilized state. It is also a task that no state (such as the United States) could perform nearly so credibly as an impartial third party.[20]

Activities of the "three UNs" and their essential INGO partners come together most closely in efforts of post-conflict peacebuilding. These efforts involve the domestic affairs of newly independent or "failed" states with little or no history of democratic government, whose economies have been devastated by civil war, hundreds of thousands, or millions, of their people made refugees, and whose social and political infrastructure has been demolished. Again, the execution of all these tasks together by the UN is a recent development, impelled by the political upheavals born of the collapse of one end of the formerly stabilizing bipolar international system. Such efforts require, in addition to some variant of peacekeeping, creation of the preconditions to hold free elections and to hope to hold democratic institutions together afterward; massive resettlement of refugees and of discharged soldiers, and insurgents; large-scale economic assistance, including support for free markets; and often the creation of new and democratically accountable legal and administrative systems (police, judiciary, military, telecommunications and postal systems). The UNDP carries on many of these activities, addressing both the elites and the general populace.

These efforts are extremely expensive, and difficult to make successful. (Examples include Cambodia, El Salvador, Namibia, and Bosnia.) The UN and its INGO associates form an extremely loose system given to administrative overlap and duplication, not to mention working at cross-purposes. Attempts to resettle combatants or create essential administrative structures may compete directly with those to bring a measure of fiscal responsibility and discipline. Peacebuilding necessarily runs into conflict with long-standing principles of impartiality and respect for sovereignty. It cannot succeed without the committed support of UN member states, the will and ability of local actors, and the capacity of local institutions (DeSoto and del Castillo 1994; Bertram 1995; Ratner 1995; Zartman 1995; Russett and Oneal 2001). It may often fail. But without such help it may be quite impossible even to imagine the creation of a security community within such a state, or in its relations with its neighbors.

Authority and legitimacy in international organizations

Most of the activities of international organizations, especially outside of the traditional scope of military security, do not represent the threat or exercise of coercive authority. The United Nations and its family of component or related organizations is hardly tightly coupled; at best it may become a very loosely coupled security community. Such organizations build the institutions of state and civil society with the more or less willing consent of most of the relevant parties within states. While international organizations frequently do intrude on states' sovereignty, typically these instances are the consequence of bargaining (as in the condition- ality of development organizations) that leaves both sides better off in the Pareto- optimal sense (Krasner 1995/96). Van Wagenen, a few decades ago, judged the consensus-forming result of international organizations as the most important result in building security communities (Van Wagenen 1965: 818).

In discussing security as well as economic matters, Robert Keohane and Lisa Martin argue,

> institutions can provide information, reduce transaction costs, make commit- ments more credible, establish focal points for coordination, and in general facilitate the operation of reciprocity . . . controlling for the effects of power and interest, it matters whether they exist. They also have an interactive effect . . . depending on the nature of power and interests.
>
> (Keohane and Martin 1995: 42)[21]

International organizations provide transparency, search for the basis of accept- able compromise or minimum common-denominator agreements, and create preferences for, and expectations of, peaceful settlement. Finally, they engage in norm building—both regulative of the international system and constitutive of its member states.

Some of the most auspicious periods of transnational creativity for changing the international system, limiting the frequency and intensity of war, and creating new international organizations, regimes, and norms to guide behavior tend to follow great wars. The Napoleonic Wars brought the Congress of Vienna and the Concert of Europe; the two great wars of the twentieth century brought the League of Nations and the United Nations (Wallensteen 1984; Vasquez 1993: ch. 8).[22] Outside the realm of military alliances they do not flourish during wartime, but when peace comes policy-makers are often ready to construct new institutional underpinnings. The more stable the peace appears, the readier are states and peoples to trust the new institutional arrangements. Perhaps the end of the cold war—an intense conflict and quasi-war even if only sporadically overtly violent—offers such an opportunity, maybe a fleeting one. Increasing interdependence, including that of the consequences of violence by state and nonstate actors, may create the demand.

No discussion of the role of international organizations in creating, however incompletely and unevenly, conditions for a security community on a global level should avoid questions about the authority structure within the United Nations itself. Those questions are doubly inescapable in an essay which has placed such emphasis on the importance of democratization within states. It has permeated much of the discussion about democracy that has been carried on at the United Nations. The introductory piece in a collection of European essays on *Cosmopolitan Democracy* asks not only whether a "democratic" international organization can thrive when most of its component states do not practice democracy at home, but also whether democratic states can flourish in a world not itself organized on democratic principles (Bobbio 1995).[23] Underlying such questions are appropriate concerns about the implications of hegemony by the global North/West.

A discussion of democracy at the level of global institutions is conceptually difficult because the same principles do not always make sense at both levels. The fundamental democratic principle of "one-person, one vote" runs into special difficulties not just from fears of another source of hegemony (roughly 20 percent of the people on Earth live in the People's Republic of China; about 80 percent are in all the developing countries). Where so many states still do not experience free elections in their domestic affairs it is impossible to imagine democratically elected representatives from those states to a global assembly.[24] The alternative principle of "one-state, one vote," as applied to the General Assembly, grossly under-represents the citizens of great powers at the expense of mini-states. It is probably tolerated there only because the Assembly is such a weak body with so little authority. The entity with the greatest authority, and coercive powers, blatantly violates both principles. The veto power in the Security Council is undemocratic in the extreme. By standard measures, virtually all voting power rests in the hands of the five Permanent members; the voting power of any nonpermanent member is calibrated in decimals, and of course the 170 states not on the Council at all have zero voting power. The Security Council probably must be undemocratic because of its need to be able to act quickly and efficaciously; it is hard enough to get enough agreement among fifteen states without trying to assemble it among most of 185.

More to the point, if decisions by the Council are to be effective, they must reflect the will and resource commitment of the great powers, the states with the muscle. No action can be taken without the active support of most of them, and none can be taken against the determined resistance of one without destroying the Organization (Russett 1997c). Therefore the Permanent Five were intended, in 1945, to be those with the greatest military and financial capacity. There was always some fiction in characterizing all Five that way, and there is far less truth in doing so now, especially on the financial side. Yet a "democratic" principle that overtly assigned voting power based on the international distribution of bombers, or of dollars, would be odd indeed. The distribution of voting rights in the IMF and World Bank, for example, is fully recognized as undemocratic, but essential to obtaining the needed resources from the big rich countries.

Thus the discourse on democratization of the UN is typically couched less in terms of voting power than of principles—part of democracy, but not all of it—of "representation," participation, and transparency. To some degree this may be served by increasing permeability of UN bodies to the influence of transnational NGOs.[25] Another element of the discourse is about subsidiarity and delegation to more homogeneous regions (though delegation to regional great powers might be extremely "undemocratic").[26] Much of the effort may have to go to facilitating loosely coupled security communities at the regional level, as well as at the global one. These principles are not irrelevant to states or to peoples. Perhaps they can be applied in ways—differently in different units—that achieve and preserve substantial legitimacy for the Organization as a whole.[27]

The search for acceptable principles of representation and participation, however, cannot come at the expense of effectiveness. Any organization's legitimacy depends as much on its effectiveness as on its principles of governance. A balance must be struck between them. And here is where some potential virtues of hegemony need to be recognized. The new North/West transnational ideological near-hegemony on democracy and free markets is surely an asset in constructing many of the necessary conditions of a security community. At the same time, that very ideology (similar to that of a security community) of pluralism and participation militates against the exercise of coercive hegemony.

Moreover, the UN lacks the constitutional machinery to enforce many decisions on its member states. There really is no "hegemonic" state with the will as well as the capacity by itself to impose order on the international system. (The United States *might* in theory be said to have the capacity, but its government certainly does not have the will to do so in most instances.) For many purposes the most that can be expected is for a "core" of powerful states, predominantly but not necessarily only rich ones, to reach agreement and act in some degree as a collective hegemon.

The idea of security community comes to mind less readily for situations of hegemonic imbalance than does that of domination. To be tolerated in any hegemonic role hegemons will have to be "nice" ones who provide collective goods as well as coerce recalcitrants. The Deutsch *et al.* praise for "strong core areas" needs to be seen in this light, and as cores of identity as well as strength. Moreover, hegemonic groups will have to respect shared norms of the global system when they do act coercively, and be seen as holding themselves to the same norms they enforce. If authoritative rules are to be issued, subordinate states will have to be able to recognize dominant ones as having some right to issue them, derived from shared norms. Some echoes of Gramscian hegemony may be audible (Russett 1985; Snidal 1985; Reisman 1993; Brilmayer 1994).

At heart, global community building is in large part a rationalist enterprise familiar to liberal institutionalists. Yet it is also in part a constructivist enterprise of identity formation, one that has substantial accomplishments among the rich and democratic states of the "West," and discernible if much weaker achievements more globally. It is difficult to see just how all these eventualities will develop, but impossible to imagine a global security community without them. And I mean constructivist very precisely as explicating the Kantian liberal internationalist principles that underlie the concept of security communities. Consistent with those principles, they will have to be grasped and put into practice not just by policy-making elites, but by their peoples. This statement cannot deny the necessity of analyzing the empirical world as dispassionately and objectively as a social scientist ever can. But neither is it ever to deny the possibility of shaping as well as describing reality, and that the description helps the shaping.[28] This latter is not wishful thinking. The kind of world envisaged here is hardly perfect, by any standards of justice or order. Nevertheless it may, considering the alternatives, be the "best" of possible worlds even a pessimist can presently imagine. In some degree, however limited, we continually create the world we desire, and deserve the world we get.

Notes

1 I thank the Carnegie Corporation of New York, the Center for Global Partnership of the Japan Foundation, the Ford Foundation, the World Society Foundation of Switzerland, and the National Science Foundation for support of various pieces of research that have fed into this overview, and Emanuel Adler, Michael Barnett, Stephen Brooks, and Alexander Wendt for comments.

2 Of ninety-six armed conflicts during the six years 1989–1994, only five were between two internationally recognized states (Wallensteen and Sollenberg 1995).

3 For a relatively early but cautiously favorable assessment of the UN as a step toward a global security community essentially as defined in this volume, see Van Wagenen (1965). The definition of security community, subsequently adapted by Deutsch, derives from Van Wagenen (1952). Two major reports on UN reform are in many ways implicitly Kantian as I use the term below. See Commission on Global Governance (1995), and Independent Working Group (1995); also Russett (1997a).

4 By Kenneth Waltz's definition, polarity is determined by the strength of the most powerful state at each pole, not by that of the alliance it leads. See Waltz (1979: 97–99).

5 A detailed historical analysis of political developments in the Soviet Union is not appropriate here. But the two most-widely used comparative codings judged that substantial movement in the direction of democracy in the Soviet Union took place between 1986 and 1991. Polity III scorings (scale of 0 to 10) assign the USSR a 0 on the institutionalized democracy index in 1986, a 1 in 1989, and an 8 in 1991; on the institutionalized autocracy index a rating of 7 in 1986, 5 in 1989, and 0 in 1991. On the Freedom House indicators the USSR received the least democratic scores (7) on the scales for political rights and civil liberties in 1986, dropped to 6 and 5 respectively for 1988, and to 3 on both scales for 1991. Gastil (1989); McColm (1992); Jaggers and Gurr (1995). Arguably Russia became less democratic after 1992.

6 Archibugi (1995b) rightly points out that this is not a fully accurate rendition of Kant, chiefly in that Kant thought of peaceful democracies primarily as a monadic phenomenon (peaceful in general) rather than a dyadic one (peaceful with one another). The distinction matters as an item of intellectual history, but it nonetheless seems appropriate to credit Kant for most of the basic insights, recognizing that more than 200 years of experience and scholarship modify them somewhat. Hence I use the term "neo-Kantian." The important consideration is whether the theoretical and empirical evidence for this vision, however one labels it, is sound. The question of whether democracies are relatively more peaceful in general is contested. The most persuasive evidence so far

indicates that whereas democracies do not behave more pacifically when they are in crises with nondemocratic states, they are less likely to get into such crises in the first place; see Rousseau *et al.* (1996).

7 For use of this term, see Independent Working Group on the Future of the United Nations (1995); Commission on Global Governance (1995).

8 Zacher (1992); Barnett (1995a). Steven Krasner, however, in an important article, shows that the principles of sovereignty as expressed in the Treaty of Westphalia in 1648 have regularly been violated, by conventions and contracts as well as by coercion and imposition, ever since then. It is also worth noting that Krasner, often considered an arch-realist, makes a critical modification to realist understanding: "At the international level, different rulers can champion different principles not only because their interests vary, but because their normative frames of reference, primarily derived from their domestic experiences, also vary." See Krasner (1995/96: 148).

9 See also Mansfield and Snyder (1996), who, referring to their earlier article in that journal, declare (196) they do not contest the consensus that mature stable democracies rarely fight each other. Several critiques are addressed by Maoz (1997); also see the exchange initiated by Thompson and Tucker (1997a,b). Good micro-level evidence is in Risse-Kappen (1995).

10 MacMillan (1995) notes both the necessity to consider peace as a condition for democracy and the need to embed a democratic peace perspective in the wider Kantian emphasis on international law.

11 For early micro-level evidence, see Russett (1963). A good review of liberal hypotheses linking interdependence to peace is Stein (1989). Because of the possibility, cogently presented by Mercer (1995), that a sense of mutual identity may well entail characterizing others as "outgroup," it is essential to recognize links of mutual self-interest that do not depend on shared social identity.

12 The importance of interdependence is illustrated in the *dependencia* literature, and dates back to Hirschmann (1945). Also note that rich countries are unlikely to fight each other. As a realist would probably recognize, the costs of fighting another rich country with a modern, highly destructive military capability now outweigh any possible economic gain in an era when national wealth depends far more on physical capital (skill, technological capacity, organization) than on land or natural resources. See Mueller (1988b) and Kaysen (1990).

13 For evidence that democracies are able to enter into longer-term commitments with each other, see Gaubatz (1996). Other versions of the link from democracy and free trade to peace include Putnam (1988); Verdier (1994); Weede (1995).

14 See Bliss and Russett (1998), for strong evidence of this, with a database and method similar to that of Kim (1988) and Oneal and Russett (1997).

15 See especially Arat (1991); Przeworski and Limongi (1993); Alesina and Perotti (1994); Burkhart and Lewis-Beck (1994); Helliwell (1994); Muller (1995) and the subsequent exchange (Muller 1995: 983–996) among Kenneth Bollen, Robert Jackman, and Muller.

16 Note that all the neo-Kantian influences (democracy, interdependence, international organization) operate independently of such realist influences on conflict behavior as relative power, wealth, and alliance patterns. In relations among states where the neo-Kantian influences are weak, the realist ones remain very important.

17 The process, however, may not result in more durable settlements by democracies; see Raymond (1996).

18 Wendt (1999: ch. 8) argues that the creation of transnational capitalist institutions in the late twentieth century creates conditions of a rule of law regime making interdependence a force for peace that did not exist in earlier periods. Also see Murphy (1994) and Ruggie (1996: chs. 5–6). Barbieri (1996) reports that in the 1870–1939 period economic interdependence was positively associated with conflict. The different results seem rooted in differences in the studies' spatial rather than temporal domains. Her analysis includes many very distant pairs of states, while Oneal and Russett limit analysis to major powers and contiguous pairs, where the great majority (75 percent or more) of disputes arise.

Without an explicit control for contiguity or distance, trade produces a spurious association between interdependence and conflict: nearby states trade more, and nearby states have a high incidence of disputes because of both opportunities to fight and issues to fight about. See Oneal and Russett (1997: 272).

19 The spatial and functional scope of these efforts is evident in Boutros-Ghali (1996).

20 For a view of this as the latest manifestation of international organizations' promotion of Western cultural prescriptions for citizenship and state building, see Thomas et al. (1987); McNeely (1995).

21 Also see the basically rationalist argument of Moravcsik (1993).

22 On the Concert of Europe, see Schroeder (1994); Ikenberry (1996) contends that the liberal founders of the UN system overtly held a concept of peace deriving from democracy, interdependence, and international organization, and that whereas this concept could not be applied to the whole world before the end of the cold war, it did substantially govern relations within the Western alliance. Weart (1998) asserts that only republics form stable leagues which help to maintain peace among themselves.

23 Deudney (1995) contends that geographically or transactionally close states need to modify their anarchy, and that republican states need to modify that anarchy on republican rather than hierarchical principles.

24 Thus Held (1995: 273) recognizes that such an assembly would have to be limited to representsatives from democratic states.

25 See, for example, Weiss and Gordenkers (1996); Willets (1996).

26 See Barnett (1995b).

27 See the effort by Archibugi (1995a) to begin sorting out some of these difficulties.

28 In commenting (Layne 1995) on my reply to his article, Christopher Layne seized on one sentence to claim I was practicing post-modernism. I found that hilarious. But some elements of constructivism I accept. See also Waever (1998), referring to the phenomenon that if states act as if there is a community, there will be one. And recall the experiments by Axelrod (1984: ch. 2), in which all the social scientists played more competitively than would have served their best interests.

9

DEMOCRATIC INTERGOVERNMENTAL ORGANIZATIONS PROMOTE PEACE[1]

Jon Pevehouse and Bruce Russett

In this chapter we take steps toward solving an empirical puzzle in the liberal institutional research program by developing a theory of interactions among democracy, international organizations, and peace. The puzzle is this: the research program has produced generally robust results on the role of democracy in reducing the risk of international violence.[2] The linkage of international trade to conflict reduction is fairly robust though still subject to more contestation.[3] But the third linkage, of international organizations to peace, has proved less robust and more problematic. A causal role of joint membership in international governmental organizations (IGOs) to violence reduction can appear strong, weak, or even negative depending on the database and statistical method.[4] In this article we propose that the puzzle stems less from methodological issues than from the need for a revised theoretical perspective emphasizing the pacific benefits of certain kinds of international organizations. We offer three theoretical processes through which IGOs populated largely by democratic states are likely to encourage peace, independently of the state-level effects of democracy. We conduct several analyses to test this new perspective.

Other interpretations

First, however, we review three theoretical reasons that might account for conflicting empirical results to date, and to which we shall return in our theoretical perspective and analyses:

1. Liberal theory is simply wrong, and the realists are right—international organizations are mere reflections of relative state power, ineffectual and at best operating only at the margins. Any effective restraint on the use of force in an anarchic world requires coercion or deterrence, and international

organizations must depend on decisions by their member states, not on the organization per se, to provide the capability and will to coerce and deter (Mearsheimer 1994/95). This position dismisses all the noncoercive functions that institutions can provide to reduce conflict among their members (for example, mediation, reducing uncertainty by conveying information, changing interests, norms, and mutual identification). Nevertheless, it makes a powerful argument and defines a null hypothesis that cannot be dismissed without persuasive theory and robust evidence.

2. Any peace-inducing effects of IGOs are obscured by the possibility that they may reflect existing conflicts or even stimulate new ones among their members. Kinsella and Russett propose this interpretation when they find joint IGO membership to be positively related to conflict. They suggest that not only are many (nonglobal) international organizations formed among states that are already salient for one another because of existing diplomatic and commercial ties, but that IGOs are likely to make those ties more salient and hence increase the likelihood that disputes will arise. Only at high frequencies of shared IGO membership, in the context of well-developed institutional capacity, would a net conflict-reducing effect emerge (Kinsella and Russett 2002).

    Relatedly, Boehmer, Gartzke, and Nordstrom maintain that not all IGOs should be expected to reduce conflict, and that only well-institutionalized organizations may have the mediating capacity to reduce conflicts among their members (Boehmer *et al.* 2004).[5] They report that over the 1950–1991 period, IGOs with greater institutional structure, especially those with a security mandate and tighter cohesion of preferences, do experience fewer violent conflicts. We agree that the idea of distinguishing among different kinds of IGOs is potentially valuable.

3. Only certain types of IGOs, defined by function and by the global-regional distinction, may have significant conflict-reducing effects. For example, global organizations with nearly universal membership may have no discernible effect, but others which, though global, have more restricted membership (for example, the General Agreement on Tariffs and Trade [GATT], World Trade Organization [WTO], World Bank, and International Monetary Fund) may exclude states already in highly conflictual relationships with one or more of their members, and so may more effectively inhibit violent conflict among those who are members.

Furthermore, both global and regional IGOs may be distinguished as those addressed primarily to military, political, economic, or social functions. Leskiw (2002), for example, looks at participation in international rivalries and their severity levels. He finds that engagement in rivalries is lower among states sharing many regional rather than universal IGO memberships, while regional organizations with predominantly political or social functions are associated with fewer rivalries— military or economic organizations have little effect. But these results run contrary to other research indicating a pacifying effect of a particular kind of economic organization—the Preferential Trade Agreement (PTA). Mansfield and Pevehouse (2003, 2006) show that PTAs provide institutional settings for dispute settlement and conflict resolution, allowing states to resolve their differences peacefully. These institutions are especially valuable when they support a dense network of commercial connections, as pairs of states that trade heavily and join PTAs are far less likely to experience militarized conflict.

Theory: densely democratic IGOs

The efforts to identify a consistent effective role for joint IGO memberships, whether by measuring overall network density (number of shared IGOs) or by distinguishing among capabilities or functions, have met with only moderate success. Here we develop a theoretical position that looks more closely at particular kinds of IGOs: those identified not as regional or global or by function, but by the kinds of states that compose them. Specifically, we analyze IGOs by the political systems of their members, focusing on densely democratic IGOs. That is, we hypothesize a kind of interaction between IGOs and democracy, and that IGOs comprised mostly of democratic states will be more effective in reducing the risks of militarized inter-state conflict among their members than will other kinds of IGOs. Dyads in these densely democratic IGOs will also have a lower risk of violence compared to dyads that share few or no joint IGO memberships. This proposition better reflects Kant's basic insight about the conditions of peace, which applied not to all states and organizations, nor to a centralized amalgamation, but to a voluntary "pacific federation" [confederation] of republics. "[W]herever in the world there is a threat of war breaking out, they will try to prevent it by mediation . . ." (Kant [1795] 1970: 104, 114).[6]

Several mechanisms have been hypothesized in linking IGOs to peace, but here we focus on three that are likely to be more influential when most of the member states of the organization are democracies. Nearly all IGOs contain some autocratic or only marginally democratic states. Therefore it is important to ask whether these violence-reducing influences apply only to the democratic members, or to both democratic and nondemocratic member states. Recall that while violent conflicts short of war between democratic states are unusual, they are not rare enough to be ignored. For example, Oneal and Russett report that when both states in a dyad are at the 90th percentile on the democracy scale, they are 43 percent less likely to have a fatal militarized interstate dispute (MID) than are two states at the median on the democracy scale (Oneal and Russett 2006). Thus joint democracy alone, independent of other influences, reduces violent conflict by less than half. So densely democratic IGOs have a potentially major role in reducing residual violence between their democratic members, as well as between their less-democratic members. We therefore begin with a prior belief that, together if not individually, democracy and IGOs can have important pacific effects.

Credible commitments

If it is true that a major reason for state conflict is the inability to make binding commitments to fulfill bargains (see Fearon 1995 and Gartzke *et al*. 2001), then IGOs can help alleviate this credibility gap. Members of IGOs who could potentially come into conflict have a ready mechanism to engender credible commitments. Because they can turn to a mutual institution to help monitor commitments, they will be more likely to overcome the commitment problem and refrain from fighting. IGOs may provide institutional mechanisms to monitor members' commitments, substituting for or supplementing member states' capabilities, and helping to ensure that the commitments will be reinforced at the institutional level. Indeed, states will often turn to external agents when creating credible commitments is difficult. Governmental leaders—especially democratic ones—face potential audience costs for not following through on their international obligations or for reneging on these commitments; this increases the likelihood of fulfilling these promises (see Fearon 1994; Leeds 1999; and McGillivray and Smith 2000, 2004). Of course, it is important that the commitment of the IGO to monitor and enforce agreements is credible. Thus, IGOs populated by democratic governments, which are more likely to uphold their commitments, enhance confidence that the institution's commitment is credible as well.

While this argument suggests why IGOs populated by democracies might have commitment advantages, what about democratic states within democratic IGOs? What is the value added in terms of credible commitment in these cases? While it is true that democracies may make more credible commitments than autocracies, ceteris paribus, IGOs may still help democratic states confront what could be labeled the "turnover problem." Because officials in democratically elected governments change, there is a possibility that a new government could undo the commitments of the previous government. In particular, they would not necessarily face the same level of audience costs because they did not enter the commitment in the first place.

Many agreements, including those between democracies, provide mechanisms of commitment. For example, trade agreements are particularly effective in serving as a promise for democracies not to renege on their commitment to liberalize trade (Mansfield *et al*. 2002; also see Goldstein 1998: 143–144 and Milner 1998: 24). A similar argument has been applied to monetary integration as well (Martin and Simmons 1998: 748). Thus, future administrations will be bound to these international commitments, especially compared to a situation where the policy change was only domestically legislated. Because even pairs of democracies face uncertainty about the nature and behavior of future administrations, IGOs can serve as an important commitment device.[7]

A related but distinct "turnover problem" is confronted by new democracies attempting to make credible commitments. Often, new regimes have difficulties making reliable commitments because others fear the potential collapse of the new government. Here again, densely democratic IGOs can assist in preventing autocratic backsliding, making these democratizers' commitment to democracy (and the agreements they sign) more ironclad. For example, densely democratic IGOs can and do make entry or continuation in the IGO conditional on being democratic and have been shown to further the consolidation of nascent democracies (Pevehouse 2005).

In particular, highly democratic regional IGOs often punish members who appear to backslide into autocracy. The European Union (EU) from its foundation had a commitment to democracy, bundling national democratic institutions and European institutions in a mutually supporting manner to solidify peace.[8] It has never had a nondemocratic member. It suspended the Greek association agreement in 1967 after a coup. It has put Turkey under heavy pressure to strengthen its commitment to democracy, and especially to tighten civil control of the military as a condition of entry. Other European institutions are also important in this regard — previously, the Council of Europe suspended Turkey's involvement in that organization after the September 1980 coup.[9]

The Organization of American States (OAS) also has the power to levy severe economic and political sanctions (such as suspension of membership, approval of military intervention by member states) after a seizure of power.[10] Its June 1991 Santiago Commitment to "defense and promotion of representative democracy and human rights . . . and respect for the principles of self-determination and non-intervention" makes it an important signaler of legitimacy for new governments. The major subregional organization in Latin America—MERCOSUR, consisting of Argentina, Brazil, Uruguay, and Paraguay — also requires its members to be democratic.[11]

Thus, even for states that are already democratic and may have an easier time overcoming the commitment problem, IGOs may enhance credible commitments by addressing the turnover problem. They may also enhance the credibility of commitments for new democracies by assisting in their consolidation. For all types of states, IGOs can be important external anchors for solving commitment problems, which can be key to preventing conflict.

Dispute settlement

Many IGOs have standing dispute settlement and mediation mechanisms to prevent political or economic differences from spiraling into military conflicts. As noted above, Kant expected that his republics would be more likely to use mediation to resolve their conflicts. Indeed, the success of his federation depended on states being accustomed to the rule of law at home, and an extension of that behavior to settling disputes with similarly lawful states.

Democracies tend to promote institutions of conflict resolution in international relations. In particular, they are more likely to employ third-party conflict management techniques such as adjudication and arbitration. In their study of legalization and dispute settlement mechanisms, for example, Keohane, Moravscik, and Slaughter contend that liberal democracies are more likely than nondemocracies to submit to transnational dispute resolution mechanisms (independent judicial bodies), rather than interstate dispute resolution mechanisms such as bilateral talks (Keohane *et al.* 2000: 478–479). Mitchell also notes that through the twentieth century, democracies have increasingly championed third-party dispute mechanisms in their regional organizations (Mitchell 2002: 753).

Indeed, the general rise in legalism in world politics finds an impetus in the increase in democratization. Kahler contends that democracy gives power to pro-legalization interests who either prefer legal frameworks for normative-legal reasoning (for example, human rights organizations) or for contractual-economic reasons (for example, business organizations): "[A]mong the industrialized democracies, law occupies a central institutional place, and these pro-legalization normative lobbies are powerful" (Kahler 2000: 671).[12] Thus, democracies are more likely to take a legalistic approach to relations with one another that can help to empower IGOs.

These dispute settlement mechanisms within IGOs populated by democracies are also more likely to succeed in ending threats of violence. Successful mediation involves promoting the exchange of concessions, encouraging the use of contracts, and reducing the cost of enforcing them (Stone Sweet and Brunell 1998). This may include commitments to enact or cement redistribution within member states (Martin and Simmons 1998). Institutions such as the European Court of Justice incorporate a degree of voluntarism in the participation of their democratic member states and do not depend on enforcement by the threat of military force. IGOs frequently mediate disputes where the capability of enforcing settlements is explicitly absent (see Miall 1992; Bercovitch and Langley 1993; Haas 1993; and Abbott and Snidal 1998). The dispute settlement capacity of regional trade agreements has been key to solving or reducing conflicts among member states, and more densely democratic regional economic organizations are far more likely to design institutions with more legalized dispute settlement frameworks (see Mansfield *et al.* 1999; Bearce 2003; and Pevehouse and Buhr 2005).

IGOs populated predominantly by democracies are thus more likely to engender respect for the institutional mechanisms to reduce and eliminate conflict, and to provide more legalistic mechanisms as part of their institutional package. This is certainly a strong reason to expect densely democratic IGOs to settle disputes among members. In fact, democratic IGOs may require their members to resolve acrimonious border disputes with their neighbors (for example, the EU's requirements for Eastern European membership candidates), thus reducing a common cause of international conflict (Bunce 1997). Manlio Brosio, as Secretary-General of NATO in 1967, helped mediate the dispute between Greece and Turkey over Cyprus, averting a widening of the war.

But again, what value added are IGOs to democracies that would already be likely to engage in conflict resolution? For two reasons, we still expect strong dispute settlement advantages for IGOs even among democratic states. First, several scholars argue that transitional regimes of liberalizing states often can and do make overt attempts to spur nationalist sentiment regarding ethnic identity.[13] If so, IGOs may play an important role in minimizing conflict between these liberalizing states or between a liberalizer and stable democracies.

For instance, in the aftermath of the 1989 revolutions in Eastern Europe, some observers feared that nationalism would be a rallying point for leaders in the region's democratizing states. One such concern was Hungarian nationalism and the fate of Magyars living in neighboring states. In the first years after the break from the Soviet orbit occurred in Hungary, the transitional Joszef Antall regime could easily have tried to legitimate itself by arousing nationalist sentiment in Hungary over the Magyar issue. In fact, Antall himself made an early statement that he desired to be the "Prime Minister of 15 million Hungarians." (There are only 10 million Hungarians in Hungary.) That statement was taken by Hungary's neighbors as "a revival of traditional Hungarian revisionist nationalism" (Kozhemiakin 1998).[14]

As Kozhemiakin argues, however, Hungarian political elites have not tried to base their legitimacy and popularity on nationalist issues. Rather, "when other sources of political legitimacy are not too difficult to find, nationalist sentiments in Hungary can be contained." IGO memberships, such as the Council of Europe or the Association Agreements with the European Union, served as a substitute for appeals to nationalism. Kozhemiakin continues, "Hungarians value their internationally recognized democratic status too much to allow their unqualified desire to protect Magyar minorities to hurt it and, by implication, impede Hungary's efforts to integrate itself fully into the West" (Kozhemiakin 1998: 82–83).

Indeed, when pressed by the EU, the North Atlantic Treaty Organization (NATO), and the Organization for Security and Cooperation in Europe (OSCE), Hungary signed friendship treaties with both Romania and Slovakia, spurring one commentator to note, "With both treaties in force, potentially explosive tensions in the heart of Europe will have been calmed."[15] Although this is just one case, it is nonetheless instructive. Especially when they are democratically dense and able to provide a "democratic seal of approval" for transitional governments, IGOs may lessen efforts by leaders to resort to nationalism and the risk of conflict with other liberalizing or newly democratic states.

Second, as we previously emphasized, democracies do have disputes—conflicts still arise between democracies, even if they do not escalate into war. Indeed, we contend that one explanation for nonescalation is the network of IGOs in general, and densely democratic IGOs specifically. Dispute settlement mechanisms within IGOs are important even for pairs of democracies. Recent history provides a case where such a situation arose.

In 1986, Colombia and Honduras signed a maritime treaty effectively excluding Nicaragua from access to a large portion of the Atlantic Ocean. Although Nicaragua protested at the time, its relations remained cordial because Honduras never ratified the treaty. Then on November 30, 1999, the Honduran legislature ratified the treaty, bringing an immediate response of trade tariffs from Nicaragua. Days later, Honduran troops opened fire across the border, while Nicaragua mobilized its forces near the border.[16] After these violent acts, both parties asked the OAS to mediate the dispute. By December 30, 1999, an agreement was signed in Miami to reduce tensions, but in February 2000, Nicaraguan and Honduran boats exchanged fire in a dispute over the possession of an uninhabited island. Again the OAS stepped up mediation efforts and began the process of monitoring and verification of the agreements, which were still in place as of 2005.

Several facets of this case are important for our argument. First, at the time of the dispute, both Honduras and Nicaragua were democracies. Second, the OAS was populated almost entirely by democracies. Third, Honduras and Nicaragua initially took their dispute to the International Court of Justice (ICJ) but eventually decided the OAS was their preferred forum due to the long decision time scheduled by the ICJ. Thus, despite all the factors that should have kept two democracies out of a bilateral militarized dispute, it took the dispute settlement mechanisms of a highly democratic IGO to de-escalate the violence once it began.

Socialization

In addition to an institutional commitment to mediation and law, IGOs may socialize member states to particular types of behavior (see Strang and Chang 1993; and Finnemore 1996). By influencing what states define as acceptable behavior, IGOs may redefine what are appropriate ways to deal with potential interstate conflicts. Socialization and norm change have long been central to perspectives on international integration, notably in Deutsch's interest in the creation of a pluralistic security community (Deutsch et al. 1957), whereby the citizens and governments of sovereign states developed a sense of mutual identity based on shared values such as democracy and a market economy that made war, and the preparation for war, obsolete among those states. Trust, driven by learning and facilitated by mutual identity, meant understanding "not just about each others' purposes and intentions but also of each others' interpretations of society, politics, economics, and culture . . ." In such a community, understanding and trust bring a condition wherein, "Decision-making procedures, conflict resolution, and processes of conflict adjudication are likely to be more consensual than in other types of interstate relations" (Adler and Barnett 1998: 54–55; also see Ruggie 1992).

But Deutsch was not much interested in institutions. They do not appear among his fourteen essential or helpful conditions for pluralistic security communities save under the larger heading of a wide range of mutual transactions, "together with the institutions to carry them out." There his discussion of institutions is limited to a page and a half with a few proper nouns, some counts, and no mention of processes (Deutsch et al. 1957: 146–147). Much the same could be said of Wendt's bow to Deutschian integration theory's discussion of creating collective identity (Wendt 1994).

Adler and Barnett—among the most important revivers of Deutschian ideas in the last decade—do, however, regard institutions as important. The more expectations of nonviolent conflict resolution "are institutionalized in both domestic and supranational settings, the more war in the region becomes improbable. . . . The institutional context for the exercise of power changes; the right to use force shifts from the units to the collectivity of sovereign states and becomes legitimate only against external threats or against community members that defect from the core norms of the community" (Adler and Barnett 1998: 55–56).[17] Since democracy appears to be a fundamental norm for a security community, and some transnational institutionalization is also necessary, it is not a stretch to believe that an interaction between the two is likely in those IGOs populated largely by democratic states.

In his study of the OSCE, Adler notes that though it is neither fully a security community nor fully democratic, it has been successful in spreading norms and trust-building practices. MERCOSUR was formed in large part to provide means for new democratically elected presidents to control their militaries. Through shared economic institutions they were able to open up each other's markets and reduce the size of their military establishments under conditions of peaceful international relations. New security-producing practices grew out of a shared Latin American identity and common democratic practices (Adler 1998; also see Hurrell 1998; and Kacowicz 1998). Finnemore and Sikkink discuss how IGOs may perform as norm entrepreneurs through phases of imitation, socialization, and internalization; densely democratic IGOs may make it possible to pass the "tipping point" to a security community earlier than would otherwise be possible. They may create new identities, and norms, unintentionally as well as deliberately (Finnemore and Sikkink 1998; also see March and Olsen 1998).

Indeed, Mitchell shows empirically how through a process of socialization by IGOs, nondemocracies become socialized to practice peaceful dispute settlement, especially regarding territorial claims (Mitchell 2002). While Mitchell concentrates on the number of democracies in the international system, causal mechanisms of norm emergence and norm acceptance give no reason to expect this process not to work at the level of IGOs, especially regional IGOs. Negotiations with NATO for admission seem to have been important in persuading Romanian officials to adopt norms of transparency and accountability in matters of defense and security, and a sense of their wider identity with NATO (Gheciu 2005; also see Zurn and Checkel 2005). Indeed, within systems of organizations, liberal democracies can represent an "Axelrod-like core of cooperators" who increase the likelihood of cooperation (Starr and Lindborg 2003).

Thus, we argue that one is more likely to find peaceful norms evolving through a process of identity transformation in IGOs that are more homogenously democratic. Risse-Kappen makes such an argument with regard to collective identity and the emergence of cooperation: "Democratic features of liberal democracies enable the community in the first place. But the institutionalization of the community exerts independent effects on the interactions. In the final analysis, then, democratic domestic structures and international institutions do the explanatory work together" (Risse-Kappen 1995: 215; also Dembinski and Freistein 2005).

Taken together, these three groups of causal mechanisms cover a range of phenomena encompassing structural, institutional, and normative explanations, sometimes competing but often complementary (Fearon and Wendt 2002)[18] in ways reminiscent of similar interpretations of the democratic peace itself. We lack the fine-grained and micro-level information to distinguish between them in our quantitative analysis below. Nevertheless, they all suggest one common observable implication: IGOs composed largely of democracies should be marked by less violence among their members. We now turn to an empirical test of this proposition.

Analysis

To test these hypotheses we need to move beyond simple counts of joint dyadic memberships in IGOs. We thus create a measure of IGOs for how densely democratic they are, weighting each IGO by the mean level of democracy (Polity IV) among its members.[19] Based on this set of weights for each IGO, we create the variable Democratic IGOs,[20] which we introduce into the following base model of fatal MIDs:

$$
\begin{aligned}
\text{FATAL MID} = \; & \beta_0 + \beta_1 \text{Democratic IGOs} + \beta_2 \text{Democracy}_S + \\
& \beta_3 \text{Dependence}_S + \beta_4 \text{Contiguity} + \beta_5 \text{Distance} + \\
& \beta_6 \text{Major Power} + \beta_7 \text{Cumulative MIDs} + \beta_8 \text{IGOs} + \varepsilon
\end{aligned}
$$

Our sample is the period 1885–2000, a longer period with more observations than in most previous analyses. We examine all dyads for which data are available. The dependent variable in this analysis (fatal MID) is the onset of a MID between states i and j in which at least one fatality occurs in year $t+1$ (see Jones et al. 1996; and Ghosn and Palmer 2003). We use Maoz's adjustment of the MID data set that corrects for the absence of fighting between sides in multilateral disputes (Maoz 2002). We prefer to focus on MIDs where fatalities occur since these MIDs are of greatest concern to members of the international system. Moreover, focusing on these violent conflicts helps to avoid possible biases in the reporting of less severe military disputes from dyads under closer reportorial scrutiny (see Oneal et al. 2003: 376; and Fordham and Sarver 2001).[21]

The first variable, Democratic IGOs, is a count of a subset of all IGOs of which states i and j are members; namely the number of such IGOs whose average level of democracy is at or above 7 on the Polity IV scale (which runs from -10 to $+10$); see Marshall 2004. We choose 7 since this is the threshold used when labeling states democracies in the Polity data. As with the individual patterns of democracy and IGOs, the number of democratic IGOs in the international system has increased greatly. Figure 9.1 shows the number of dyad-years with at least one membership in an IGO whose average is at or above 7. As shown in the graph, the number of states involved in democratic IGOs grows immensely over time, especially late in the twentieth century.

Other variables tap Kantian processes that may correlate with both the onset of fatal MIDs and the nature of IGOs joined by states. Democracy$_S$ represents the Polity IV scores of each state, sorted by whichever state is the less democratic state in the pair, since more emphasis is placed on the less constrained actor. When

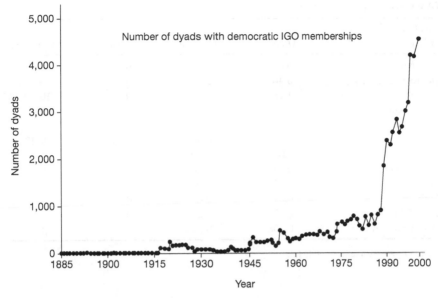

FIGURE 9.1 Trends in democratic IGO membership over time

testing our hypothesis it is essential to ensure that any effect of democratic IGOs is not simply a proxy for the peaceful effect of democracy alone. By including this variable we control for the general influence of states' democracy at the dyadic level, so that the estimate for Democratic IGOs taps only the effect of the degree to which members of the IGOs are democratic.

We capture the effects of economic interdependence by introducing Dependence$_s$. This measures each country's imports and exports with its partner, divided by each state's gross domestic product (GDP). The lower of these ratios identifies the dependence of the less constrained state.[22] To control for opportunities to use force against one another as well as the opportunity to join regional IGOs, we need variables for contiguity and distance. Contiguity is coded 1 if the pairs of states in the dyad share a land border or are separated by less than 150 miles of water. Distance is the natural logarithm of the great circle distance between state capitals.[23] We already know that democracy is clustered, probably causally, by region, and so is peace among democracies (Gleditsch 2003). Since many IGOs are regional in their membership, a failure to control for proximity might exaggerate the peace-inducing effects of democratic IGOs. It is also important to control for the presence of major powers, whose military capabilities can be effective even at great distance. Major Power is coded as 1 if either state i or j is called a major power by the Correlates of War (COW) project.

One other theory-driven variable for the analysis stems from the fact that a small minority of dyads account for the great majority of disputes in the global system (see Diehl 1998; and Maoz 2004). It is thus likely that past dispute behavior influences current dispute behavior (see Oneal *et al.* 2003; and Boehmer *et al.* 2004)

TABLE 9.1 Descriptive statistics

Standard variable	Mean	Deviation	Minimum	Maximum
Fatal MID	0.001	0.03	0	1
Democratic IGOs	0.46	2.38	0	46
Democracy$_S$	−4.18	5.93	−10	10
Dependence$_S$	0.001	0.004	0	0.26
Contiguity	0.04	0.20	0	1
Distance	8.20	0.80	1.61	9.42
Major Power	0.09	0.29	0	1
Cumulative MIDs	0.17	1.16	0	39
Joint IGOs	21.77	11.90	0	108
Allies	0.01	0.08	0	1
EU-EFTA	0.07	0.25	0	1
Democratic dyad	0.108	0.310	0	1

Note: For each variable, N = 454,380.

and also depresses the number of IGOs shared by disputatious dyads. Conversely, states may join IGOs (or democratic states join densely democratic IGOs) primarily with those states with whom they already have a predominantly peaceful relationship. We thus calculate a running sum of militarized disputes between peaceful relationships. We thus calculate a running sum of militarized disputes between states i and j for the entire period, and label this variable Cumulative MIDs.

To ensure that any relationship between our weighted IGO variables is not simply a reflection of pairs of states that are members of many IGOs, we use Joint IGOs, the number of IGOs of all varieties in which both members of the dyad share membership.

As is now customary, to control for the possibility of temporal dependence in the onset of fatal MIDs we create a counter of the years between each onset and use this measure as the base of a cubic spline function with two knots (Beck *et al.* 1998). We omit the estimates of these in the tables, but each term is statistically significant. Finally, ε is a stochastic error term. Table 9.1 shows the descriptive statistics of these variables.

Results: democratic IGOs matter

The first column of Table 9.2 shows the estimates of our base model with only the core variables. Our key variable, democratic IGOs, is negative and highly statistically significant. Thus, the more joint memberships in IGOs composed of democracies, the less likely it is that the states in a dyad will engage in fatal MIDs. It is important to note that this effect is independent of and in addition to the effect of democracy in the dyad. Consistent with past research and the weak-link hypothesis, Democracy$_S$ is also negative and statistically significant, suggesting that the higher the level of democracy for the less democratic state in the dyad, the less likely is a fatal dispute. Taken together, these findings provide strong support for a Kantian interpretation of interstate relations—democracy and international institutions building a more peaceful international system together.

This relationship between democratic IGOs and conflict is not only statistically significant, but substantively significant as well. As the number of joint democratic IGOs for the pair of states rises from the mean to a one standard deviation increase, the probability of a dispute drops by about 21 percent. Clearly, IGOs composed

TABLE 9.2 The effects of democracy, interdependence, and IGO membership on fatal militarized disputes, 1885–2000

Democratic variable	Base model	Dyads	Allies	Base model 1	EU–EFTA
Democratic IGOs	−0.079**	−0.072**	−0.079**	−0.073***	−0.073***
	(0.037)	(0.036)	(0.037)	(0.027)	(0.044)
Democracy$_S$	−0.063***	−0.052***	−0.063***	−0.058***	−0.063***
	(0.014)	(0.017)	(0.014)	(0.014)	(0.014)
Dependence$_S$	−52.011***	−52.110***	−51.915***	−51.705***	−51.670***
	(18.272)	(18.407)	(18.051)	(18.047)	(18.229)
Contiguity	1.635***	1.632***	1.638***	1.631***	1.635***
	(0.263)	(0.264)	(0.270)	(0.264)	(0.263)
Distance	−0.693***	−0.695***	−0.693***	−0.690***	−0.694***
	(0.104)	(0.104)	(0.104)	(0.104)	(0.104)
Major Power	1.348***	1.347***	1.348***	1.361***	1.350***
	(0.190)	(0.191)	(0.191)	(0.191)	(0.189)
Cumulative MIDs	0.118***	0.117***	0.117***	0.119***	0.117***
	(0.015)	(0.015)	(0.015)	(0.014)	(0.014)
Joint IGOs	−0.001	−0.002	−0.001	0.001	−0.001
	(0.007)	(0.007)	(0.007)	(0.007)	(0.007)
Democratic dyad	—	−0.393*	—	—	—
		(0.301)			
Allies	—	—	−0.011	—	—
			(0.183)		
EU–EFTA	—	—	—	—	−0.480
					(1.300)
Constant	−0.939	−0.846	−0.942	−0.961	−0.938
	(0.836)	(0.853)	(0.833)	(0.839)	(0.836)
Pseudo R^2	0.27	0.27	0.27	0.27	0.27
N	454,380	454,380	454,380	454,380	454,380

Notes: Parameters are estimated using logistic regression, after including a cubic spline function with two knots. Entries in parentheses are Huber standard errors clustered on the dyad. All significance tests are one-tailed: *** $p \leq 0.01$; ** $p \leq 0.05$; * $p \leq 0.1$.

Democratic IGOs includes IGOs with composite democracy scores at or above 6.

of predominantly democratic members lessen the probability of conflict. This is true while controlling for a host of factors that have traditionally explained interstate peace, several of which are correlated with membership in democratic IGOs.

The remaining variables have the expected signs. Higher levels of economic interdependence reduce the propensity of states to engage in violent interstate disputes. Contiguous dyads and dyads containing a major power are more likely to engage in fatal disputes, and dyads of states some distance from each other are less likely to do so. Each of these is consistent with previous work on the Kantian peace.[24]

Two other estimates are worthy of note. One is that Joint IGOs has no effect in any of these models; that is, when controlling for how democratic the members of the IGO are, the institutional density between the states does not matter. This suggests that the political character of its member states strongly affects what the institution is able and willing to do by way of reducing conflict among its members.

This should not, however, be read as implying that nondensely democratic IGOs make no contribution to preventing militarized disputes. Many such IGOs are quasi-universal organizations that include nearly all states and so cannot be densely democratic. With so few dyads outside these organizations, we cannot establish a reliable baseline level of conflict in the absence of any IGO membership. Also, we will show below that membership in all kinds of IGOs does contribute to preventing the escalation of lower-level MIDs to fatal ones.[25]

The other estimate of interest is that dyads with greater experience of violent conflict (Cumulative MIDs) show a much higher risk of a fatal MID. Conversely, the absence of previous violent conflict lowers the risk that a fatal MID will occur. Yet that independent effect of prior history supplements but does not erase the independent effect of democracy or the independent effect of densely democratic IGOs in reducing conflict. Jointly democratic IGOs reduce conflict not merely because they may have a prior history of peace.

In sum, these initial results suggest that IGOs do play an important role in mediating conflict between member states, but this effect emerges systematically only in IGOs composed largely of democracies. If it were only democracy and not the institutions leading to peace, only the state-level measure of democracy would be statistically significant. So democratic IGOs serve as instruments to enhance the effects of democracy.

Table 9.3 compares the marginal effects for variations in several variables in the model. Note that while the effect of democratic IGOs is quite strong, other Kantian variables are just as influential. Indeed, raising democratic IGO, democracy, and dependence by one standard deviation simultaneously yields a 57 percent decline in the probability of a fatal MID. Non-Kantian variables are important too, such as a history of conflict between states. Raising the number of past MIDs within the dyad by one standard deviation from the mean yields a 14 percent increase in the probability of a fatal dispute. Still, higher levels of democratic IGO membership, trade, and democracy can account for a significant reduction in serious violence between states.

TABLE 9.3 Changes in predicted probabilities of a fatal militarized dispute

	Percent
Percentage change in dispute risk from one standard deviation increase above mean for:	
— Democratic IGOs	−21
— Democracy	−36
— Dependence	−20
— Democratic IGOs, democracy, and dependence	−57
— Cumulative MIDs	+14
— Distance	−43

Notes: Predicted probabilities are computed based on column 1 of Table 9.2. All continuous variables are initially set at mean values, Contiguity is set at 1, and Major Power is set at 0.

Robustness checks

We want to ensure that our finding is neither the result of model underspecification nor a statistical artifact. To this end, we conduct several robustness checks. First, some might object to our attempt to hold democracy constant in the previous model since we directly control for the regime type of only the less democratic in the dyad. That is, despite our theory suggesting the contrary, it could be that for pairs of democracies, IGOs provide little value added when it comes to peace. To control for this possibility, we reestimate our model including an indicator variable coded as a 1 if both states in the dyad are democracies. Again, if democracy is leading to peace and there is little value added to the process by IGOs, we expect this new variable to reduce any conflict-mediating effect of democratic IGOs. But as seen in the second column of Table 9.2, this is not the case. While this new variable is negative and statistically significant, democratic IGOs is still statistically significant.

In addition, limiting our estimation sample to only dyads in which both states are autocracies yields similar results—the estimate of democratic IGOs is negative and statistically significant. These findings strongly suggest that democratically dense institutions help all states keep peaceful relations. Our finding is not simply an outgrowth of democracy itself, but that international institutions of democracies do matter for peace.[26] Second, it is important to include other realist-oriented factors that may influence the relationship of IGO membership to MIDs. Alliances are especially crucial in this regard because they form a small but important subset of IGOs for which some have hypothesized that similar political systems and similar security concerns may suppress intra-organizational conflict in alliances more than in nonsecurity IGOs (for example, Farber and Gowa 1997). Though little by way of consistent results for the influence of alliances has been found in other studies (for example, see Bennett and Stam 2004: ch. 5; and Leeds 2003), in this instance it remains necessary to identify any particular effect security-oriented IGOs may have above that of all types of IGOs.

We regard similarity of preferences, including alliance when conceived as a preference measure, to be a mediating variable rather than a direct influence on conflict, and thus not appropriate in a parsimonious model (see Achen 2005; and Ray 2005). We do, however, add it as a robustness check on our findings. To this end, we add a measure of alliances (Allies) (Gibler and Sarkees 2003) to the initial model. The estimates for this model are in the third column of Table 9.2. There it is clear that alliances (security-oriented IGOs) neither reduce nor increase the risk of violent conflict between their members, and this finding is largely consistent with most previous research. Moreover, including this variable does not alter the estimate of the effect of democratic IGOs on conflict.[27]

We also want to ensure that our findings are not the result of measurement decisions. Thus, in the fourth column of Table 9.2, we reestimate our initial model but relax our definition of democratic IGOs. While our previous threshold was 7 to be counted as a democratic IGO, we move this threshold to 6 to ensure our definition alone is not responsible for our findings. The result is entirely consistent with our earlier estimates.[28] Our key theoretical variable is negative and highly statistically significant at both the 6 and 5 thresholds for defining a Democratic IGO.

One concern when discussing the influence of IGOs is that the results may really depend on the impact of just one or two large and democratic IGOs, notably the European Union and the European Free Trade Area (EFTA). The final column of Table 9.2 introduces a dummy variable for IGOs composed of European dyads in either the EU or EFTA. Since all those states are also democracies, and in the region with the greatest number of democracies, we need to ensure that the apparent effect of densely democratic IGOs is not merely a European phenomenon. It is not. The EU-EFTA variable has no effect, while the strong effect of Democratic IGOs is unchanged.[29]

Next, because fatal MIDs are rare events, to avoid bias in our statistical models we utilize King and Zeng's rare events logit (King and Zeng 2001), reestimating the models of Table 9.2. The results are consistent and change very little from the initial estimates, giving us confidence that there is little bias in our existing estimates.[30] In each model, Democratic IGOs remains negative and statistically significant.

We are also wary of the possibility that our findings are time-bound. We want to ensure that our findings are not an artifact of the recent post-cold war rise in democratic states and organizations during a time of relative peace. Moreover, Kant himself hypothesized that the effect of federations of republics would not be constant over time, but increase in a process that suggested positive feedback. To this end, we estimate our initial model on three subsamples of our time period: 1885–1945; 1945–2000; and 1945–1989. Interestingly, although we do not find strong support for Kant's supposition, it is because the influence of Democratic IGOs appears strong in each of these subsamples.

Indeed, in the 1885–1945 subsample, there are no fatal disputes between states with at least one membership in a democratic organization.[31] For the other subsamples, Democratic IGOs remains negative and statistically significant. This is particularly important for the 1945–1989 sample since excluding the post-cold war period has little influence on our findings. Again, while we cannot confirm Kant's expectation that the pacifying effects of confederations of republics would grow stronger over time, we can be confident that the influence of IGOs is consistent over time and not an artifact of one particular time period.

Finally, and perhaps most importantly, we examine a possibility raised earlier: that democratic IGOs are really endogenous to conflict. One competing explanation of our findings, for example, would be that states that are on good terms and/or unlikely to fight (especially because they are democracies) are members of democratic IGOs. To guard against this possibility, we led the dependent variable in each model. In addition, we conduct an additional test for reverse causality. We estimate a negative binomial count model, where democratic IGOs (in year $t+1$) is the dependent variable, and fatal MID becomes an independent variable along with the remaining control variables from the base model.[32] These results yield no evidence that fatal MIDs reduce membership in democratic organizations. The estimate of the parameter is not statistically significant at the $p < 0.05$ level, alleviating concern that the causal arrow might run in the direction opposite to that stated by our hypothesis.

Democratic IGOs and escalation?

Given our choice of the dependent variable (fatal MID), there is a possibility that some selection bias is occurring. That is, we have shown a consistent and robust relationship between democratic IGOs and a lack of fatal disputes, but could this be because members of democratic IGOs have fewer tensions generally? Before entering into disputes that create fatalities, surely states begin their differences with less intense levels of hostility, later escalating to fatal MIDs. It is important to control for this possibility since, for example, if states in democratic IGOs are generally less likely to dispute in nonfatal MIDs, then we are mistakenly inferring a relationship that does not exist—we have an upward bias in our estimate of democratic IGOs.

To understand the influence of democratic IGOs more fully, we ask whether violent MIDs can be prevented by these institutions, when a MID already exists in the dyad, while controlling for the possibility that IGOs lessen the possibility of a MID generally. To this end, we estimate a Heckman selection model, where the first stage tests for the influence of democratic IGOs in preventing the onset of *any* MID, and the second stage examines whether MIDs that do occur become violent with at least one death. The two equations are:

$$\text{DISPUTE} = \alpha_0 + \alpha_1 \text{Democratic IGOs} + \alpha_2 \text{Democracy}_S + \alpha_3 \text{Dependence}_S + \alpha_4 \text{Contiguity} + \alpha_5 \text{Distance} + \alpha_6 \text{Major Power} + \alpha_7 \text{Capability Ratio} + \alpha_8 \text{IGOs} + \varepsilon_1$$

$$\text{FATAL MID} = \beta_0 + \beta_1\text{Democratic IGOs} + \beta_2\text{Democracy}_S +$$
$$\beta_3\text{Dependence}_S + \beta_4\text{Contiguity} + \beta_5\text{Distance} +$$
$$\beta_6\text{Major Power} + \beta_7\text{Cumulative MIDs} + \beta_8\text{IGOs} + \varepsilon_2$$

Again, for the second equation, a fatal MID is observed only if MID equals 1. By simultaneously estimating both stages, we ensure that any correlation between the onset of a dispute and its escalation to a fatal dispute (correlation between ε and ε_2) is modeled. As previously noted, if the two processes are correlated, failure to account for this relationship can lead to biased inferences (as shown by Reed 2000). This test is important for discovering if democratic IGOs inhibit dispute escalation since if dyads with high numbers of democratic IGO memberships engage in fewer MIDs overall, sampling on disputes could risk bias.

For identification purposes, we add capability ratio to the dispute model since past studies have linked the balance of forces in a dyad to the onset of militarized disputes, yet a great disproportion may more inhibit the initiation of a militarized dispute than its escalation to a fatal dispute under the uncertainties of crisis decision-making.[33] Similarly, we exclude cumulative MIDs from the dispute model for identification purposes, as we have found this variable to be related to fatal disputes, yet there is much less theoretical reason to expect it to be related to the onset of all militarized disputes.

Table 9.4 presents the estimates of this new model.[34] Note that for both the dispute and fatal MID portions of the model, democratic IGOs is negative and highly significant. Higher numbers of memberships in democratic IGOs reduce the propensity to enter MIDs, and then also prevent those MIDs which do begin from escalating to fatal MIDs. This result makes the pacific effect of democratic IGOs clearer and more persuasive, even when controlling for unobservable factors influencing the onset and escalation of disputes.

A few of the remaining estimates are worth noting. Regime type appears to strongly influence the onset of disputes, but not their escalation—a finding that parallels Reed (2000). Interdependence (Dependence$_S$), however, has a strong conflict-reducing effect for both processes. Trade linkages seem very important in dispute prevention and restraining dispute escalation thereafter.

Interestingly, the Joint IGOs variable is positive and statistically significant in the first stage. Again recall that democratic composition of IGOs is controlled for, thus this variable is likely capturing the influence of the institution itself. Perhaps pairs of states with a high level of interaction join some IGOs to manage many conflicts of interest with the potential of escalating to a serious MID. This interpretation is consistent with the strong positive impact of all IGOs on the onset of any MID, but the strong negative impact of all IGOs on fatal MIDs. Thus, when examining IGOs in an undifferentiated manner, they may appear to promote conflict generally, but to inhibit more violent disputes—a finding consistent with past empirical work.[35]

The error correlation term (ρ) for this model is positive but not statistically significant, suggesting that the two processes of onset and escalation are independent,

TABLE 9.4 Heckman selection model of militarized disputes and fatal militarized disputes, 1885–2000

	Dispute	Fatal MID
Democratic IGOs	−0.022★★★	−0.063★★★
	(0.007)	(0.018)
Democracy$_S$	−0.023★★★	−0.004
	(0.003)	(0.010)
Dependence$_S$	−11.863★★★	−24.867★★★
	(5.223)	(9.596)
Contiguity	0.856★★★	−0.370★★★
	(0.074)	(0.131)
Distance	−0.184★★★	−0.094★★
	(0.032)	(0.054)
Major power	0.934★★★	−0.353★★★
	(0.066)	(0.111)
Capability ratio	−0.086★★★	—.—
	(0.019)	
Cumulative MIDs	—.—	0.021★★★
	(0.008)	
Joint IGOs	0.010★★★	−0.006★★
	(0.002)	(0.003)
Constant	−0.914★★★	0.545
	(0.253)	(0.472)
ρ		0.040
		(0.088)
χ^2	88.21★★★	
N	454,380	
N (uncensored)	1,754	

Notes: Parameters are estimated using Heckman's probit, after including a cubic spline function with three knots in the first-stage equations and a cubic spline with one knot in the second stage. Entries in parentheses are Huber standard errors clustered on the dyad. ★★★ $p \le 0.01$; ★★ $p \le 0.05$; ★ $p \le 0.1$. All significance tests are one-tailed.

and that adding the selection portion to the model of fatal MIDs adds little information to the model.[36] So we can be reassured that our initial estimates of the influence of democratic IGOs on fatal disputes are not biased.

Since there appears to be no statistical reason for a selection model for the onset of disputes and their escalation to fatal disputes, we reestimate the second equation, for the onset of fatal disputes, using only those cases where a MID onset has occurred. Thus, we can see whether, conditional on the existence of some conflict, hostilities escalate to the point of creating fatalities. Recall that one of our hypothesized causal mechanisms dealt with dispute settlement mechanisms, many of which are designed

TABLE 9.5 The effects of democracy, interdependence, and IGO membership on the escalation of militarized disputes to fatal militarized disputes, 1885–2000

	Base model	Democratic dyads
Democratic IGOs	−0.118★★★	−0.122★★★
	(0.040)	(0.040)
Democracy$_S$	−0.006	−0.012
	(0.017)	(0.020)
Dependence$_S$	−46.905★★★	−46.865★★★
	(18.656)	(18.419)
Contiguity	−0.654★★★	−0.651★★★
	(0.176)	(0.176)
Distance	−0.087	−0.088
	(0.081)	(0.081)
Major power	0.751★★★	−0.752★★★
	(0.157)	(0.176)
Cumulative MIDs	0.020★	0.020★
	(0.012)	(0.012)
Joint IGOs	−0.010★★	−0.009★★
	(0.006)	(0.006)
Democratic dyad	—.—	0.231
		(0.656)
Constant	1.123★★	1.083★★
	(0.650)	(0.656)
Pseudo R^2	0.07	0.07
N	1,754	1,754

Notes: Parameters are estimated using logistic regression, after including a cubic spline function with two knots. Entries in parentheses are Huber standard errors clustered on the dyad. ★★★ $p \leq 0.01$; ★★ $p \leq 0.05$; ★ $p \leq 0.1$. All significance tests are one-tailed.

with this explicit purpose in mind. Evidence that democratic institutions inhibit severe disputes once tensions are already high would provide strong support for that particular causal path linking IGOs to peace.

Table 9.5 shows the estimates of these models, which consistently support the idea that democratic IGOs engender peace. In all the models, Democratic IGOs is negative and highly significant statistically. Again, this is true when controlling for joint democracies, as shown in column 2.[37] To examine the substantive significance of these results, we compute the predicted probability of a fatal MID based on simulations of the parameter estimates in column 1 of Table 9.5.[38] Figure 9.2 shows the results. The top and bottom lines represent 95 percent confidence intervals around the center line which represents each predicted probability. Moving from no common democratic IGOs to 5, for example, yields a sharp decline of nearly 40 percent in the probability of escalation to a fatal MID. The effect of common membership in democratic IGOs comes through strongly even for dyads belonging to only a few such institutions.

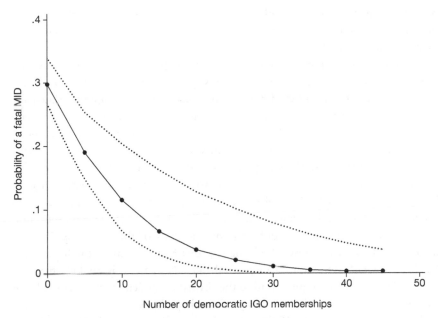

FIGURE 9.2 Predicted probabilities of escalation to fatal MIDs

Note: Dotted lines are 95 percent confidence levels.

Consistent with the estimates of the second stage of the Heckman model (in Table 9.4), democracy alone has little influence in preventing the escalation of lower-level MIDs to fatal disputes. Rather, democracy seems to work through the instruments provided to democratic states by international organizations. Economic interdependence, however, continues to play a strong and independent role in suppressing violence between states during times of crises. Again the effect of joint IGOs is negative and usually statistically significant at the $p > 0.05$ level, suggesting that even when controlling for the nature of the IGOs in the dyad, the sheer number of joint memberships influences the prospects for conflict escalation.

Finally, it is worth noting that higher numbers of previous MIDs increase the likelihood of escalation to fatal MIDs, as does the presence of a major power in the dyad. In addition, Table 9.5 shows that directly contiguous states are actually less likely to escalate the violence after they have become involved in a dispute. The shift of this variable from strongly positive in past studies of all MIDs to strongly negative here, when moving to the escalation framework, suggests that while neighbors may be far more likely to engage in conflict, they may be more careful about which conflicts escalate.

Conclusions

We are now more confident in rejecting the realist hypothesis that IGOs are fundamentally irrelevant to reducing violent international conflict. Rather than focusing on all IGOs in the world system, attention to a particular theoretically informed subset proves productive. To paraphrase a previous US president: "It's *democratic* IGOs, stupid."

We found consistent evidence to support our hypothesis that a particular kind of IGO is conflict reducing, and that those IGOs produce their effect in conjunction with the regime characteristics of their member states. IGOs comprised principally of states with democratic governments are strongly and consistently associated with a lower risk of fatal militarized disputes among their constituent states. Peace among democracies depends in part on their ability to use conflict-reducing mechanisms associated with those IGOs populated mostly by democratic states. The effect of densely democratic IGOs is in addition to any separate effect either of joint democracy or of joint IGO membership, and it operates on both democratic and nondemocratic dyads. This result holds up well under a variety of robustness tests for different measurements or different specifications of the equations. Densely democratic IGOs help to lower both the risk that MIDs of any sort will arise, and that lower-level MIDs will escalate to fatal ones. Notably, it is unlikely that low frequencies of previous disputes lead to the formation of densely democratic IGOs and thus reverse the causal relationship of our hypothesis.

Since densely democratic IGOs reduce both the frequency of MIDs and their escalation, the direct Kantian causal arrow from a particular kind of IGO to peace seems clear, operating both on democratic and nondemocratic members. Other research points strongly to a positive role for democratic IGOs in promoting and consolidating democracy (Pevehouse 2005). In combination with the evidence for joint democracy sharply reducing the onset of militarized conflict, this indicates an additional, indirect influence running from democratic IGOs through democracy in the Kantian triangle and then to peace.

These strong statistical results of course cannot tell us exactly how democratic IGOs work to prevent conflict among their members, nor can they sort out the effect of the different causal processes we suggested as operating. We lack the kind of case study process tracing that would illuminate the conditions under which these statistical results might occur. We do not have the kind of rich, detailed measures of IGOs by function or institutional structure that might provide useful explanations. We require good micro-level evidence of the ways in which institutions work, and such micro-theories of behavior as the principal-agent rational models that have illuminated the democratic peace and even the liberal peace of economic interdependence. We need to know precisely how democracy matters, in different contexts.[39] Other characteristics of IGOs may also have independent effects.

A focus on densely democratic IGOs may allow other methods and models to dispel some important remaining shadows within the still-unfolding Kantian peace research program. It is likely that densely democratic IGOs contribute in various ways to the uneven learning process by which Kant expected his confederation of republics to form, deepen, and expand.[40]

Notes

1　We thank Robert Axelrod, Erik Gartzke, Edward Mansfield, Thomas McCarthy, and Nicholas Sambanis for comments, the Ford Foundation and the University of Wisconsin Research Foundation for financial support, and Ann Fishback and Courtney Hillebrecht for research assistance.

2　For this conclusion, see Bennett and Stam (2004: ch. 5); Chernoff (2004); and Reuveny and Li (2003); for a contrary view, see Rosato (2003); but then Kinsella (2005).

3　Bennett and Stam (2004: ch. 5) confirm robustness; for varied views, see Schneider *et al.* (2003); and Mansfield and Pollins (2003).

4　Oneal and Russett's work is illustrative. An IGO effect was significant among politically relevant dyads: Russett *et al.* (1998); Russett and Oneal (2001); but not all dyads: Oneal and Russett (1999). The IGO-peace link appears using one kind of statistical correction for duration dependence, GEE: Russett and Oneal (2001: ch. 5); but not with peace years in Oneal and Russett (1999) as specified by Beck *et al.* (1998). The link appears among all dyads with peace years correction when the dependent variable is wars, but not for lower-level disputes: Kinsella and Russett (2002); Oneal and Russett (2006). IGOs may be formed by states that already have peaceful relations with each other: Russett and Oneal (2001: ch. 6) find causal arrows in feedback loops running in both directions. Oneal *et al.* (2003) resolve some of these issues in a distributed lag analysis to address both duration dependence and reciprocal causation. Even among all dyads they find a strong conflict-reducing effect for IGOs on all militarized disputes and on fatal MIDs (militarized interstate disputes resulting in at least one fatality).

5　For another attempt to differentiate IGOs theoretically, see Haftel and Thompson (2006).

6　A useful commentary is McCarthy (1999).

7　A sizable literature—for example, Cowhey (1993); Gaubatz (1996); Martin (2000); and Lipson (2003)— shows that ratification requirements allow democracies to commit more credibly to international agreements. This suggests that densely democratic IGOs should be well suited to enforce commitments. While one might argue that this means IGOs are not needed for democratic states to engender credible commitments, in every empirical investigation of this topic the ratification-commitment linkage involves IGOs or international regimes, suggesting there is some value added to signing international commitments versus relying only on the potential bilateral "promising advantages" of democracies.

8　Eilstrup-Sangiovanni and Verdier (2005) contend that the EU institutions were carefully designed as a means of committing a temporarily weakened West Germany not to use its future power to pursue military ends in Europe.

9　On Greece, see Whitehead (1994: 154); on Turkey, see Phillips (2004); and Karaosmanoglu (1991).

10　See Donno (2008), for an analytical typology of various IGO action options against democratic backsliders.

11　*Washington Post*, April, 30 1996: A13.

12　It is true that Kahler then argues that because of turnover in democracies, they may have an interest in not legalizing their relations with other states. While this is possible, our discussion in the previous section suggests it is equally likely that states will legalize their relations with one another so as to bind future governments.

13　Mansfield and Snyder (2002) and (2005) find that states liberalizing from autocracy to somewhere in the anocratic range of Polity scores (not into the democratic range) evidence increased conflict. Even so, Oneal *et al.* (2003) report that a full democratic transition from autocracy to democracy brings the risk of conflict with a democracy down to that between two well-established democracies. Also see Rousseau (2005: ch. 6).

14　According to Batt (1994: 183), the question was not "whether nationalism will play a role in Hungarian politics, but whether it will be nationalism of a more moderate variety which can coexist and support the transition to democracy."

15　*New York Times*, March 26, 1995: D4.

16 On the likelihood of war between Nicaragua and Honduras, see *Christian Science Monitor*, December 27, 2001: 5; and *Miami Herald*, February 22, 2000: A1. On this case generally, see Pratt (2001).

17 Dembinski *et al.* (2004) fear that mutual identity, especially as fostered by a democratic alliance, may create greater willingness to use force against autocracies outside the alliance. Such a phenomenon may be consistent with a "clash of civilizations" thesis— see Huntington (1996)—but does not appear for Western civilizations versus others outside of the cold war context. Russett and Oneal (2001: 258–260).

18 In focusing on democratic IGOs, our first two mechanisms can incorporate many of the rationalist variables mentioned by Boehmer *et al.* (2004), and our third includes but goes beyond their interest in preferences.

19 All references to "democraticness" of an institution refer to the level of democracy among member states. We do not address issues of whether the rules or procedures of particular organizations are judged as democratic—an issue beyond our scope here.

20 The IGO data are from Pevehouse *et al.* 2004. From 1965 forward, all data are annual observations. For 1885–1965, where the original COW IGO data measures membership in five-year periods, membership data are filled in for as many organizations as possible. Where this was not possible, membership was interpolated based on the five-year observations bracketing the year in question.

21 Despite examples such as Senese (1997), we are not satisfied that the whole MID scale is truly ordinal; that is, a threat to use military force or demonstration of force (such as a threat to use nuclear weapons, or visibly putting them on alert) is not necessarily less serious than some uses of force without violence (such as seizing a fishing boat). Escalating a use of force to where it results in a fatality, however, seems a more defensible indication of a step-level jump.

22 We use an extended version of the data from Oneal *et al.* (2003), who rely on multiple sources of trade data including Gleditsch (2002b).

23 We include both distance and contiguity since some states may share a border yet have distant capitals (Russia and China), while others may be in close proximity but have no common border (Gambia and Guinea-Bissau).

24 We also estimate a model substituting a variable controlling for the average number of democratic great powers in IGOs shared by states *i* and *j*. The estimate of this variable does not achieve statistical significance, suggesting it is not large, democratic powers exerting a peace-enhancing effect.

25 One simple test is to compute the rate of fatal disputes for dyads who share zero, one, and two IGO memberships in any given year. Those states that share no IGO membership are more likely to engage in fatal MIDs than those dyads who have at least one or two joint memberships. This difference is statistically significant.

26 We do not show these later estimates but they are available from our website: http://users.polisci.wisc.edu/pevehouse/research1.htm. We also reestimate our original model on only a sample of democratic pairs. Democratic IGOs remains negative and highly statistically significant.

27 We also ran a robustness check on similarity of preferences as measured by UN voting agreement, applying the Signorino and Ritter (1999) similarity measure of *S* to UN voting patterns (data concern only the post–World War II era). The estimate of *S* is negative but not statistically significant, with no systematic relationship to the probability that states engage in a fatal MID. Moreover, the democratic IGOs variable remains statistically significant at the $p < 0.1$ level. While Signorino and Ritter show *S* to be a more useful measure than the traditional Tau-B measure, we generated similar estimates using Tau-B. It does attenuate the influence of democratic IGOs somewhat, but not for the results presented in the next section. Since joint democracy is one of the principal influences on UN voting patterns—see Russett and Oneal (2001: 228–237)—it is preferable to use it as a direct influence on conflict. We also added a variable for the balance of military capabilities, but it has no effect on our independent variable of interest.

28 To conserve space we show only the threshold 6 estimates, but changing the threshold to 5 yields similar results.

29 This result stays consistent if only the EU is counted in the indicator variable. In addition, defining our Democratic IGOs variable as including only regional organizations generates similar findings—the recomputed variable remains negative and statistically significant. We define regional organizations as IGOs whose members are in the same geographic region, thus excluding universal organizations such as the UN.

30 Similar checks show unchanged results in Table 9.4. Results for all the robustness tests discussed but not shown here are available on the website.

31 Farber and Gowa (1997) claim little evidence of peace among democracies before the cold war, which led them to conclude that the democratic peace was an artifact of structural-realist variables. Our results dispute their contention that Kantian variables had little influence before World War II.

32 Our model of IGO membership is similar to Russett et al. (1998: 461); Russett and Oneal (2001: ch. 6); and Mansfield and Pevehouse (2006). It includes all the control variables in column 3 of Table 9.2, in addition to a measure of international hegemony and an indicator for the post-cold war years. On the addition of these later variables, see Mansfield and Pevehouse (2006).

33 We rely on the COW Capabilities data for the ratio of material capabilities. Each state's political-military capacity is measured by averaging its share of the international system's total population, urban population, military expenditures, military personnel, iron and steel production, and energy consumption. Capability ratio is the ratio of the capabilities of the larger state to those of the smaller state: see Singer (1987); and Singer and Small (1993).

34 To estimate these models, we use the "heckprob" routine in STATA 8.0.

35 On the former finding, see Kinsella and Russett (2002); on the latter, Oneal et al. (2003).

36 This is counter to the findings of Reed (2000), but there are important differences in model specification. In particular, Reed examines escalation to wars, not fatal disputes.

37 We also re-ran earlier robustness checks on the presence of military alliances, the presence of EU-EFTA states, and adjusting the democracy threshold to 6 and above. All results are consistent with our initial findings.

38 Simulations are based on 3,000 simulations of parameter estimates using CLARIFY. See King et al. (2000).

39 A complementary enterprise would unpack the variable democracy. For example, Minnich (2005) finds that certain kinds of democracies (notably parliamentary systems with incentives for multiparty representation) are more likely to join IGOs.

40 Efforts to model this as a systemic learning process include Cederman (2001); Cederman and Penubarti Rao (2001); and Rousseau (2005: ch. 7).

10

SECURITY COUNCIL EXPANSION

Can't, and shouldn't

"Reform" of the Security Council has been a popular goal, an old dream, and an understandable ambition for decades. Reform typically means expanding the Council's membership to make it, in the words of the Report of the High-level Panel (2004) to the Secretary General, more "representative," "democratic," and "accountable" (para. 249). The Panel aims to increase its "objectivity," (para. 197), "credibility" (para. 248), and especially "legitimacy" (para. 204). There is much precedent for these concerns. The only amendments to the United Nations Charter, adopted in 1963 and coming into force two years later, were principally to Article 23. That change expanded the membership of the Council from 11 to 15, with all the increase going to the nonpermanent (and thus nonveto-wielding) members. The motivations behind that change were similar to those of the Panel. The change came in the process of decolonization and admission of some states that had initially been barred from membership because they were on the wrong side of the victors in World War II. The wish to expand in order to accommodate this new diversity was appropriate and widely shared.

Such a wish is even more popular now, with near doubling of the number of member states in the UN between 1963 and now, reflecting the essential completion of decolonization and the break-up of many states at the end of the cold war. Four of the five permanent members are from North America and Europe, rich countries of predominantly white citizens from North America and Europe. The other is a rapidly developing Asian country. None is really poor, and none is from Latin America, Africa, or the Middle East. The world's population does not look like that. Further complicating matters, some states that were weak in the early years of their UN membership now are powerful and virtually necessary to the success of any Security Council action (e.g., Germany, Japan, perhaps India).

Though the term is vague, a necessary though not sufficient condition for "legitimacy" in a world body is widespread participation and voice. In its discussion of the conditions under which the Security Council might legitimately authorize the use of force (para. 209) the Panel lists five that spring to mind, in spirit if not in exact wording, standard criteria from international law and the normative principles of the just war tradition. The conditions are: serious threat, proper purpose, last resort, proportional means, and balance of probable consequences. Conspicuously missing, however, is the principle that the war must be declared or sanctioned by a legitimate authority. Historically this authority was a monarch or president, but the role is one that many states and theorists have tried to pass to the Security Council. Of course the Panel assumes that the Council is the proper bestower of legitimacy on the military action, and so it doesn't have to say that this is so. But the Panel is concerned that the Council itself may not have the necessary stock of legitimacy to bestow.

The normative arguments for these changes in the composition of the Security Council demand respect. The Panel accords that respect, and makes two proposals for change. That it offers two proposals—only one can be adopted—shows the inability of the Panel itself to settle on a single recommendation. It is a very bad omen, signaling that achievement of their goal will be extraordinarily difficult politically.

It should also signal that the normative grounds for expanding the Council are both ambiguous and conflicting. None of the six concepts mentioned in the first lines of this chapter is defined in the Report. They are not synonyms. Furthermore, the effort to achieve them may be seriously at odds with other normative goals of the Panel, most importantly with their quite proper concern not to impair whatever "effectiveness" (para. 249c) the Council has. But the Report does not at any point analyze what effectiveness means or how it is to be assured.

These ambiguities, even confusions, warn about both the feasibility and the desirability of the effort. A tilt too far in the direction of representativeness or democracy could undermine effectiveness, which in turn would endanger the institution's legitimacy from another direction. In this chapter I will first point out the huge difficulties in getting *any* reform proposal adopted, and then address the question of whether it would really be a good idea even if it were feasible.

Feasibility: been there and not done that

An immediate clue to the feasibility question arises from the fact that virtually all of the dozens of serious proposals for reforming the UN have called for expansion of the Security Council in the name of some or all of the six nonsynonyms. Such proposals are *de rigueur* for any international commission making reform proposals, not least because such commissions virtually always include members from the chief states aspiring to Council membership. So the Panel can hardly be faulted for following such powerful precedent in trying. Yet none of these previous commissions' proposals have ever even come to a vote of the first body that must address Charter reform: the General Assembly.

Most of those proposals have come to grief through their attempts to change the number, composition, or statutory powers of the permanent members of the Council. In this Paul Kennedy, James Sutterlin, and I can speak from our experience as staff for the Report of the Independent Working Group (1995). The Report recommended expansion of the Council to approximately twenty-three members, of whom up to five would be new permanent members not specified by name. Because of the competing interests of our commissioners, it fudged the question of whether the new permanent members should have veto power. While some of our Commission's many recommendations were implemented, those on the Security Council certainly were not. Nor, speaking for myself, did I expect or even want them to be implemented, most especially if veto power accompanied the new members. But we were (somewhat) faceless staff, not signing commissioners.

James Sutterlin and I tried to make amends for this in a subsequent book (Russett 1997c) and in the role of informal advisors to the Malaysian Representative to the UN, Mr. Razali Ismail. The Ambassador was a smart and decent man who devoted his time before, during, and after his 1996 term as President of the General Assembly to trying to broker a compromise formula that could gain assent from sufficient member states. Politics and the structure of the institution thwarted him.

The structural situation is that the composition of the Security Council can be changed only by amending the UN Charter. First, two-thirds of the UN's member states must vote in favor of any amendment in the General Assembly.[1] This majority must include all the permanent members of the Security Council. Then, two-thirds of all the member states of the UN must ratify the change, again including all the permanent members of the Council. Given the greater diversity of governments and goals in the UN than in the United States, Charter amendment sounds, and is, even harder than amending the US Constitution. It has been done once, as noted above, but that was in an era with a much smaller membership and one more malleable by the super-powers in those situations where they were in agreement. The 1963 amendments succeeded with help from a superpower deal that brought in comparable numbers of allies from both sides.

Despite much public rhetoric from all sides, private preferences have stymied all subsequent efforts to broker a compromise satisfactory to all the blocking points implied in the structural constraints. The problem of new permanent members has been the most obvious sticking point, one deeply enmeshed in regional rivalries. Pakistan and China have adamantly opposed any package that would give India a permanent seat; Mexico and especially Argentina have made it clear they would not permit a permanent seat for Brazil; Japan was opposed by China and others in East Asia with long memories. Even closely integrated allies could be opposed: Italy conducted an extended and vigorous campaign against Germany, partly a result of long memories and because a German permanent seat would reduce the chances for Italy even to have frequent access to a nonpermanent one. If Nigeria is in Africa, then what about Egypt and South Africa? Nor are the permanent five necessarily enthusiastic about adding institutional equals. The previous illustrations mention China, but all of the others have serious reservations about one or most of the chief aspirants.

The politics and politicking are more complex and arcane than these illustrations, but they all boil down to this: a coalition of minorities has always been able to defeat any such proposal even before it could be brought to a vote. Each member might accept certain kinds of changes, but any package always seemed to carry a poison pill to which the status quo was preferable. To supplement our verbal analyses for Mr. Razali we conducted a session with diplomats in consultation with a specialist in the computer analysis of coalition formation, Professor Bruce Bueno de Mesquita. His model has an excellent track record of predicting what coalitions will form on the basis of experts' judgments on the intensity and preferences of each actor. In this case his model also produced the negative forecast: no successful coalition can form—and he too was proven right.

The coalition-of-minorities problem is especially acute regarding any assignment of veto power to new permanent members. The majority of member states feel that the veto is already abused by the current five, and to extend it to others (especially though not only their regional rivals) would merely increase the impotence of everyone else. Most resistant to extending the veto to new permanent members, however, are the current five, because to do so would dilute their own power and make it harder than ever for them to get any resolutions through the Council. All of the new permanent members would need to be persuaded to favor or at most abstain on a resolution. Whether by persuasion, threats, or favors, the diplomacy becomes immensely more complicated, especially when dealing with powers of near-equal wealth. For them both threats and favors would have to be much bigger than with the typical state in a nonpermanent two-year seat. The problem stems from the dual character of power in any parliamentary body: the power to pass a resolution and the power to block a resolution. The more veto-wielding members the harder it is to pass, and the easier to block. This relates directly to the matter of the Council's effectiveness, and I will say more about that below. It is obvious that blocking power, for themselves or for a trusted ally, could be the more important.

While all the permanent members have a clear interest in not having more procedural equals on the Council, the position of the United States has some particular interest. During the cold war era it had to support publicly its allies, Germany and Japan, in their persistent efforts to achieve permanent member status with veto, while nonaligned India was quite another matter. Privately, however, the enthusiasm for German and Japanese membership was much more muted. Could they be trusted in the long run to follow US leadership? After all, once a veto wielder always a veto wielder. The present configuration of world power does not help the prospect. Is it reasonable to expect the current US administration, or any US Senate with less than a full two-thirds Democratic majority (itself virtually unthinkable) to extend equal status to Germany after the experience over Iraq?

In short, for general and particular reasons there can be no increase in the number of permanent members with veto power. The Panel clearly recognizes that, as their proposed Model A calls only for five new nonvetoing permanent members. That avoids the problem of multiplying potential veto points and the diplomacy around them, but probably will not satisfy the desires of the major aspirants for whom equality and prestige, not to mention the power of the veto, remain important. For similar reasons their regional rivals are unlikely to acquiesce in the permanent status upgrade of even the nonveto role. The Panel's Model B adds nothing to that category, instead settling for the addition of eight new four-year seats with renewable terms, and a single new two-year nonrenewable seat (which is the current alternative to permanent membership). Eight new four-year seats (cleverly assigned equally two each to the four big regional groups) might assuage some regional rivals who could hope to alternate occasionally if not regularly with the biggest players. But in compensating the regional rivals of permanent seat aspirants, it removes even more incentive for the powerful aspirants to settle for what would be continued long-term status in a downgraded second class.

A potentially intriguing issue, completely neglected in the Panel Report, is what the voting rules would be. If a resolution is to pass in the current Security Council a majority of at least nine of the fifteen members (60 percent) must vote in favor, with no permanent member voting against. (In the original Council of eleven members, the action threshold was seven, or 63.6 percent.) If all the permanent members do vote in favor, that means they need only gain the acquiescence of four of the ten nonpermanent members. That is very easy, given that many of the nonpermanent members are de facto allies of one or more of the permanent members. Moreover, the permanent members can readily play the mostly weaker nonpermanent members against one another. By some combination of favors, threats, and persuasion, the necessary four can be found. (By contrast, when the United States and the UK wanted Council sanction for their invasion of Iraq in 2003, they failed to bring along the other three permanent members, and so could not even persuade a symbolic if legally ineffective seven other states to give approval.) The ease with which the necessary supplementary votes can usually be found means that the formal rule of one state one vote hugely exaggerates the actual political power of each nonpermanent member. Because of the heavy competition for the favor (or to avoid the disfavor) of the permanent members, the others acting individually have essentially no real voting power at all if voting power is defined as the probability of actually changing the outcome of the resolution (O'Neill 1997). Being a nonpermanent member of the Council does have its rewards: the opportunity to express views, to interact with the real powers on the world stage, some fleeting element of prestige, and the possibility for ambassadors to garner approval back in the home country. But true voting power is not one of them. This holds major implications for the Panel's two models. Model A, with five new permanent seats but no veto power, would leave Germany, Japan, India, etc. down with the masses in terms of near-zero voting power. Model B would add to this injury the insult of denying them even whatever prestige a nonveto permanent seat might hold.

Two developments, however, might modify this harsh statement. If a sufficient number (seven of the ten nonpermanent members in the current Council) were deeply committed to similar policy and tightly bound in honor not to break ranks, they could constitute what has been called a "sixth veto" player. Such a tight bloc has never emerged and has been unlikely to do so, given that the provisions for geographical representation across the globe virtually ensure that the nonpermanent members will be quite diverse in their preferences. But it could be more likely if a larger Council weighted more than at present to Africa (to six seats) were combined with a voting rule that required a much higher percentage of the Council membership to pass a resolution. The higher the threshold, the greater the power accorded to the group of less-developed countries known as the G-77 (actually now constituting well over a majority of the UN members). If, for example, in the twenty-four-member body the Panel proposes the bar were set at eighteen (75 percent), requiring the permanent five to attract at least thirteen of the remaining nineteen votes, the leverage of the nonpermanent members would increase somewhat. But a threshold of 75 percent is not really imaginable. The big five are not fools enough to greatly dilute the power they already have—and they also have a veto to prevent such dilution.

The Panel does not mention a proposed action threshold at all. The current percentage is 60; fifteen out of twenty-four would amount to a mild bump upward to 62.5 percent, and is the most prominent solution. That would require ten dissenting states to act as a sixth veto player. One could in principle imagine a bloc of ten veto-less states, perhaps led by India and the two African states in the role of new permanent members (Model A) or in renewable four-year seats (Model B). Even so, a diverse coalition of ten mostly weak states without the resources of a big industrialized power to bankroll it would be very hard to hold together. On inspection, the ten-state bloc possibility seems to have little substance. And to suggest any possibility of a higher threshold returns us to the question of why *all* of the big five would permit such a dilution of their current power.

Possibly some wide-ranging deal could be struck to corral the large coalition required to pass a Charter amendment, but I am very skeptical. Moreover, just to discuss the above possibilities raises the critical issue of trade-offs between effectiveness and legitimacy (and the other nonsynonyms). Anything that adds another veto point in the Council and increases the number of players that have leverage in its negotiations throws one more bucket of sand into the wheels of rapid and decisive action by the Security Council. Most observers regard fifteen seats on the Council as too few to make it sufficiently representative. And most observers would probably agree that a Security Council as big as the fifty-four-member Economic and Social Council, though more representative, would be too big to take the kind of prompt and decisive action necessary to deal with an international security crisis. But how to choose between those limits, given that we don't even know how rapidly the curve of effectiveness falls or rises as more members are added? The Panel proposes twenty-four as a compromise. But that compromise would be political, not informed by careful analysis, and it might make the Council unable to act in some major crises.

How one judges such a compromise depends on where one sits, and what one thinks the Council most needs. It is very hard to have it both ways. As a world citizen I might favor the legitimacy side, and welcome what might curb further the ability of certain great powers to extract Council approval for their own visions of how world order might be enforced. Yet world citizens, as well as those great powers who have been frustrated in the Council, should be very reluctant to weaken whatever capacity the Council has to act. The coalition favoring effectiveness ought also to include some not-so-great powers chastened by such egregious failures to execute humanitarian intervention as the Rwanda affair.

A trade-off between effectiveness and legitimacy?

Unlike wealth, military power, or even intelligence, legitimacy is an ascribed quality and not readily subject to measurement. Moreover, different actors bestow legitimacy on the same object in widely varying degrees. For many Catholics Pope John Paul II is the legitimate leader of their church; for many Muslims, Osama bin Laden is their most legitimate political/religious leader. Neither group accords much legitimacy to the other's figure. Making the Security Council more representative and "democratic" would likely increase its legitimacy in the eyes of many people in the poor and "southern" countries of the globe, and even many in Europe and Japan as well. But would it have the same effect on other Europeans, or on many Americans? The answer may be no, for two reasons that would apply to two different groups of observers.

First, legitimacy and effectiveness are partly complementary, not polar opposites. While a body that proved ineffective might lose legitimacy widely, an effective body might readily lose legitimacy in the eyes of those regularly on the wrong side of its decisions. There is a difference between approving a sanction against a member state of the UN and having the capability to make that sanction effective. Nothing can happen without the capability or power to do it, and the willingness to exert that power. In the global arena, major UN activities must have the approval, and usually the active participation and support, of the most powerful states in the system. Although the World Bank and the International Monetary Fund owe their existence to the needs of economic justice, they cannot violate the wishes of the states that provide their principal funding. The Security Council cannot, given the veto, embark on an operation against the wishes of a permanent member. Nor should it do so without assurances of financial and military commitment from the major powers whose active participation in some form will be necessary. Power talks, and acts. No action in the absence of adequate power will be effective. And power will not act in a particular case unless the most powerful states in the UN deem the action to be worthwhile by their definition (broad or narrow, immediate or long term) of its national interest. We learned that during the cold war.

Second, if it is also to be effective, the Security Council will never be very "democratic" if democracy is defined either as one-state one-vote or, over the whole world, one-person one-vote. It is no coincidence that the Security Council, with the potential and some history of exerting strong powers of enforcement under Chapter VII of the UN Charter, is probably the least democratic UN organ. The Security Council can, when its members so choose, make or break states. The powerful states represented on the Council, and who would bear the brunt of carrying out enforcement action, are unwilling to be committed by a vote that does not reflect their economic and military differential. By contrast, the General Assembly, often derided as a talk shop and certainly with no formal power of enforcement, is one of the most democratic (one-state one-vote) organs.

Voting power is the power to authorize action; it is also the power to block action. Veto power and provisions for super-majority voting (requiring "ayes" well over 50 percent, as in the Security Council and the US Senate) give a minority the power to block, at the expense of the power of a simple majority to act. Such provisions are meant to protect certain rights and privileges of the minority from "majority tyranny." They are part of the US Constitution, of many states with large ethnic minorities, and of the UN Charter.

Majoritarian democracy can succeed within a country only where there are serious limitations on the exercise of coercive violence by the state and limits on the concentration of economic power (income and wealth). Additionally, democratic government requires some community of basic values among the populace, or at least some protection for the rights and values of minorities. The international system, however, lacks all these conditions. Military power for state violence is concentrated overwhelmingly in the hands of the five permanent members (with nuclear weapons) or a single superpower with global reach (which accounts for more than half of all world military expenditures). The 20 percent of the world's population living in the wealthiest countries receives 85 percent of global income— a concentration far higher than within any single country, rich or poor. Despite some convergence on values, one cannot talk persuasively about a community of basic values in the world. Under such circumstances—and I lament them—the rich and powerful will not surrender real power to any organization controlled by a "democratic" majority of states or individuals. One can perhaps hope for greater consultation and transparency, and greater deference to the needs of the poor and weak. Democratization of the Security Council in the form of majority rule could happen, if at all, only in a Council deprived of the capacity to accomplish anything.

But democratization is not really the problem at hand for the Security Council. The United States can always veto any Council action, and it is now evident even in this post-cold war "hegemonic" era that if the United States over-reaches sufficiently the Council can withhold its approval of any US action. In much of the world the Security Council gained, not lost, in perceived legitimacy by its refusal to endorse US military action against Iraq in 2003. It could not, however, prevent that action by an administration determined to act unilaterally. Thus the US administration derided the Security Council (and by extension the UN generally) as wrong-headed, ineffective, and illegitimate.

Given its institutional structure and the distribution of military capability in the world, the problem for the Security Council is that it cannot pull together the resources for major effective action without US support, let alone in the face of US opposition. There is not as yet, and will not be for at least a couple of decades more, a number two state with the power of the old Soviet Union. The principle of collective action, and experience, make it clear that the notion of restraining US power by a coalition of the chilling is a dream only, of desire without ability. US power can, and will, be restrained only by the weight of its own failures.

For these reasons, it would be unwise to press ahead with a reform agenda that was opposed by the UN's most powerful members, and particularly by the United States. And it would be even less wise to press so far that US opposition took the form of an outright rejection of Charter revision by the administration or, still worse, of a job left to the US Senate. That would lead to a further decline of UN legitimacy in the eyes of many of the powerful in Washington, and to an even greater willingness of the United States to go it alone. I do not wish that for either the United States or the United Nations.

Conclusion: Let it be

The High-level Panel deserves credit for creativity and ingenuity in coming up with a plan for Security Council expansion that might appeal to a wide range of UN members. Just possibly its proposals might, in an extended process of negotiation, lead to some agreement that can be adopted. But the odds against that happening are very high, since a coalition of minorities constituting only one-third of the members, or even just the United States alone, could kill it. Should it somehow be adopted, that success would be blemished by major and foreseeable problems in how it would play out in institutional diplomacy over subsequent decades. Constitutions are made hard to change for very good reasons. The system needs to be really "broke" to make the risks of a "fix" worth taking. Is the UN that broken? I don't think so. Better to concentrate on the many other constructive and more feasible proposals in the Report.

Note

1   Two-thirds of the members, not just two-thirds of the Assembly. Article 109 of the Charter provides a little wiggle room in its provision for a General Conference called by two-thirds of the General Assembly and *any* nine members of the Security Council. A two-thirds vote of the conference—which conceivably could be boycotted by up to one-third of the UN's member states—would suffice at this stage. The other requirements, for approval by all the permanent members of the Council and ratification by two-thirds of all the member governments, would still apply, however. No such conference has ever been held.

11

LIBERALISM

The most important transformation in world politics over the past sixty years derives from the concurrent and interlinked expansion of three key phenomena associated with liberalism and its emphasis on the potentially peace-promoting effects of domestic and transnational institutions. One is the spread of democracy throughout most of the world. A second is the multiple networks of communications, trade, and finance often summarized as globalization. The third is the multiplication of intergovernmental organizations, especially those composed primarily of democratic governments. Each of these supports and extends the other in a powerful feedback system envisioned by Immanuel Kant. Moreover, each creates a set of norms and interests which dramatically reduce the risk of violent conflict among the countries so linked. Contemporary Europe constitutes the prime example of these processes at work, but they are not limited to Europe or to developed economies.

The world is full of testimony to tragedy. Governments oppress their own people and commit aggression against their neighbors. World politics is conducted in a condition of anarchy as that term was used by the Greeks: not chaos, but "without a ruler," having no overarching authority to enforce order. There is some order, but on a globe far from ready for world government most order is not something imposed from above.

Realists say that every country is potentially an enemy of every other—intentionally or not, a threat to their security and very existence. In the absence of a world state they are caught forever in this precarious condition of freedom and risk. This tradition, like the anarchy that underlies it, has a history from Thucydides, Niccolo Machiavelli, and Thomas Hobbes, and shapes the perspective of many policy-makers. Yet there are restraints on the use of force. States do not fight all others even when purely realist principles dominate; they are constrained by geography, the coincidence of national interests expressed in alliances, and the balance of power. Deterrence forms the heart of survival, but deterrence—and especially nuclear deterrence— is an uncertain and dangerous way of avoiding war. Treating all international politics as unending struggle, and everyone as a potential enemy, risks becoming a self-fulfilling prophecy.

A competing perspective deserves equal attention. This perspective, sometimes labeled liberal-institutionalist, is associated with classical analysts like John Locke, Hugo Grotius, and Immanuel Kant. Kant proposed that "republican constitutions," commercial exchange embodied in "cosmopolitan law," and a system of international law among republics governed domestically by the rule of law would provide the basis for sustained peace. The alternative would be the peace of "a vast grave where all the horrors of violence and those responsible for them would be buried" (Kant [1795] 1970). Peace was not simply an ideal to Kant. He believed that natural processes of self-interest could impel rational individuals to act as agents to bring a just peace. He was also realistic in acknowledging that nations must act prudently until a "federation" of interdependent republics is established.

Key "liberal" assumptions in Kant's framework include belief in the rational qualities of individuals, faith in the feasibility of progress in social life, and the conviction that humans, despite their self-interest, are able to co-operate and construct a more peaceful and harmonious society. Liberal internationalism arising from Kant has transposed these beliefs to the international sphere by emphasizing the fact that war and conflict can be overcome, or mitigated, through concerted changes in both the domestic and international structures of governance.

The Kantian perspective has frequently been characterized as antithetical to realism. That is an error. Kant accepted Hobbes's description of conflict among many of the nations, but went far beyond it. The pacific federation he envisioned is more accurately a confederation, and not a world state. Its members remain sovereign, linked only by partially federal institutions as in Europe today, or by collective security alliances. The difference between the two traditions is that Kant sees democratic government, economic interdependence, and international law and organizations as means to overcome the security dilemma of the international system.

Kant contended that the three elements of his pacific federation would strengthen over time to produce a more peaceful world. Individuals desire to be free and prosperous, so democracy and trade will expand, which leads naturally to the growth of international law and organization to facilitate these processes. He held that peace among republican states does not depend upon a moral transformation of humanity if even devils understand how to promote their own interests in cooperation. Kant was an empiricist who taught anthropology and geography; he drew on the history of his native Königsberg—once a member of the Hanseatic League of trading states in Northern Europe. He knew that the achievement of durable peace is not mechanical, nor is the outcome determined. Human agents must learn from their own and others' experience, including the experience of war.

ILLUSTRATIVE THEORY BOOK

In *Ways of War and Peace*, Michael Doyle traces the development of IR theory starting with Thucydides on the Peloponnesian War nearly 2,500 years ago. Doyle was one of the first IR theorists in the modern era to advance the Kantian idea of a liberal peace. In his book Doyle not only provides a detailed account of classical liberal thought, he shows how it developed alongside two historical alternatives—that of realism and Marxism.

Classical realists such as Thucydides were aware of the primacy of power politics. As he argued in *The History of the Peloponnesian Wars*, it was the growth of Athenian power and the fear this aroused in the Spartans, that led to war between the two most powerful Greek city states. This classic realist statement focuses on the inherent vulnerability of independent states in any anarchic system. Yet it is not just a statement about shifting power balances, but is also about agency: how individual leaders interpret the shifts and choose the actions they take to protect their security. Personality and domestic politics are part of his story. Statesmanship requires good judgment, and morality resides in a commitment to the safety of one's own people. Hobbes, writing in seventeenth-century England after a vicious civil war, emphasized the need for a powerful leader to enforce order so as to protect his rule at home and his ability to defend his state in the anarchic international system. Nearly all states then had such powerful leaders, or if not suffered from their absence.

Subsequent realist theorists, such as Jean Jacques Rousseau in 1756, experienced more variation in how states were governed, and thought carefully about how democracy, revolution, and cultural differences might affect the ability of states to survive internationally. Kant in part built on this view, developing it much more fully in his concern with republican government and commercial relations. Kant's difference was in his strong rationalist view that leaders could perceive and even create a different system of rules and incentives for cooperation by which, in their own self-interest, they might be able to tame the threats inherent in international anarchy. By the twentieth century, Marxist thinkers like Lenin developed a sharply different view. They held that economic imperatives would create states controlled by monopolistic commercial interests, whose states would inevitably fight bitterly as they sought ever-expanding markets abroad. Joseph Schumpeter, by contrast, believed that industrialization would produce more democratic leaders and that rising international commerce would tame militaristic imperialism.

Doyle makes us aware of how classical accounts of realism, liberalism and Marxism developed in the minds of important theorists and activists in the context of very different political and economic conditions. The legacy of these competing schools of thought, along with changing global economic and political realities, continues to shape contemporary theory and policy concerned with our own and others' interests.

Four big changes in the world

As background for the following discussion four graphics show key changes in the world over the past century and especially over recent decades. Figures 11.1 and 11.2 illustrate the long-run decline in battle deaths from violent conflicts in which one or more states were participants. Figure 11.1 shows the pattern since 1900, with the huge peaks of violence during the two World Wars. This graph controls for the growing number of people in the world, showing that in each of the worst years of World War nearly 0.2 percent of the people (two out of every thousand) in the world died in the war. The highest total since then was about 0.025 percent shortly after World War II, and then fell substantially afterward to a point that is almost undiscernible in the scale of this graph. Figure 11.2 shows total annual deaths during the post-World War II years more clearly, with progressively lower mountains continuing downward before and after the cold war. It also shows that the decline in deaths occurs in all types of war: interstate, intrastate, and extrasystemic (wars of colonial liberation). It's essential to keep a longer perspective to understand that the most recent decline is not just a temporary spike downward.

The big drop in world conflict is not widely recognized. Conflict always draws media attention. The graph does not include terrorism by nonstate actors, but while

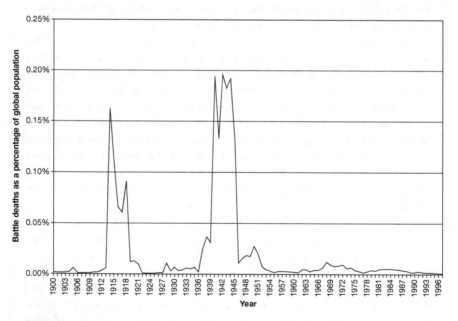

FIGURE 11.1 Average individual's risk of dying in battle, 1900–2008

Civilian and military battle deaths in state-based conflicts, divided by world population.

This graph was not in the original version of this chapter. Data from Lacina and Gleditsch (2005) updated at: www.prio.no/CSCW/Datasets/Armed-Conflict/Battle-Deaths/The-Battle-Deaths-Dataset-version-30/.

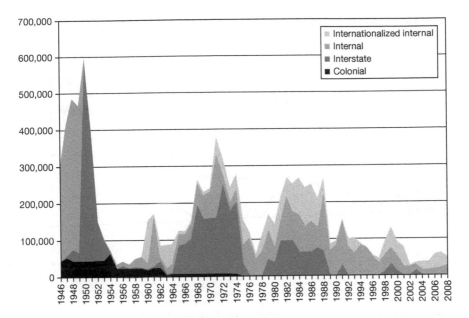

FIGURE 11.2 Battle deaths by type of war, 1946–2008

This graph replaces an earlier one in the original version of this chapter. Data from Lacina and Gleditsch (2005) updated at: www.prio.no/CSCW/Datasets/Armed-Conflict/Battle-Deaths/The-Battle-Deaths-Dataset-version-30/.

that has risen recently, the total number of deaths worldwide from terrorism 1998–2008 is about 5 percent of the battle deaths in all wars during that period (Human Security Research Project 2011). Even a big terrorist attack with weapons of mass destruction could not approach the level of death and destruction had there been a cold war nuclear exchange.

No single cause can account for the decline in global conflict deaths. However, this chapter makes a case that major contributions to that decline in destruction have been three great advances associated with liberalism in the post-World War II era, and especially since the end of the cold war. Two more graphs illustrate these trends. Figure 11.3 shows the drastic decline in the number of autocracies (dictatorships) in the world, and the even greater increase in the number of democracies as defined by the degree of free political competition permitted by their institutions. (The dotted line is for "anocracies," a category between the extremes.) By the mid-2000s, and for the first time in history, more than half the countries in the world were governed democratically.

Figure 11.3 plots the percentage increase in the number of democracies since 1946, along with lines for two other major developments. One is the very great increase in international trade, measured as constant (noninflated) value.[1] This trend of widespread economic interdependence has been building steadily, with ups and downs corresponding to the state of the world economy. The growth in countries' membership in intergovernmental organizations (IGOs), including both global and

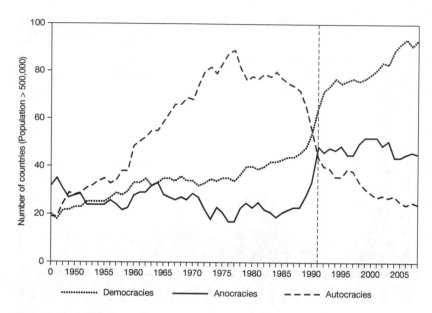

FIGURE 11.3 Global trends in governance, 1946–2008

This graph is updated from the one appearing in the original version of this chapter. Data are from Polity IV Project, Center for Systemic Peace.org/polity4.htmt.

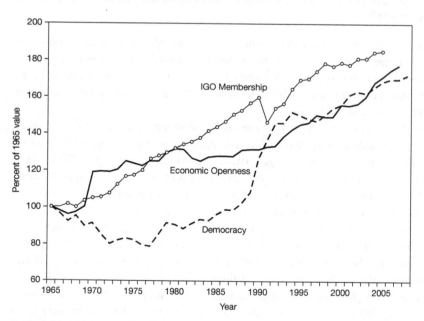

FIGURE 11.4 The growth of liberal influences since 1965

Trendlines show the average level of democracy (Polity IV scale), economic openness (trade/GDP), and IGO membership (Pevehouse *et al.* data as in Chapter 9). This graph is updated from the one appearing in the original version of this chapter.

Source: Kinsella *et al.* (2012).

regional institutions has also been building for a long time, especially in recent decades. Figure 11.4 shows the post-1965 increase in all three of these.

There are other possible reasons for the decline in world combat deaths (for instance, nuclear deterrence or US hegemony), but there is a strong case that these three trends deserve particular credit. That case rests on research designed to discover the effect of key liberal Kantian variables—democracy, economic interdependence, and international institutions—on peace.

The "epidemiology" of international conflict

The research draws on an analogy between the way medical scientists try to understand the causes of disease and the way some social scientists try to understand the causes of conflict. Medical researchers seek, by a combination of theory and empirical research, to identify the conditions that promote or prevent fatal diseases. Much of their research is *epidemiological* in character. They look at the distribution of particular diseases in large populations to discover why some individuals contract a disease while many others do not. Huge databases—about who dies where and when of various diseases, and about the life experience of those individuals—help researchers to uncover the causes, and to advise on prevention or treatment.

An epidemiological study of the causes of heart disease might show that smokers run a much higher risk of heart attack than nonsmokers. So too do those who consume a diet high in saturated fats, or who engage in little physical exercise. No single risk factor is a perfect predictor. Many people who do not smoke have heart attacks. Many smokers live a long time without a heart attack. The predictions are probabilistic, about greater and lesser risks. Each influence operates somewhat independently of the others. That is, smoking increases the risk of a heart attack regardless of diet. So a doctor might say:

> Based on your age, sex, family history, and lifestyle, statistically you run a four percent risk of having a heart attack in the next year. You can't totally eliminate that risk, but if you will quit smoking (or go on a diet, or get off the couch) you can cut it in half. And if you will quit smoking, go on a diet, *and* get off the couch—you can cut the risk by three-quarters.

Similar conclusions can be derived by analyzing countries' behavior in war and peace.

The following analysis uses an information base on international relations, analogous to the life histories of individuals. It consists of data on relations between virtually all countries in the world in each year over the period from 1885 to 2001. It can consider the expansion of democracy, economic interdependence, and international organizations over time and their effects in different historical periods.[2]

Countries can in principle fight any other country, but they typically fight only a few, so the data are organized by pairs of countries, or *dyads*. For example, it looks not at Germany in general, but rather its relations with Austria, Italy, Japan, Sweden, and so forth. It asks which kinds of dyads are prone to conflict and which are apt to remain at peace. Looking at dyads over more than a century gives nearly half a million cases, where a case is the experience of one *pair of countries in one year*. From them one can compute the likelihood that a pair of countries sharing a certain constraint on conflict (such as a common alliance, or both being democracies) experienced the onset of a serious militarized dispute in a particular year.

The analysis uses information compiled independently by many scholars and organizations, from standardized sources. The conflict data include all militarized interstate disputes, not just wars. Wars are (fortunately) rare events and, as with rare diseases, it is hard to find general patterns for where and why they erupt. Including all uses of violence between countries gives a better chance to find general patterns. Here we consider the results for *fatal* disputes, in which at least one combatant died. These incidents are far more common than wars. Other analyses show that the constraints on war do not differ much from those on militarized disputes. The influences, and their measures, include the following:

Realist constraints

Power ratio. One way to reduce the likelihood of going to war is to deter it by military strength. Most deterrence theorists argue that conflict is best prevented by a great predominance of power for one side. When power is unbalanced the outcome of conflict is usually predictable, and the weaker side generally will not fight because it knows it will lose. In Thucydides' words, "the strong do as they will and the weak do as they must." To assess the effect of power on the likelihood of conflict, we use information about states' material capabilities—economic, demographic, and military. Together they tap a combination of elements that can be used immediately for military purposes (soldiers and expenditures) and longer-term military potential that matters in a protracted conflict. It is a reasonable measure of power over a century-long period. The power ratio is the stronger state's capability index divided by that of the weaker member.

Allies. Allies share important strategic and security interests. If they have military disputes among themselves, they risk weakening their common front against a country each perceives as an enemy. During the cold war, NATO allies (save for Greece and Turkey) did not fight each other.

Two other realist influences are distance and size. Distance makes it harder and more expensive to exert military power. Neighbors can readily fight, and are more likely to have competing interests for territory, control of natural resources, or common ethnic groups that may provoke conflict. Great powers typically have strong military forces able to exercise force at a distance, and wide-ranging—even global—interests to fight for.

Kantian constraints

Liberal institutionalists, however, insist that the realist perspective does not exhaust the list of constraints on war over which states can and do exercise some control. States do not fight all others at all times and places where the realist constraints are weak. To the realist influences we add the three Kantian influences: that democracies will refrain from using force against other democracies; that economically important trade creates incentives to maintain peaceful relations; and that international organizations can constrain decision-makers by positively promoting peace.

Democracy. The first Kantian influence suggests that democracies will rarely fight or even threaten each other. Democracies may also be more peaceful with all kinds of states. Many studies support the first proposition. But the claim that democracies are more peaceful in general is much more controversial. Two plausible explanations for why democracies at least do not fight each other are as follows (Russett 1993).

One explanation is about norms. Democracies operate internally on the principle that conflicts are to be resolved peacefully by negotiation and compromise, without resort to the threat or use of organized violence. Democratic peoples and their leaders recognize other democracies as operating under the same principles in their internal relations, and so extend to them the principle of peaceful conflict resolution.[3] Negotiation and compromise between democratic states are expected, and the threat of violence is both unnecessary and illegitimate. Dictatorships, by contrast, are expected to operate more on Hobbesian principles, making threats, taking advantage of weak resolve, and using force. Thus dictatorships in their relations with dictatorships, or with democracies, will not be subject to the same restraints.

The other explanation is about institutions. Democratic leaders who fight a war are held responsible, through democratic institutions, for the costs and benefits of the war. The costs often outweigh the benefits, and many of the costs are borne by the general public. Democratic leaders who start wars risk being voted out of office—especially if they lose, or the war is long or costly. In anticipating this political judgment, democratic leaders will be reluctant to fight wars, especially wars they are likely to lose. When facing another democracy, both sets of leaders will be restrained. Dictators, however, are better able to repress opposition and to stay in power after a war. By repression they can keep more of the benefits and impose more of the costs on their peoples than can democratic leaders. So they may be less hesitant to fight anyone, either a democracy or another dictatorship.[4]

Likely both explanations operate, depending on circumstances. In our database, the measure of democracy incorporates several restraints on government, notably institutions and procedures through which citizens can express their preferences in truly competitive elections, and institutional constraints on the exercise of executive power. No democracy is perfect, nor are even the most totalitarian governments totally without restraints on arbitrary rule. Many states combine some mixture of democratic and authoritarian features. So we use information from the source cited in Figure 11.2, which ranks each country on a full scale of +10 to −10. An international conflict can result from the actions of either state. Nonetheless, the likelihood of conflict depends primarily on how undemocratic the less democratic state is. The greatest risk is between a dictatorship and a democracy, and the least between two highly democratic states.

International trade. Commercial interaction has a solid place among parents of the liberal tradition, as well as in Kant. Sustained commercial interaction becomes a medium of communication whereby information about needs and preferences are exchanged, across a broad range of matters ranging well beyond the specific commercial exchange. This may result in greater mutual understanding, empathy, and mutual identity across boundaries. A complementary view stresses the self-interests of rational actors. Trade depends on expectations of peace with the trading partner. Violent conflict endangers access to markets, imports, and capital. It may not make trade between disputing states impossible, but it certainly raises the risks and costs.

The larger the contribution of trade between two countries to their national economies, the stronger the political base that has an interest in preserving peaceful relations between them. We measure the importance of trade for each state in a dyad as the sum of its imports from and exports to the other state, divided by its gross national product (GDP). A given volume of trade will exert greater economic and political impact on a small country than on a big one. Similar effects can be expected from international investments.

International organizations. IGOs include both almost-universal organizations like the United Nations or the International Monetary Fund, and those focused on particular types of countries or regions. They may be multi-purpose, or "functional" agencies directed to specific goals like military security, promoting international commerce and investment, health, environmental concerns, or human rights. The means by which they may promote peace also vary greatly, on a range that may include separating or coercing norm-breakers (UN peacekeeping is an example), mediating among conflicting parties, reducing uncertainty by providing information, expanding members' material interest to be more inclusive and longer-term, shaping norms, and generating narratives of mutual identification. IGOs vary widely in effectiveness.

The network of international organizations is spread very unevenly across the globe. Some dyads in Europe share membership in over 100 IGOs; other dyads share few or even none (e.g., the United States and China during much of the cold war). Our measure is the number of IGOs to which both states in the dyad belong. This crude index equates all types and strengths of IGOs in a simple count. Using such a crude measure is likely to under-estimate the conflict-reducing effect of IGOs. Later we consider a more refined measure, taking into account the kind of countries which constitute IGOs' membership. Other refinements could consider the degree to which IGOs built strong institutions, or their different purposes.

Almost all of these influences are measured on scales. They propose, for example, that the more trade or democracy between countries the less chance they will fight each other. So these are probabilistic statements, not absolute or deterministic laws; for example, that democratic countries will never fight each other. International relations are not so simple.

Analyzing the global experience of a century

To uncover the relative importance of these various influences on the risk of interstate conflict we use a statistical technique like that employed by epidemiologists. It estimates the independent effect of a change in any one variable while holding the effect of all other variables constant. Analyses must minimize the danger of wrongly imputing causation. For example, trade may promote peace, but also peace may enhance trade. So one must get the sequencing right. Statistical methods cannot *prove* causation, but theory helps strengthen causal inference. After more than a decade of vigorous debate, many social scientists of international relations generally accept the following results.

Table 11.1 shows how much lower the risk of a fatal militarized dispute would be if the two countries were allied, or if both were both democratic, and so forth. It gives the percentage change in the risk associated with a change in each variable that might be affected by political action. (It controls for the effects of the "background" influences—geographical proximity and size—but does not show them because they are not readily affected by policy.) The percentages show the effect of changing the value of each separate influence, from what it would be if the dyad were at the average level for all states to the 90th percentile for that influence. This shows the relative impact of each one individually. Finally, we see the effect if all the Kantian influences were together at the 90th percentile. The changes shown here should not be taken as precise, but they do approximate those of other research. The average annual risk of a fatal dispute is about six in 1,000, meaning that most

TABLE 11.1 Percentage change in risk that a pair of countries will experience the onset of a fatal militarized dispute in any one year, 1886–2001

	Percent
Keep all influences at mean or median values, except:	
— Make the countries Allied	−9
— Increase Power ratio to the 90th percentile	−61
— Increase both Democracy scores to the 90th percentile	−43
— Increase higher Democracy score to 90th percentile, and decrease lower Democracy score to 10th percentile	+197
— Increase Trade/GDP to the 90th percentile	−56
— Increase number of IGO memberships to the 90th percentile	−31
— Increase Democracy, Trade, and IGOs together	−83

dyads avoid fatal disputes most of the time. But the risk varies substantially depending upon both realist and Kantian factors.

Unequal power generally does deter weak states from challenging strong ones. If the power of the stronger state is increased from a near-even balance to the 90th percentile of imbalance, the chance of a militarized dispute emerging is cut by 61 percent. But that demands a forty-fold growth in relative power. Since our measures include such basic determinants of power as population and industrial capacity, that big an increase is really unattainable for any nation. Alliance, the other realist influence, has little effect (9 percent) in reducing the risk of a fatal dispute.[5]

Although a Kantian perspective does not contest the influence of power, it predicts relationships that realist theory does not predict, and these predictions are confirmed. If both states are in the 90th percentile on the democracy scale rather at the average level, the risk of fatal violence conflict is much lower, by 43 percent. Disputes between very authoritarian states (both in the 10th percentile) are much more common: an increase of 39 percent from the average level. Conflicts are by far most likely if one state is in the 90th percentile and the other in the 10th one: a risk increase of almost 200 percent.[6] Economic interdependence also has a very strong effect. If both states are in the 90th percentile of trade dependence rather than in the middle, the chance of violent conflict goes down by more than half. In this analysis the effect of IGOs appears somewhat weaker, but still reduces risk by nearly a third when both states are in the 90th percentile. When all three influences operate together, they reduce the risk of a fatal dispute by 83 percent. This is strong support for Kant's liberal propositions.

We also tested whether Samuel Huntington's (1996) famous "clash of civilizations" thesis made a difference. Using his categorization of eight civilizations, we asked if dyads of countries from different civilizations were more likely to get into disputes than were those from the same civilization. The answer was no if the realist and Kantian influences were included—they did all the explanatory work, and differences in civilizations added nothing more. The same answer emerged when we asked whether disputes were especially likely between Islamic and Christian countries. The answer was no, both during the cold war years and the following years up through 2001. The clash of civilizations could become a self-fulfilling prophecy, but it had not yet done so.

The benefits of the Kantian variables are not just phenomena of the bipolar nuclear era of democratic capitalist states against their communist rivals. Similar relationships existed in the pre-cold war era, both before World War I and in the interwar years. Furthermore, they continued to operate in the post-cold war era after 1989.

Are democracies peaceful in general?

A dyadic perspective, however, does not tell us whether democracies, or even fully Kantian states, maintain more peaceful relations with all other states. In a world of countries with very different political and economic systems, they may still come into conflict with some of them. In fact, any statement that democracies are especially peaceful monadically (more peaceful in general) must be carefully qualified. A sweeping claim that democracies are peaceful in general ignores the dangers democracies face in the realm of power politics in an incompletely Kantian world. The dyadic claim by definition includes both the dynamics of domestic political interactions between leader and potential opposition, and the interactions between two independent states. The monadic claim completely ignores the latter.

One important refinement of the simple relationship arises as follows. Suppose that democratic states comprise only a small minority of states in the entire system. That was in fact true of the nineteenth and twentieth centuries until after the end of the cold war. Add to that some evidence that the most peaceful dyads are democracies with each other, with autocratic dyads being more conflict-prone and mixed dyads (democracies-autocracies) even more so. The combination of many mixed dyads in such a system and greatest hostility between mixed dyads means that the average difference in total conflict involvement by democracies and autocracies may appear slight. Perhaps we might see a stronger monadic effect in a system where democracies were a strong majority. We do know that geographical neighborhoods in which democracy is the predominant form of government are especially peaceful (Gleditsch 2002a).

Another big qualification concerns which side starts or escalates the fight, raising a largely peaceful diplomatic dispute up to a militarized one, or a low-level militarized dispute to full-scale war. Here the evidence is stronger: even when democracies are involved in diplomatic disputes with dictatorships they are less likely than the dictators to initiate the use of violence and less likely to escalate any violence to a high level (Huth and Allee 2002). Thus the dictator's action tends to produce the fight. Sometimes, however, great powers—even democratic ones—may take "preventive" military action to defeat potential challengers before they become big threats.

All great powers are war-prone. Their power and interests may draw them into fights far from home. They must rely on their own power to protect themselves. Small or weak states, however, can contribute little to the chance that a strong state will win a war. Thus small states have great incentive to free-ride on a big ally's military efforts. A big state, by contrast, can make all the difference for the survival of a weak one.

Moreover, great powers are less constrained by trade and IGOs. Mutual trade in a dyad less constrains the political system of the bigger state than of the smaller one, since that trade represents a lower percent of its GDP. For example, US-Guatemala trade is a 500 times larger share of Guatemala's GDP than of the US economy. Also, great powers depend less on regional or functional IGOs for their security than do many middle and smaller states. So the difference in total conflict involvement between democratic and autocratic great powers may be small. Just five countries—United States, United Kingdom, France, plus regional powers India and Israel—account for nearly 80 percent of the violent conflicts by democracies.

A similar pattern emerges for dictatorships, with the Soviet Union and China at the high end.

Finally, democratic political systems vary greatly in how, and how effectively, they can restrain their leaders (Geiss *et al.* 2006). Nor should one forget the influence of particular leaders' personalities and perspectives, such as a "we–versus–them" attitude or a belief that peace is served by forcibly transforming other states' regimes. Untangling this complex interplay of influences is necessary to comprehend why a monadic democratic peace may be hard to identify in a world that still contains many autocracies.

A self-perpetuating system?

This is only part of the Kantian perspective on world politics, which is about an interdependent system of influences, in a series of "feedback loops" with each of the major forces strengthening the other. This understanding is expressed in Figure 11.5, which appeared first in Chapter 8. The relationships so far discussed are represented by the arrows running from each of the apexes of the triangle toward the center, directly promoting peace. Reverse arrows run back from the center. Each represents a relationship that is supported by theory and some evidence. Democracy is easier to sustain in a peaceful environment. States in conflict with other states restrict information about government activities and limit public

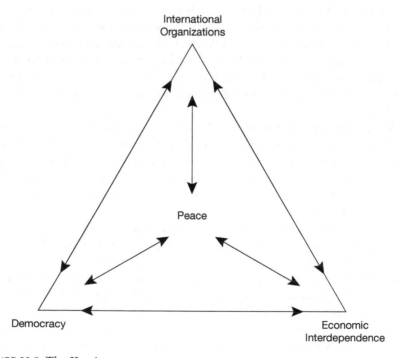

FIGURE 11.5 The Kantian system

criticism, but states at peace need fewer restraints on democracy. Trade and peace are reciprocally related. Traders are reluctant to trade with, or invest in, countries with which political relations may be disrupted at any time. While many IGOs are created to reduce or manage tensions between adversaries, most IGOs depend on peaceful relations among their members to be effective, and are most often formed when peace seems probable.

The arrows around the sides are also important. Along the base of the triangle, democracies trade more with each other, knowing that trade agreements are more likely to be kept, and foreign property rights respected, under a stable rule of law. In turn, trade typically promotes mutual prosperity, which contributes to the development and stability of democracy. Along the right side of the triangle, open trading systems require institutions and rules to make government and commercial actions predictable. In turn, the institutions encourage commerce by helping to lower barriers and resolving conflicts of interest.

The two arrows on the left indicate not only that democracies join and utilize international organizations, but that IGOs increasingly are involved in promoting democracy. Some of this activity is carried out by global organizations, notably the UN. Much more is done by regional organizations like the European Union, the Organization for Security and Cooperation in Europe, and the Organization of American States. These regional organizations are especially important because they are composed mostly of democracies. They possess a range of powerful carrots and sticks to attract new member states who want to become democratic, and to support member democratic governments against overthrow from within. IGOs composed mostly of democracies are also especially effective in maintaining peace among their members—even with whatever nondemocratic governments may be within the organization. They help to mediate conflicts, help governments make credible commitments to peace and democracy (by being able to apply sanctions against governments that would break their commitments), and socialize elites to norms of democratic practice and peace. At least half of the peace-promoting influence of all IGOs identified earlier can be attributed to the regional IGOs composed mostly of democracies. And they have an indirect impact on peace by promoting democracy—first down the left side of the triangle, and then from the democratic corner into the center (Pevehouse 2005; Pevehouse and Russett 2006).

Over the past sixty years this full set of influences has become an increasingly broad, deep, and stable set of relationships among many countries. It is most evident among the members of the European Union. The case study gives more detail. Yet it is not limited to the EU, also encompassing nearly all economically advanced democracies and many poorer democracies (most institutionalized in Latin America). Democracy cannot be created as rapidly in the Middle East as it was in Europe, Latin America, and parts of Asia with some democratic experience. Current governing elites will certainly resist it, and given the depth and endurance of bitter conflict, it is too much to expect new democracies there to be inherently peaceful, especially with Israel. But in the long run the peace and prosperity of the Kantian community can peaceably attract new governments and peoples.

CASE STUDY: THE EUROPEAN UNION

Sometimes a vicious circle of conflict and violence can be broken by deliberate policy. The most prominent reversal occurred in Western Europe after World War II. With tens of millions dead, their economies in shambles and cities in ashes, the new European leaders, including Konrad Adenauer, Alcide de Gasperi, Jean Monnet, and Robert Schuman, decided to break the old pattern. Informed by a set of classical liberal insights, they set up an intricate system of mutually reinforcing political, economic, and social elements, creating a set of virtuous circles to promote peace.

Democracy. They believed that the breakdown of democracy had played a key role in destroying peace. World War II could readily be blamed on authoritarian or totalitarian states, especially Germany, Japan, and Italy. So the initial task was to establish stable democratic institutions and to root out old nationalist and authoritarian ideologies. In this they were aided by the total defeat and discrediting of the old leaders (some of whom were executed for war crimes) and by institutional changes put in place by the allied occupation of western Germany.

Economic integration. Dictatorships had arisen largely because of the breakdown of the world economy in the 1930s and the Great Depression. Governments tried to protect their citizens' income by the competitive imposition of tariffs and other trade barriers. They preferred to preserve jobs at home rather than to import goods produced by foreign workers. This kind of economic policy has a basis in eighteenth-century practices of mercantilism, to strengthen a state's security by promoting exports, discouraging imports, and bringing an inflow of gold and foreign currency that the state could tap to build its power. In Germany, the Weimar Republic, established in 1918 after the forced abdication of Kaiser Wilhelm, was distrusted by supporters of the old autocratic system. Millions of Germans who were impoverished by unemployment and inflation in the 1930s turned away from democracy and toward Hitler, who promised prosperity and glory.

After World War II, Europe's new leaders understood that real prosperity would require the efficiencies of a market bigger than that of any one European country. A complex network of economic interdependence would underpin democracy, and also strengthen peace directly. War would be economically irrational: businessmen, companies, and workers would suffer, and would use their political power to oppose it.

Economic integration began with industries important to an economy's war potential. In 1951 the leaders formed the European Coal and Steel Community to ensure that Germany could not again turn its heavy industries into a war machine. A similar plan for the nuclear industry (Euratom) followed. American

continued

Case study: The European Union—continued

policy-makers supported integration. They insisted that Marshall Plan aid for European recovery from World War II be coordinated by a new institution, the Organization for European Economic Cooperation. That ultimately became global, as the Organization for Economic Cooperation and Development (OECD) with members around the world, including several newly industrialized countries.

International institutions. Economic interchange required organizations empowered to make rules that encouraged and protected it. All the benefits of free trade could not be achieved if member states had radically different labor or social policies. That meant dismantling regulatory barriers to free movement not just of goods, but of services, capital, and people. Then the legal gaps had to be filled by new regulations. Common environmental policies and health standards were needed so producers in countries with lax standards would not have a market advantage over those in countries with strict controls. Economic policies had to be coordinated, and fluctuations in the relative value of national currencies brought under control. One form of economic liberalization led to others. The European Common Market became the European Community and ultimately the European Union. At each stage the institutions assumed broader functions. The process was so successful that other countries wanted to join, in time bringing the EU to its current total of twenty-seven members.

The EU has some supranational powers (Moravcsik 1998). It collects taxes (called fees) from all its member states. The European Commission enforces a wide range of common regulations. The Council is an executive body where important decisions are made by a weighted-voting scheme, so that a small minority of Europe's population or countries cannot block action. The European Parliament is directly elected by the citizens of member states (though its powers are limited). The European Court of Justice settles conflicts between different institutions of the EU and takes referrals from states for the inter-pretation of EU regulations, and EU laws prevail over national ones. A non-EU institution, the European Court of Human Rights, has elaborated a bill of rights to which citizens may appeal against their national governments. Court rulings have required Britain to permit gays to serve in its military and to restrict the use of corporal punishment in its schools. With the achievement of the Economic and Monetary Union among some of the EU members on January 1, 1999, a European Central Bank took over in the vital area of fiscal and monetary policy.

Yet in many ways the EU acts as an intergovernmental body, with its member states retaining important elements of their traditional sovereignty.

continued

Case study: The European Union—continued

Despite some steps toward a limited European military force for crisis intervention, the member states still do not have a common foreign policy nor,
in significant form, common defense institutions (Howorth 2007). Citizens
feel loyal to their separate states and local units (like Scotland, or Catalonia)
as well as to Europe. But the system has produced stable peace among those
states—an extraordinary achievement compared with centuries of catastrophic
warfare.

All this began in the cold war, when the United States urged its allies to
be more integrated and thus stronger. However, integration outlasted the cold
war, expanded far beyond the initial cold war allies, and became far deeper.
Growth rates for democracy and IGOs in Europe were similar to those for the
world in Figure 11.3, from starting points about twice as high. Intra-European
trade started lower than for the world, but its growth rate was very much
higher. Europe's experience shows how virtuous circles can solidify peaceful
relations while states retain many of their traditional characteristics.

That does not mean it will inevitably include all states in the system, or that
the process cannot be reversed. A severe economic shock, like a global depression,
could reverse its momentum. The immediate effect would be felt in trade and
finance, which, magnified by a rise in protectionist policies, would sharply weaken
economic restraints on international conflict. International organizations would
find it harder to defend free trade, and democratic governments could fall—as
they did during the depression of the 1930s. All this could lead to greater
international conflict and war, continued deterioration in economic conditions
and international institutions, and a feedback reversal of the world's hard-won gains.
An economic downturn could also be started by major war or really massive terrorist
attacks. Nonetheless, the system now has a great deal of institutional and normative
resistance built into it.

The continuity and stability in this system suggests another way to think about
how these restraints work—by changes in the international system as a whole. Global
increases in the average level of democracy, interdependence, and IGO involvement
represent not just what is happening to pairs of states that share those characteristics, but to the dominant norms and institutions of the whole system. States at
the low end on these characteristics may be peacefully induced, by threats or rewards,
to observe international norms. Even dictatorships can find it in their interest to
do so. (Libya's renunciation of nuclear weapons in 2003 was achieved by
negotiation rather than by military action.)

The world is not as Hobbesian as in previous eras. It was once common for
aggressors simply to eliminate states. Twenty-two internationally recognized states

were forcibly occupied or absorbed during the first half of the twentieth century, but no state has permanently lost its sovereignty through external conquest since World War II. Democracies with democratic neighbors feel less threatened. When democracies fight dictatorships they usually fight well—winning nearly 80 percent of all their wars, and more than 90 percent of those they choose to start (Reiter and Stam 2002). So as the proportion of democracies in the international system grows, autocracies must be more concerned about weakening themselves in war. If most great powers become democratic, peace among them would reduce the incentive for wars with nondemocratic states across great power spheres of influence. If international norms and institutions for resolving disputes grow, even nonliberal states may be impelled to use regional or international organizations to help settle their disputes rather than accept the political and economic costs the liberal community could impose on them for using force.

Promoting order in anarchy

This analysis has implications for a particularly dangerous and important pair of countries: the United States and China. First, we can calculate the mid-1960s risk factors for a fatal dispute from all the influences at that time. The two countries were not geographically close or contiguous, reducing the risk. But since both were big powers, with wide interests and power projection capability, that raised the risk. America was predominant in power over China, but not hugely so, implying a moderate risk. None of the Kantian influences helped reduce the risk. Mao's China was very totalitarian on the political scale (–9). US–China trade was nil; as were shared IGO memberships (China was not even in the UN).

By comparison, some influences at the beginning of the twenty-first century were still unchanged: same geographical location, both great powers. But with the very rapid growth of China's economy relative to that of the United States, the power ratio had moved substantially closer to equality: a dangerous development by our analysis. However, all the liberal Kantian influences had come into play. China had liberalized somewhat, moving from up to –7 on the political scale. Chinese-American trade flourished. Their trade is a smaller part of the US GDP than of China's—but even the US trade/GDP ratio is in the 90th percentile. Finally, they now share membership in many IGOs. China is in virtually all the universal organizations, and in many smaller functional and North Pacific regional organizations to which the United States also belongs. On this basis we can revise the risk factors. Even controlling for the more dangerous power balance, we find more than a 50 percent reduction in risk under current conditions from what it was in the 1960s.

Engagement is working. Yet its success cannot be assumed, and some elements of deterrence remain. China's political liberalization lags appreciably. Demands for democratization may be brutally suppressed once again or, alternatively, get explosively out of hand. Major environmental degradation may create extensive political and economic problems. Finally, the status of Taiwan remains a major threat to peace, requiring careful statesmanship by China, Taiwan, and the United States. A big war between the world's two biggest powers would be a tragedy, but it is not impossible.

Some countries, though not all, do learn to live peaceably with each other despite a centuries-long history of violent competition. There is order to be discerned and nurtured within the anarchy. The assumption that everyone is a potential enemy, not anarchy itself, is what drives the Hobbesian security dilemma. Many countries can and do get along with many others, rarely threatening to use military force. They operate substantially by principles of negotiation and compromise, in an order of cooperation and reciprocation broadly consistent with basic precepts of moral behavior. This kind of order does not demand a moral transformation of humanity so much as it requires a careful structuring of relationships to channel self-interest in directions of mutual benefit.

Of course, not all states are at present part of this order. Those not bound by mutual ties of democracy, economic interdependence, and international institutions have a much weaker basis for cooperation. Where Kantian linkages are still weak, the Hobbesian dilemma may remain (perhaps with Iran and North Korea). Yet even with such states more stable relationships may be created, perhaps stumblingly, as in the early days of US–China relations.

Conclusion: power, hegemony, and liberalism

The United States is sometimes described as hegemonic, with the burdens, benefits, and temptations dominance implies. It does not always behave as a Kantian state. With military spending nearly as great as all the rest of the world, it is tempted to rely on the armed force that money and high technology create. But hegemony cannot last forever. A Kantian liberal perspective on world politics can provide means for sustaining a stable peace when military advantage fades. Promoting democracy (but rarely imposing it by force, and then only in response to aggression), deepening linkages of international trade, and extending the multilateral network of IGOs offers the possibility of strengthening existing peaceful relations and expanding their scope to most of the world. Doing so depends less on the material elements of power than on soft power, on perceptions that the United States is acting on legitimate principles and following agreed rules. Doing so can serve both American interests and those of many other states and peoples.

Being the strongest power in the world does not mean being able to dictate all the important political, military, or economic outcomes. Moreover, predominant power can stimulate a "balancing" reaction against itself. Fear of domination is an obvious motivation, but for other members of the Kantian community it is probably less important than distrust of American judgment and behavior. Many Europeans do not fully trust Americans to act according to Kantian principles of negotiation and compromise. Nevertheless, a power-balancing alliance cannot easily be formed. Europe is not yet ready to act as a single foreign policy actor. Because of the great gap in power between the United States and even the biggest second-tier states, any such alliance would require many members. That raises the problem of collective action among members of an alliance without a strong leader, and consequently the temptation for each member to pursue its separate interests.

This "free-riding" problem existed even in the great cold-war alliance epitomized by NATO. Indeed, NATO's success in deterring the outbreak of conflict in Europe was a direct cause of its collective goods problem. So long as the US nuclear deterrent seemed reliable, other NATO members had little incentive to contribute large forces of their own. Consequently the US spent twice as large a percentage of its GDP on defense than the average of all other NATO members (Russett 1970: ch. 4). This suggests the difficulty of achieving common action when collaboration might be in the common interest.

Incentives to free-ride on international security continue. The more US policy in the "war" against terrorism seems unwise, or in the narrow interest of the United States and a very few of its allies, the more other states will resist it. Some may not want to be protected as the Americans intend. Others, especially European states, have conflicting interests. One is the demographic and economic pressures that limit their willingness to spend on defense rather than care for aging populations. Another is the presence of tens of millions of poorly assimilated Islamic workers and their families. The incentives to avoid doing anything that might inflame Islamic sentiments are very real. All this implies the possibility of an inadequate response to global terrorism. Yet a broad US defeat, abetted by the indifference of other states, could bring down the whole global economy and Kantian system.

This chapter is not about predictions, but about possibilities. Democratic liberties can be debased, the inequalities of capitalism may run wild, a global authority could become a leviathan, peace does not always mean justice. Nor can we take for granted the continued growth of liberal influences. Real people—leaders, elites, voters—make choices. They can discover constructive patterns of behavior and act accordingly. We are not condemned to choose between being passive victims and being caught in endless cycles of violence. Openings exist for actions that can be other-regarding while still self-interested. In the daylight we can see Hobbes's realist vision as the nightmare it is, and Kant's liberal one as the partial reality it has become.

Notes

1   Trade is controlled for inflation and graphed as the natural log of trade increase to approximate its impact in an expanding global economy.
2   The sources, definitions, and decisions needed to turn concepts and hypotheses into measures for statistical analysis are discussed in a comprehensive report (Russett and Oneal, 2001), and more recent results are in Pevehouse and Russett (2006).
3   MacMillan (1998) discusses liberal pacifism as an evolving tradition.
4   This is basically the argument of Bueno de Mesquita et al. (2003); also see Rousseau (2005). A different and also plausible argument about democratic institutions is that by permitting open debate before using force or concluding international agreements a democracy's commitments become more credible to both friends and adversaries. See Lipson (2003) and Schultz (2001).

5 The effect of alliances is not statistically significant, but all the other percentages are highly significant, meaning that the odds that the sign should be the opposite from what we find are less than one in 1,000.

6 Mansfield and Snyder (2005) continued to narrow their earlier claim that states in transition from autocracy toward democracy are war-prone, limiting it to incomplete transitions far short of full democracy when combined with other conditions such as weak central authority. Even so, wars fitting their causal model are extremely rare, almost non-existent in the twentieth century (Narang and Nelson, 2009).

12

NO CLEAR AND PRESENT DANGER

A skeptical view of the United States' entry into World War II

Preface to the 1971 edition

It has been a long trip, and is not yet complete. Nevertheless I have come far enough to want to give a report on the vivid scenery to be viewed from this prospect. I began, as a child in World War II, with a firm hatred of the Axis powers and a conviction that America was fighting for its very existence. After the war, Stalinist Russia merely replaced Hitlerite Germany as the insatiable aggressor. With most Americans I accepted without much question the need for active resistance to Communism, and the necessity that such resistance would often have to be military in character. Though as a young scholar I did become very concerned about arms control and the risks of nuclear war, my faith in the requirement for military assistance to threatened members of the Free World remained essentially unshaken. I was fairly hawkish on Vietnam, and saw only in early 1967 that the war had been a mistake. In retrospect, I am not proud of having taken so long. Even then, I considered that the sole mistake was having chosen a conflict where the essential conditions of victory were absent.

In the past few years, however, I have slowly begun to question my earlier easy assumptions. Once some began to fall, others became far less tenable. Here really was a row of intellectual dominoes. If Vietnam was unnecessary or wrong, then where else? How distorted were our images of the origins of the cold war? What has been the role of economic interests in promoting foreign involvements by the United States government?

This is an exciting time in which to be a scholar. Some of these questions were forced on me directly by observing events; others were in substantial part impelled by the questioning of students who had been less thoroughly indoctrinated in the cold war myths than I, and thus rejected them more easily. In this reexamination I am, of course, not alone. Many Americans of all generations have come to question their former assumptions. Still, the results differ among us. I find the New Left's emphasis on foreign investment and trade interests to be stimulating and overdue; in the anti-Communist hysteria of the first cold war decades such matters were all too thoroughly ignored. Nevertheless I am still unconvinced that such influences should be elevated to the role of a primary explanation, and while in this book I sometimes suggest their relevance to pre-World War II policy preferences I do not emphasize them. But I am interested in the work of others on these questions, and consider them with a mind more open than before.

And although there are finally some rumblings on the New Left, and occasionally elsewhere, about the propriety of American participation in World War II, they have yet to surface much in public. The situation is curious. A few writers, I among them, challenged the prevailing interpretation about war with Japan some time ago (Russett 1967), but with little impact beyond a small circle of professional scholars. Participation in the war against Hitler remains almost wholly sacrosanct, nearly in the realm of theology. Yet it seems to me that many of the arguments against other wars can also be applied, with somewhat less force, to this one too. Hence I came to rethink, and to write while still in the process of rethinking.

Preface to the twenty-fifth anniversary edition (1996)

Re-publication of a controversial book allows the author, as well as readers, the opportunity to look both backward and forward. Looking backward offers a chance to root the text in the author's personal intellectual biography and in the context of the particular historical period and place in which the book was written. How reasonable, given that context and subsequent developments, was the argument? How might the argument have been presented differently, and how well has it held up? However one might judge it flawed, did it say something that was worth hearing at the time? Looking forward presents the chance to wonder whether elements of the argument, recognizable as such though perhaps not stated clearly or explicitly then, have something useful to say about contemporary world politics and the conditions we might reasonably expect to apply in the coming years. Both the backward and the forward look ask, in effect, does this book still have legs?

To permit a useful discussion, we must begin with the text itself. We reprint it here without any changes. Both the main body of the book and the original preface are untouched; even typographical errors have been left alone. What you see now is what you got then.

This was a controversial book, and likely remains so. It is clearly a brash book by a then relatively youthful scholar (age 35 when the writing was completed at the end of 1970). Being older now should make me more sensitive to the negative reactions that the book could be expected to elicit from many readers and that I might have anticipated and at least partly avoided. Yet if "mature caution" had overridden "youthful folly," preventing me from writing the book at all, it might not have been for the better.

First, where did the book come from in my personal history? As I stated clearly in the original preface, it stemmed from my experience, as a scholar of American foreign policy, of the Vietnam War. Published at the height of the war, it originated from my disgust and represented my effort to understand why the war had happened and persisted. I believed then, and still do, that such standard interpretations as bureaucratic inertia on Pennsylvania Avenue, economic interest on Wall Street, or anticommunist ideology on Main Street, constituted at best partial explanations that missed a broader kind of ideological underpinning. I would characterize that ideological underpinning as a particular kind of "realist" view of international power politics that exaggerated both the necessity and the possibility of effectively exerting American military power all over the globe.[1] A shorthand label for such a view now comes under the expression "imperial overstretch." And I believe that view was, for many Americans, born out of the experience of World War II.

World War II was in many ways a "good war," in that it had many desirable outcomes that by my Western perspectives on human rights and democracy represent the "just cause" associated with the normative criteria for a just war. It destroyed Nazi and fascist power in Europe—perhaps forever. Although the victory over Nazism came too late to save millions of victims from Hitler's racist viciousness, it at least prevented the accumulation of millions of additional victims. It permitted the institution of democratic governments in the former Axis states and allowed for their subsequent admission into a peaceful Western community. Arguably it set in motion the events and policies that led first to the containment and ultimately to the collapse of Soviet power. If so, it was the first step toward the creation of a globe-straddling community of democratic and economically interdependent states. These are impressive if partly unforeseen gains that would make the human costs of the war more than "proportionate."

Furthermore, I accept most of this evaluation as essentially correct, with the exception of the weakening of Soviet power. That might equally have been achieved by the German army, perhaps in some sort of grinding stalemate. Would that have been preferable to the Soviet victory in the East, with its creation of a somewhat different list of millions of innocent victims? It is hard for me to find much to like either way. A recognizable cold war with the Axis—maybe even ultimately a hot one—seems probable from a stalemate outcome as well. It is also possible that, with a stalemate, the United States would have emerged even earlier as the world's single superpower.

My point then was not that the outcome of World War II was on balance undesirable—far from it. But it was not quite the clear-cut good outcome that some observers assumed. Some results that would have been good were not achieved, and some results that were bad by most people's standards were not avoided and were even magnified. Even with such a strong effort by the most powerful country on earth (the United States), the ability to reshape the post-World War II world in desirable directions was limited. To think about alternative outcomes (e.g., what if the United States had avoided overt military participation) is an exercise in "counterfactual" reasoning, trying in hypothetical fashion to imagine what difference such a decision would have made in a historical process that of course cannot be remade except in some imagined alternative universe. It can become merely a parlor game. Or, if carried on in disciplined fashion, it can become an illuminating if always inconclusive intellectual exercise (Tetlock and Belkin 1996).

The fundamental problem with the World War II experience—rightly judged in some degree to be a success—was, in my view, that it led to an exaggerated sense of American power and wisdom; *hubris*, in effect. It seemed such a success that the limits and the particular circumstances of that success were ignored in subsequent policy. And that hubris led to the intervention in Vietnam, a military expedition for which the motivation and the need were far less clear than in World War II. Consequently, the national will for a total commitment in Vietnam was, properly, lacking, and thus the prospects for that intervention were poor. In other words, the construction put upon the World War II experience was an invitation to subsequent failure; to understand that failure, and to avoid repeating it, required some deconstruction of World War II's lessons. It required speculating about whether active American participation in the war could have been avoided, and if so, what the costs and benefits of such an alternative might have been. It was a task for historical evaluation as well as a practically oriented form of theoretical discussion. So I entered the lions' den with this book. (Perhaps it was no coincidence that we named our son, born while I was gestating this book, Daniel.)

In writing it, I hoped to contribute to bridging two sets of critics of the Vietnam War and the overstretched policies that underlay it. One set was of course the left, the extremely heterogeneous and vociferous critics of the war. I considered myself to be of the moderate left, "progressive" but never "Marxoid." But I did not believe that a sufficiently large or stable coalition against those policies could be put together from the left alone. Another audience, therefore, was that subset of libertarians who disliked big government and were prepared to be critical not just of its domestic role but of the expansive foreign policy attributable to the "military-industrial complex" and many of its conservative allies. Since there were also big differences between these two groups (the left and some libertarians), especially on domestic policy, this was not an easy coalition to put together. And it never really was built. Still, it pleased me that this book did find receptive audiences in both groups.

What I did not welcome was one other group sympathetic to a message they mistakenly took from the book—the supposed message that "Hitler was not so bad after all." This group, often expressing thinly disguised anti-semitism, was not part of my target audience. Here perhaps youth and ignorance cost me; I should have been more emphatic, in the book, in disavowing such views and such possible company.

So much for retrospect. Does the book have legs for contemporary policy? The world twenty-five years later looks quite different. With the end of the cold war, the United States is, in the cliche, now the world's only superpower. If this country cannot shape the international system and bring peace and stability to much of the world, surely no other state can. Yet the will to create a broadly internationalist foreign policy, and in some degree the objective means to support it as well, cannot currently be found in the United States. The near-consensus that ranged across foreign policy elites before the Vietnam War has never been restored, in any form. Maybe that's just as well. But I hold to much of the basic perspective of this book as offering some guidance for fellow "cooperative internationalists." The power to shape international affairs is limited; military intervention is a costly, blunt, and dangerous instrument. The five questions I ask on page 108 of the 1996 edition remain appropriate—even though the answers to them must in every case be contested and uncertain.

I do believe there are appropriate circumstances for military action in international affairs, and it is somewhat easier to evaluate those circumstances from the vantage of an additional quarter-century of superpower experience. In most circumstances I do not believe that it is desirable, effective, or just to try to spread democracy or other American values by force of arms. I believe, however, that much more could be done, by way of financial assistance as well as consistent ideological and technical support, to create a more democratic and interdependent environment within which peace can be secured (Russett 1993).

There is a great need for an active, engaged American foreign policy. Isolationism is not viable. Yet given the limits of American power and wisdom, an engaged policy has to be conducted in a multilateral framework, informed by criticisms as well as agreement from other countries, and carried out with their active cooperation in multilateral institutions. If the Vietnam War derived in substantial part from an overconfident and unilateral interpretation of history, that is a mistake from which we can still learn. If this book still has even short legs, that's the original lesson I hope they support.

Note

1 Subsequently, working in the mode of empirical social scientist rather than essayist, I found substantial evidence for this evaluation (Russett and Hanson 1975).

13

DEMOCRACY, HEGEMONY, AND COLLECTIVE ACTION

> Think . . . of the great part that is played by the unpredictable in war: think of it now, before you are actually committed to war. The longer a war lasts, the more things tend to depend on accidents. Neither you nor we can see into them; we have to abide their outcome in the dark. And when people are entering upon a war they do things the wrong way round. Action comes first, and it is only when they have already suffered that they begin to think.[1]

The great power disparity emphasized in Chapter 1 shows that American hegemony still remains in substantial degree, though it is also under significant strains that seem likely to weaken it as the twenty-first century continues. Serious threats to its continuation exist. This chapter gives a partial overview of a huge topic. Many questions are inherent in the political and economic constraints under which efforts to retain hegemonic status must operate. The first section of the chapter raises some big questions about the conditions for sustaining systems in general, and the second section asks more specifically about what particular economic and political conditions (including democracy) in the hegemonic state affect that state's ability to maintain its leading role. Both categories include a range of questions including the following, often with ambiguous or conditioned answers.

- Does hegemony lead to peace and cooperation, or to violent conflict?
- Does hegemony encourage collaboration against common threats, or free-riding by weak allies who are protected by the hegemon's power?
- What is the role of "softer" economic power in managing hegemony?
- What conditions affect the hegemon's ability to sustain its own productivity?
- How may democracy support or undermine a hegemonic foreign policy?
- In turn, how may hegemony support or undermine democratic governance?

Further sub-questions are embedded in each of those above.

Is hegemony sustainable internationally?

Hegemony and the balance of power

Does hegemony bring greater peace and cooperation, or greater violent conflict? Since the end of the cold war in 1989 there have been no fatal militarized disputes between big powers (China, France, Germany, India, Japan, Russia, Britain, USA), whereas in the preceding forty years fatal disputes between such states were relatively common, and included several major wars and near-wars.[2] If American hegemony has reduced interstate violence in the world, the strongest effect is on relations among the great powers. Even there, however, it is hard to give too much credit to hegemony, given that six of the eight big powers are democracies, and the wider and deeper disincentives that other Kantian influences (commerce and IGOs) have provided during the past two decades.

Hegemony may deter some violent conflicts but not others. Statistical tests of the effect of the largest state's share of power in the international system on the overall frequency of militarized disputes (fatal or otherwise) in the system show no relationship over the past 125 years (Russett and Oneal 2001; Bennett and Stam 2004; Oneal 2006). This test can't be definitive, however, since the international system did not previously experience a hegemony as strong as that of the United States in recent decades.

Some answers emerge in debates about whether a balance or a predominance of power serves best to deter conflict, and how that plays into specific kinds of international conflict. One side of that debate claims that predominance deters the outbreak of violence, by providing a high level of certainty about the probable outcome of a war. By this reasoning, the weaker state would be deterred from provoking a conflict that it would likely lose, and the strong state, knowing its superiority is recognized, usually will not actually need to use military force in order to get its way. This perspective on high certainty about the outcome as deterring the outbreak of violence is found, for example, in the realist analysis of Wohlforth (1999). It is also consistent with power transition theory as discussed in Chapter 7 of this book, when a challenger catches up to the dominant power and threatens to surpass it. The transitional years, when the power balance is close and the power trajectory and intentions of the challenger are uncertain, are said to increase the likelihood of war. These theories about the dangers of power balance are directly opposed to Waltz's (1979) version of realism that regards a balance of power and consequent uncertainty about the outcome of a war as deterring both sides from taking the risk of using force.

Most systematic empirical research supports Wohlforth's version, with by far the strongest risk of conflict being close to the point of equal power (Russett and Oneal 2001; Oneal 2006). Yet this conclusion, based largely on the frequency of MIDs rather than wars, needs to be qualified because militarized disputes short of war can be seen as tests of adversaries' power and determination in a developing crisis of deterrence. Competing states of somewhat equal power may gain important

information from threats, force deployments, and minor skirmishes. That information can reduce uncertainty and thus avoid escalation to a real war. Also, the
expected cost of war, not just the balance of power, must be considered. Power
disparities may not prevent war if the stronger state thinks it can cripple or eliminate a potential rival at low cost. But if war looks technically "winnable" yet sure
to be very costly even to the prospective victor (e.g., conventional or nuclear war
to Europeans after the experience of World War II; general nuclear war to the
United States against the Soviet Union) the stronger power as well as the weaker
one is likely to be restrained.

Precisely this concern was at the heart of nuclear deterrence theory about first-
and second-strike capabilities. If both states have nuclear forces capable of surviving a first strike and retaliating, the expected cost of war to both is very high,
and both may be deterred. But if one side is weaker in a key aspect—vulnerability
to a first strike—its adversary may see conducting a first strike as a low-cost option.
This situation can emerge when a powerful nuclear-armed state suspects a small
state of having nuclear weapons or becoming capable of acquiring them. A
"preventive" war by the powerful state to eliminate that possibility may seem
to be a low-cost option. To the degree that members of the George W. Bush
administration truly believed in 2006 that Iraq had or was close to having weapons
of mass destruction, that might have been a powerful motivation.[3]

Hegemony may have different consequences when it arises from a deliberate
design for power rather than a sudden and dramatic shift in the balance of power.
The latter situation developed when Germany and Japan were defeated and
disarmed following World War II. European states, including the victorious United
Kingdom, were devastated and drained, though the Soviet Union was able to establish imperial control over Eastern Europe. The United States was left as the world's
greatest economic and military superpower, and hegemon of the "West."[4] While
strong economic and political forces in the United States welcomed the opportunity for expansion, arguably the more powerful motivation was to preserve the
new status quo in the face of an emergent threat from the Soviet Union.[5] This
was consistent with the containment policy—waiting for the eventual decay of the
Soviet threat—advocated by George Kennan. The United States settled into a largely
defensive posture resisting regime change on its side of the Iron Curtain but not
actively seeking rollback or regime change on the other side. Yet mere containment
was always contested by Americans with more ambitious aims, and the fear and
often the exaggeration of communist power meant that a status quo hegemon could
not always be distinguished from a revisionist one. The Sino-Soviet rift in the 1950s
ultimately led to Nixon's opening to China, a too-good-to-resist opportunity for
a permanent shift in the global balance of power. During the Reagan administration,
US assistance to insurgencies in communist-controlled states, most notably
Afghanistan, did seek to roll back Soviet gains.

The collapse of the "evil empire" in 1989 made American hegemonic status
incontestable. Emergence of the threat from radical Islam, especially with the 9/11
attack, provided the impetus to shift from merely defending the status quo to policies

of preventive war and regime change. The temptation to over-reach is built into any great power, and especially so for a hegemon. A superpower able to intervene widely may see distant events as dangerous not just in themselves but as likely to trigger similar behavior in nearer and more important areas. Great military power then gives the apparent ability both to put down immediate threats and to discourage subsequent ones from emerging. Some of the currency of power thus needs to be spent, not just hoarded. But what happens if the currency becomes devalued, both in reality (military power truly is over-stretched) and in the perceptions of friends as well as foes?[6]

This brief review brings mixed results. Hegemony may reduce the chances of a war between big powers and deter many smaller powers from threatening others. The hegemon is nevertheless likely to become an enforcer of peace, sometimes by an act of so-called preventive war against a regionally revisionist power. Over-reach is a danger.

Hegemony and collective action

Does hegemony encourage collaboration against common threats, or instead does it encourage free-riding by weak allies who are protected by the hegemon's power? Hegemony raises the problem of collective action to provide collective goods, which is a frequent problem in international relations. Theories about public and private goods predict incentives for smaller powers to free-ride on the leading power or hegemon, but also difficulties in cooperating with other small powers in actively balancing against the biggest power. Thus a collective goods perspective gives intellectually rigorous insights into the competing realist claims about balancing versus bandwagoning in the presence of a dominant power. This question appeared early in Chapter 1, again frequently in subsequent chapters, and applies in several ways here. The Kantian Peace in part constitutes an alternative to such realist views, but it too is illuminated by propositions about the difficulty of collective action.

Nation-states often engage in cooperative behavior to secure public goods. As noted earlier, public goods are those for which the supply of the good to one actor does not diminish the supply to others, and for which it is hard to exclude particular actors from the benefit. Examples include protecting the regional or global environment, founding trade cartels to restrict production and thus raise prices, applying economic or military sanctions against a common adversary, or forming a military alliance for joint security.[7]All such activities, however, create incentives for members to break the group policy for "private" gain; that is, to pollute, to exceed production quotas, to sell covertly to the adversary, or to save on the military budget.

Promoting common action is difficult because in the real world of international relations there are few pure public goods. Most are impure because neither of the conditions is fully met. Deterrence, for example, may be a relatively pure good. During the cold war, United States nuclear forces were designed to deter the Soviet Union from attacking North America, but with only relatively minor additions and modifications they could also deter a Soviet attack on Western Europe—though still at a substantial risk to the United States. However, defense, as in holding territory against invasion, is more mixed. Large forces can be deployed to provide some protection to all members, yet defense must always be somewhat selective. There can never be enough forces to defend all territory and borders equally, so some states will be more at risk and perhaps need to spend more for their own defense.

The problem is most acute in groups where one or two members are very large and many are very small, and where institutions able to promote or even compel payment of dues or taxes are weak. Small states have the greatest incentive to undercontribute, since proportionately they can gain more by violating the norms and yet continue to receive most of the collective good provided by the big states. The more actors, and the smaller many of them are, the more acute collective goods problems are likely to be. The larger the group, the harder it is to negotiate, monitor, and enforce commitments to cooperate. Big alliances may limit the opportunities for direct observation of members' behavior, and dilute pressures for conformity to norms typical of small group behavior. Free-riding on the hegemon means that smaller states will underspend on many collective goods like defense, or environmental protection, and the largest will spend more. Together, these effects tend to produce suboptimal effort overall; that is, less than the total amount all the states might spend as unallied individuals. Yet suboptimal in NATO was good enough, which can be interpreted as a success. The smaller states believed that the alliance really was providing enough deterrence, and that they did not need to spend more.

Strong international institutions can mitigate the free-riding problem, by creating an organizational culture of collaboration, making the size of national contributions more visible, and perhaps making commitments legally enforceable. Strong institutions have another advantage. To the degree they succeed in their ostensible goals, they may attract new member states. These may be states that would not initially have wished to join or did not expect a welcome, but subsequently found themselves falling behind and no longer able to carry on alone. Similarly, even member states that have gained much less than they hoped from the institution may still be better off than if they were to secede—assuming secession is permitted (Gruber 2000).

Both the EU and NATO have shown continuing great ability to expand their membership, and no member has permanently left the alliance. Beginning in 1959 president Charles de Gaulle did withdraw all French military forces from NATO's joint command, and ordered all other NATO troops to leave France. Nevertheless, France retained its membership in the alliance, with planning and cooperation in a wide range of military activities, and it returned to the joint command in 2009. Greece left in 1974 but returned in 1980. No country has left the EU either, and even some states whose economies have suffered from adopting the euro have found the costs of returning to their own currency unacceptable. Members of the IMF, the World Trade Organization, and the World Bank do not leave.

Even in strong institutions, small states may try to make just enough effort to keep the largest engaged in their own security, and perhaps to influence its policy.

They may pursue private security goods not sought by the hegemon (e.g., in NATO Portugal had high military spending to pay for its colonial wars; Greece and Turkey to deter each other in ways not provided by NATO). Small states may not entirely trust the hegemon, nor always want what purports to be the collective good because it brings private bads. For example, open cooperation in a "war against terror" may draw fire to cooperating countries, enflame their own Islamic populations, and weaken their ties to Arab oil suppliers. States may limit their exposure to such risks by avoiding participation in overt military action, yet still cooperate through covert acts like sharing intelligence with allies. Information from friends has in fact proved of great importance to the United States. A hegemon therefore may enlist greater cooperation by limiting its demands for cooperation to those actions that are most acceptable to its partners.

Different states make different kinds of contributions, not readily measurable in a single metric of manpower, munitions, or money. Norms about what is a fair share are always subjective and contested. "For more than half a century NATO members have been more or less continually at odds on how the costs and risks . . . should be apportioned . . . just about every member believes it is doing more than its fair share while the others are not"(Thies 2009: 19). Kagan (2002) makes some good points about Kantian Europeans' continuing ability to shelter under US realist hard power in the post-cold war environment. Yet that may actually lead to a useful division of labor. The United States typically does the nasty part of forcible intervention and the Europeans do more of the heavy lifting on human rights, peacekeeping, and development. This pattern is evident both within particular operations (in Afghanistan, and largely so in the former Yugoslavia) and in the choice of operations in which to participate. Together, both sides may benefit from the more benign image of democracy (and economic and institutional integration) that is projected by Europe.

The United States and European countries are of course not the only ones attempting to increase their influence globally. Both China and Japan have developed careful strategies for influence through soft power. Both—like many other states—direct their foreign trade, aid, and investment to serve political as well as economic aims. For example, Japan has long used such enticements to help its effort to obtain a seat on the UN Security Council, and China to procure votes to deny membership for Taiwan in the UN and other IGOs. As for less overt exercises of soft power, Japan's effort is less politically centralized and more diverse than China's, and that may make it more attractive. Japan's use of hard power is still hobbled by constitution and memory (though less than in previous decades), while China's hard power is more evident in fact (naval buildup in big ships, numbers, and deployment) if not in rhetoric, and is being noticed. Despite the attractiveness of China's far more impressive growth rate, the costs of that growth (environmental, and in political freedoms) are more evident to those who yearn for transparent and accountable political systems.[8]

In the full international system, lack of balancing may be a result of collective action phenomena. If opposition to a hegemon requires the cooperation of several smaller states to provide sufficient weight, the multiple "allies" may not be able to fully depend on each other not to defect. So forming and sustaining a balancing coalition is hard (Brooks and Wohlforth 2008). Insofar as the hegemon's influence depends less on military power and more on the soft power of common culture and norms, smaller states may feel less need to balance against it. Peacefully promoting democracy, for example, may be an attractive aspect of soft power. (Soft, that is, to those who like it, but not benign to states and leaders who fear democracy and especially that a democratic regime will be imposed from outside).

Overall, incentives to free-ride favor the hegemon by inhibiting collective power-balancing against it, especially if most other states see the hegemon as a fundamentally nonthreatening user of soft power and general provider of collective goods. Within an alliance or coalition for collective action, strong institutions may promote burden-sharing and partially offset incentives to free-ride on the hegemon.

Economic power

What is the role of "softer" economic power in managing hegemony? To be legitimate, a hegemon's power needs to be perceived as defending values shared by other countries. But cultural and economic hegemony brings an ability both to satisfy and to threaten others' interests. Economic power, and specifically the power of capitalism in global competition, can bring both prosperity to winners and poverty to losers, satisfaction to those who have new cultural values and frustration to those who hold old ones. A Kantian perspective sees commerce as a builder of interests and norms for peace, but not everyone regards capitalism as a relatively benign source of soft power.[9] If free-market capitalism is a constructive force, it constructs by destroying the entrenched interests and cultures that obstruct it. For a hegemonic power with a need to be perceived as restrained in its exercise that is a problem.

Certainly economic strength can provide means to coerce others, or to resist their coercion. Economic power may come close to hard power in the area of financing international debt. The weakness of some deeply indebted European countries has limited their real sovereignty to resist very strict reforms and retrenchment imposed by other European states and bankers. Fears have been expressed that China, with its vast holdings of US government securities, might someday challenge United States foreign policy by threatening to dump those debt instruments onto the market, undermining the American economy and government finance. Perhaps more plausibly, the "too-big-to-fail" phenomenon means that China would be shooting itself in the foot.

Here too the United States is in a stronger position than is often realized. Its GDP, adjusted for purchasing power, amounts to about 27.5 percent of the world's, and still about three times China's. The US portion is thus substantial, though less than its 41.5 percent share of world military expenditures. A more accurate measure of potential coercive power over other countries reflects its position as a strong, diverse, continental economy. Despite a substantially free-trade policy, the United States is proportionately less dependent on international trade than its competitors are. For example, in 2007 exports and imports combined amounted to only 29 percent of US GDP. Of the other seven major powers, Japan was second at 33 percent and the remaining six (China, France, Germany, India, Russia, Britain) averaged 61 percent (Heston *et al.* 2009). If interdependence is seen as a potential restraint on coercing or fighting other states—as the Kantian perspective contends—then the United States is the least restrainable.

On the edge between hard military power and "softer" economic power is the international weapons trade, especially for the kind of high-tech weapons in which the United States specializes. This highly integrated global market is dominated by US firms both by the size of their own production and their ability to choose which foreign firms they will use as subcontractors. Of all sales by the world's 100 top arms-producing companies in 2007, US firms accounted for 61 percent (Perlo-Freeman 2009: 262). That kind of economic dominance facilitates American global political influence (Caverley 2007).

Two of the key influences for peace are the Kantian relatively soft powers of democracy and the capitalist market system underlying economic interdependence. They are related empirically and reinforce each other, but each makes an independent contribution. Democracy should not be subsumed as merely a correlate or consequence of capitalism. Theories that a capitalist peace subsumes the democratic peace have yet to produce convincing evidence.[10] The complexity of causal relations is inherent in the Kantian Triangle, with its six arrows showing mutual influence among the three forces, and another six for each both causing peace and benefiting from it. Gat (2005) contends that representative institutions are best produced by the wealth and culture of modernity in republics of recent centuries. That culture of modernity assuredly includes capitalism and high income, but also such elements as the control of debilitating disease, free expression, the sexual revolution and women's rights, property rights, and broader conceptions of human rights. While capitalism assuredly buttresses this culture, the culture in turn promotes both capitalism and representative government. Liberal ideas and institutions are both subjects and objects of international relations.

Economic strength supports a hegemon's ability to influence other states in both hard and soft ways. It is part of a continually evolving system of liberal influences that adapt to one another and to changes in their institutional and ideational environment.

Is hegemony sustainable domestically?

Economy and hegemony

What conditions affect the hegemon's ability to sustain its own productivity? Hegemony is expensive. Sustained hegemony depends upon economic strength at its core. Chapter 4 of this book contended that while the United States paid significant costs to maintain its predominance during the cold war years, it also achieved substantial economic benefits through policies of promoting free trade and investment. The cost-benefit ratio may well have been positive. Lenin maintained that monopolistic finance capital enriched nineteenth- and twentieth-century empires to the detriment of their colonies, but led directly to wars among the capitalist powers. Schumpeter, writing in opposition to Lenin and other Marxists, contended that Lenin had it all wrong, and capitalism—unlike the atavistic influence of a militaristic landed aristocracy—was a force for both peace and development. Studies of specific empires (including that of the Soviet Marxist-Leninist state) often conclude that while empires may turn a profit initially, eventually the costs mount up. Costs include not only the security expenditures to maintain control, but the degree to which elites at a bloated imperial center may use the receipts to live in high luxury rather than to promote productive enterprise. By this reading, Spain benefited initially by extracting precious metals from the Americas, but at the cost of a stunted economy that could not compete with rising commercial powers. The British empire at first gained a rapidly growing market for its industry, but from the middle of the eighteenth century onward could not muster the resources needed to retain its politically and economically self-confident colonies in North America.[11]

Athens and some recent empires could extract tribute from subject allies and colonies, but an alliance among freely associating states lacks the coercive power to enforce payment. The theme of overstretch and its economic costs has been common to many writers, including Gilpin (1981) and Kennedy (1987). Hegemons do inevitably decline, but they can take a long time to do so. The United States has achieved some real economic benefits, by protecting a global economy with low barriers to its exports, stable markets for American investors, and reliable supplies of strategic imports. The United States still dominates the global institutions of world economic power. It retains, through weighted voting rules, a virtual veto over IMF and World Bank decisions. Even now, it is able to run a foreign trade deficit by being a net importer of capital because US capital markets provide a safe haven when other countries suffer economic or political instability. The US dollar—not the euro, or the yen, or the renmimbi—remains the most important reserve currency for most countries. Taking this money out of active circulation helps keep the exchange rate for dollars high.

Maintaining a hegemon's military capacity is not cheap. US military spending, including that in the Defense Department and military-related spending in the Department of Energy and elsewhere, is estimated at $676 billion for 2009. That amounted to 4.5 percent of the US GDP; well below the 6.5 percent typical of the Reagan years but well above the 3.0 percent of 2000. If the US economy could sustain cold war military spending one might expect it can do so at current levels and conditions. A problem, however, is that current economic conditions are not the same as even in 2000, as the burden on public budgets and the full economy has grown. Over the decade the military budget has gone from 16.5 percent of GDP and 48.0 percent of federal discretionary spending to 21.7 percent of GDP and 55.4 percent of discretionary spending. Meanwhile national debt as a share of GDP went from 58.0 percent to 69.3 percent.[12] A comprehensive estimate of the US cost of the war in Iraq through 2017 (Stiglitz and Bilmes 2008) is $3 trillion.

The US debt/GDP ratio is not nearly as high as that of some profligate European states, but Greece, Ireland, and Portugal are not trying to police the world. Projections of the US debt/GDP ratio vary widely from varying assumptions, but virtually everyone agrees it will get worse before it gets better, and that federal spending will take a serious hit. Given military spending's share of all discretionary expenditure, it will take part of that hit. Unless, of course, America's international security situation decays dramatically in response to unpredictable but imaginable shocks. Either way, a hegemonic foreign policy will become more difficult.

Some current work (Nordhaus *et al.* 2010) on comparative military spending over time and space can help to explain why some countries spend more than others. In our work we confirm that bigger and richer states generally spend more on their military establishments than do smaller and poorer ones: GDP is the best single predictor of military expenditures. Another but weaker prediction comes from knowing the recent and current *experience of international* conflict by a state. Not surprisingly, more violent conflict, measured either as number of fatal MIDs or of fatalities suffered in war—usually does produce higher military spending. So by both size and experience of international conflict we might expect the United States to spend more than other countries. And it does, but that is not the end of the story.

To create a plausible objective measure of the *level of threat* each country faces we employ what we now call our liberal-realist model (LRM) of international relations. That model is essentially the same as the statistical model used in Chapters 9 and 11 of this book, and includes each country's relative power, distance from other countries, alliance relationships, its degree of democracy or autocracy, and its degree of integration into the global economic system. The LRM turns out to be a rather strong predictor of most countries' military spending—better than the actual experience of conflict. Still, the model omits some other plausible influences. We find, for example, that the United States may spend much more on its military than our model predicts.

We are not sure why. Some of the explanation probably lies in the American experience in international affairs, which has become not only an experience of conflict, but an experience of continued expectation of conflict.[13] Countries may subjectively *perceive* different conditions and periods as more threatening than others. For example, the United States was long protected from foreign threats by the span of the Atlantic and Pacific oceans and the economic and technological barriers they posed to European and Asian states trying to exert their power against it.[14] By the twentieth century, however, those barriers provided less security objectively, and the shock of isolationism's failure to keep the United States out of World War II against the Axis dictatorships contributed to a greater subjective sense of threat. That diminished sense of security carried over into the cold war and threat of transcontinental nuclear war and a long and very dangerous arms race. The United States created large complex organizations with a lot of bureaucratic inertia to maintain their budgets and missions, and an ideology to support them (Sylvan and Majeski 2009; Ackerman 2010; Bacevich 2010). It is institutionally and politically easier to build such organizations than to shrink them—"peace dividends" almost always fall short of the pre-conflict spending levels. And the United States has experienced the practices, burdens, and temptations of hegemony.

Rather than a general answer that hegemony is usually self-sustaining or self-destroying, the clearest lesson is that for each case the cost-benefit analysis requires careful scrutiny. The security costs of retaining control over distant lands matter, as do the distribution and deployment of resources by the political economy of the hegemon.

Democracy and hegemony

How may democracy support or undermine a hegemonic foreign policy—and in turn, how may hegemony support or undermine democratic governance? This discussion takes off partly from Chapter 2's treatment of how the type of political system matters. On balance, does American democracy encourage a hegemonic foreign policy, or does it importantly limit the prospects for such a policy to succeed? Do democracies have a better chance of winning the wars they fight? Do they do as well in fighting insurgences as in conventional international wars? Can they sustain the economic and political costs of hegemonic deterrence and hegemonic war-fighting? If the attractiveness of democracy to other peoples around the globe constitutes an element of American soft power, is that soft power enhanced or diminished by the hard power it can deploy? Can American hegemony last a long time, and what are its limits?

Democratic institutions can enable their countries to be effective security seekers and war fighters. Some power rivalries go on for decades, with arms races and long or repeated wars. It is expensive to carry on such struggles, and governments may not be able or willing to tax their citizens enough to pay the costs at the time. Alternatives are just to print money, or to borrow from their citizens or from other countries. But lenders want to be repaid, and the more they fear that the borrower will default on the loan the higher the interest rate they demand to take that risk. Schultz and Weingast (2003) consider the two-century rivalry between Britain and France, and the United States and the USSR during the cold war, in each case pitting a relatively democratic country against an authoritarian one. They conclude that representative institutions impose fiscal restraints and responsibility on the state authorities, making repayment of their bonds more likely and allowing them to borrow at lower rates than were available to their rivals. The consequence was more rapid economic growth and growth in military power, contributing importantly to victory in the security competition.

Economic costs are evident in the share of GDP going to national "defense" spending. Is the United States able to raise the taxes and make the cuts in non-military spending needed to pay the sustained costs of hegemony? Are democracies politically too sclerotic to maintain economies whose economic growth rates are not weighed down by domestic and especially foreign debt? Specifically, can a fractious democracy like the United States sustain the economic costs of hegemony —especially the military costs—in a domestic political system that prioritizes the distribution of benefits to a wide electorate? When a growing part of the electorate (those over age 65) has shown its power to acquire health and security entitlements? (A guns versus hospitals trade-off?) The 2010 debt crisis in the Eurozone suggests how difficult this can be, and it is relevant also for the United States. After all, the US constitution was designed to protect liberty and minority rights, with a division of powers and checks and balances intended to resist their disruption by temporary majorities.

Fighting wars can be costly in lives as well as money, and these costs are likely to be felt more acutely when a war is not won. Democracies may have some advantages over dictatorships. Chapter 2 noted that democracies win most of their wars, especially of those they initiate.[15] Their leaders can be held accountable by democratic institutions, as they or their parties risk being turned out of office in elections.[16] Leaders of democratic states may benefit from more diverse and more accurate information than dictators, and so may be able to choose their adversaries carefully, picking those that are weaker and easier to defeat. Chapter 2 also suggested that democracies gain war power by having more reliable and better-motivated troops, and by sharing the gains from warfare as well as its costs with the mass population. It is not clear whether in general democracies are able to mobilize their economic resources better than dictatorships, but since on average democratic states have historically had higher per capita incomes than dictatorships, they may have more resources to deploy. For the past century or so, many democracies have frequently been allied in big wars against one or more dictatorships. Their coalitions have usually included some autocratic states (in the two World Wars; less so in the wars with Iraq), but the coalitions they confronted rarely included democratic states. And their coalitions were usually bigger than their adversaries'. So, collectively the democratic alliances were able to bring more sheer power to bear. The combination of democratic government and developed economies means that democracies typically face weaker opponents.

The implications for hegemony are particularly murky when the experience of democracies and autocracies in fighting counter-insurgency wars is carefully compared, and those wars have become especially problematic and important. Lyall's (2010) very sophisticated analysis looked at 286 counter-insurgency wars, including controls for whether the wars were conducted by a state against domestic insurgents or by external occupiers, and for whether the insurgents had received material support or sanctuary from a neighboring state. In this comparison, occupiers did significantly worse than governments fighting insurgencies at home, as did governments facing insurgencies that had outside support. But for neither type of insurgency did democracy make a statistically significant difference in either the likelihood of success or the duration or war duration. So democracies are not necessarily inferior fighters against insurgents.

Governments may be under pressure to minimize wartime casualties, to themselves if not to their adversaries. The record from various wars is mixed. World

War II was fought at high levels of intensity, with both inadvertent and deliberate attacks on civilians. Both sides engaged in heavy strategic bombing, against military targets and to undermine civilian support for the war, long before the atomic bombs were dropped. The Axis powers often inflicted terrible casualties on the peoples they occupied, and were not limited to the horrors of the Holocaust. The war in the Pacific was fought with particular savagery (Dower 1986). But revulsion against deliberate killing of civilians built up over subsequent decades, a revulsion expressed in liberal political theory about how wars could be fought "justly" and found more explicitly in international law. These developments led to strong policy commitments to try to spare Iraqi civilians in the two Gulf wars. In Afghanistan American and NATO forces feel required to limit civilian casualties, expecting to lose support by the populations they want to defend if the casualties are perceived as indiscriminate or disproportionate.

Do democracies systematically suffer or inflict fewer casualties than dictatorships? One might reasonably expect democratic governments to avoid casualties to their own peoples so as to maintain public support, and to avoid inflicting unnecessary casualties on their adversaries in accordance with "liberal" moral and legal norms. An early study of this question (Siverson 1995) concluded that democracies suffered fewer fatalities than did dictatorships, notably when it was a democratic government that initiated the war. But a closer analysis requires making several distinctions. Recent work benefits from a greatly expanded database, and the ability to draw some more detailed conclusions from it.

Overall, type of government matters much less than several other influences. Certain types of wars—of insurgency, of attrition, and that threaten the very existence of a state, bring out the worst. More desperate governments become readier to inflict greater casualties on their enemies—and especially readier to target civilians. Under these circumstances democracies may be more willing to inflict high casualties on their opponents if by doing so they can better limit the casualties they themselves incur. Rich states, able to fight with high technology weapons to exercise power at great distances, can more readily limit their own casualties by carrying greater human costs to their adversaries' home territory (Sechser and Saunders 2010). In many of their wars democracies have been not only richer but also distant from their enemies. That combination can allow them to reduce political costs to their leaders and maintain higher civilian and military morale. Dictators may take fewer wartime fatalities by vigorously repressing dissent before it erupts into overt rebellion with a lot of war casualties. Democracies tend to initiate international wars that they can expect to win quickly, with lower casualties to themselves. Under such a complex and changing set of influences it may not be surprising that up through 1945 democracies inflicted no fewer casualties, and possibly more, than did dictatorships. Since then, however, and especially since about 1970, democracies have fought several wars with fewer casualties, especially when they were quick and decisive.[17] Long wars with high economic costs and extended fatalities are more problematic.

It is no wonder that governments try to minimize public awareness of wartime casualties. Building and using a capital-intensive military force may be especially important in a democracy with high income inequality. During the 2000s the United States had one of the most unequal income distributions among the developed economies—exceeded only by Portugal, Turkey, and Mexico of the thirty members of the OECD (OECD 2008: 25). Poorer and less educated groups in the United States pay a disproportionately high cost in human life. Lower-income individuals may have little enthusiasm for war, but military service in a volunteer force can give them substantial economic and social opportunities. They are more likely to serve in the military, and more likely to become wartime casualties. The price is felt also in their communities, by their families, friends, and neighbors. The results among these groups include lower levels of participation in politics, lower trust in government, and lower levels of support for the war (Kriner and Shen 2010).

It has been widely believed that democratic publics will turn against a war involving high casualties, but the full picture turns out to be more nuanced. Casualty trends matter as well as do casualty totals. So too does the public's subjective evaluation of the prospects for war to succeed in its aims, whether it was right to go to war in the first place, and their perception of the ratio of casualties between their side and their adversaries'. These influences frequently interact, and of course are subject to manipulation depending on how the government and opposition succeed in framing the discussion in the public media.[18]

Does a decline in public support translate into a decline in support at the higher levels of the political system? The strategic situation in the field obviously matters, but so too does the political environment in Washington. Presidents may wish, in their perceptions of the national interest and their own political interest, to maintain military efforts that they started or continued. That is probably easier to do early in their term of office than later. Members of Congress can make their own political cost-benefit decisions about whether to challenge a president. They have the potential—especially if the opposition party controls at least one house—to exercise budgetary restraint and conduct embarrassing investigations into the political and military conditions in the field, wasteful spending, and ill-treatment of combat veterans. A Congressional majority may not be able to force a president to abandon a war abruptly, but it may shorten its duration. At the least it can require a president to spend a lot of his political capital defending his military campaign, making it harder for him to accomplish anything else. This effectively was George Bush's fate, as an especially lame duck after the 2006 elections (Kriner 2010).

It is a mistake to think that democracies, and especially the American democracy, will never be able to support long wars. Indeed, as of 2010 two such wars continued, with a costly win or maybe a draw in one (Iraq since 2003) and one still with no decision (Afghanistan since 2001). But it is equally a mistake to think that sustaining such wars will be politically easy, and that presidents will not have to take those difficulties into consideration in making decisions to initiate a serious military action. Some new work (Scheve and Stasavage 2010) finds that democracies that must mobilize their mass populations for long wars face strong political pressures to raise taxes on the wealthy and thereby distribute the burden of the war effort more equally. The strongest case is the experience of World War I. Whether the same pressures would arise during a long period of nearly constant engagement in smaller wars may be a different matter.

Economic development, economic interdependence, and the destructive power of modern technology have raised the costs of war relative to its likely gains, not only in past experience but in anticipation of the use of weapons of mass destruction. Real-time global communication makes violations of international human rights principles readily apparent, and gives impetus to humanitarian interventions. Yet humanitarian interventions, unlike interventions justified by realpolitik motives where the national interest seems to be engaged, will rarely be supported if they are long or costly in the lives of a liberal state's own citizens.

Mutilateralism formed the basis of successful policy in regional alliances like NATO and in the UN and the global financial institutions. A hegemon can do necessary bilateral deals costing a few $100 million here and there, buying off the most relevant actors and pushing around or ignoring the rest. But a liberal hegemon needs an institutional structure of negotiation and legitimation, for peaceful conflict prevention and resolution. Multilateral diplomacy, with give and take, is hard work, and diplomacy alone, without the threat of force, may fail when dealing with persisting adversaries. The test then becomes whether liberal international institutions can act effectively without losing their liberal character.[19]

If a liberal hegemon is to underpin its hegemony by supporting democracy elsewhere, its own democracy must be a source of its legitimacy. Wars, cold wars, and terrorism typically lead to curtailments in civil liberties and free expression. Even before World War II, Harold Lasswell developed the construct of a "garrison state" experiencing perpetual crisis and dominated by the military, police, and national security bureaucracy.[20] As suggested in Chapter 11, objectively the dangers from terrorism are far less than those from full scale war. Yet Americans who, unlike most peoples, have not suffered war fatalities in their home country in almost a century and a half, may be hyper-sensitive to terrorism. They may be prepared to sacrifice liberty when their fears are stoked by opportunistic bureaucrats and politicians (Mueller 2006; D.W. Davis 2007; Donohue 2008). An ideology of counterterrorism can become a tool for legitimating repression abroad as well as at home.[21] Similar effects may arise from exaggerated fears of nuclear proliferation (Gavin 2009/10). The cost would not be only to American democracy, but to American hegemony if the soft power attributable to democracy became eroded by regularly practicing a form of state terrorism with torture, and other deprivations of human rights at home.[22]

A democratic hegemon may be more able to borrow, and less able to exercise fiscal austerity. A democratic hegemon may be able to fight harder and win more of its wars. Democracies are not particularly handicapped in counter-insurgency wars. But they face serious incentives to minimize their own casualties, and if possible those of civilians among their adversaries. A democratic hegemon will be stronger if it acts like a democracy.

A conclusion with more questions

For the big picture, one can imagine three scenarios for the next several decades:

1. *American hegemony turns into something like an empire*, widely imposing a negative peace with heavy use of military force and long-term occupations of adversary or failed states. This may be the least likely outcome, since the United States appears to lack the collective will, and even more the resources, to carry it off.
2. *Chaos.* The United States cannot sustain its hegemony, and its allies and client states run for the exits. Islamic extremists sweep to power in the Middle East and Asia, and create severe instability in many places they cannot actually control. The global capitalist economy goes down the tubes as terrorism gets much worse, the cost of fuel and raw material skyrockets, and governments effectively go bankrupt. The West loses, but the Islamists can't rule the world, so no one wins. Something like this might be a more likely outcome.[23]
3. *The United States lasts as a democratic hegemon*, with substantial support from its allies and other partners in a large coalition that shifts somewhat from issue to issue. No coherent coalition arises against it, and Islamic terrorism loses most of its support.

If many states were prepared to accept a relatively benign hegemony based substantially on Kantian principles, the Hobbesian choice between Leviathan and chaos in the international system could be evaded. Can American hegemony last a long time?

Is it the next best bet for peace? And maybe even for justice, to the degree that hegemony is based on accepted institutions and norms of justice both domestically and globally? In his *Perpetual Peace* Kant said how he feared the soulless despotism of a universal state. But a decade earlier (Kant [1784] 1991: 47) he expressed hope for a "great federation" arising "from a united power and the law-governed decisions of a united will." Most importantly, "The problem of establishing a perfect civil constitution is subordinate to the problem of a law-governed external relationship with other states, and cannot be solved unless the latter is also solved." Maybe the best summary is to say they must be solved together.

Both problems remain unsolved. A democracy trying to sustain its hegemony will have different advantages and disadvantages from those of a dictatorship. The limits a democracy imposes on a hegemon's effectiveness may prevent it from turning hegemony into a global empire. Disregard of those limits will diminish its democracy. The complexity of how democracy and hegemony affect one another precludes any confident answers to the really big questions. Social science can take us only so far in guiding or predicting the future. Meanwhile, the United States and the world are experiencing a vast experiment to determine whether a democratic hegemon can preserve its own security and values, at home and abroad.

Notes

1 Athenian ambassadors' speech to the Spartan assembly (Thucydides 1972, I:78).
2 The United States, Britain, and to a lesser degree France vs. China in the Korean War; China vs. India twice; Soviet Union vs. China in 1967.
3 This paragraph benefits from a discussion with my colleagues Alexandre Debs and Nuno Monteiro.
4 In some ways the US may have been more powerful as a hegemon of its region (the "free world" minus a few nonaligned states) before the end of the cold war than of the globe afterward. A common perception of Soviet threat encouraged consensus in the West to the degree that more amorphous (and arguably less capable) Islamic terrorism cannot.
5 Lundestad (1990) referred to this development as an "empire by invitation" from Europe.
6 Jervis (2006) has some good points to this effect.
7 The canonical text on collective goods theory in alliances, with application to NATO, is Olson and Zeckhauser (1966); on the phenomenon in enforcing sanctions, see Martin (1992).
8 Heng (2010) makes an interesting comparison of the two states' efforts.
9 Ikenberry (2000/01) regards capitalism as predominantly an instrument of soft power; others disagree. The literature is vast and inconclusive. Two rigorous empirical studies point to mixed results. Vreeland (2003) has strong evidence that the conditions made by the International Monetary Fund to its aid recipients reduce growth and increase income inequality. De Soysa (2003) contends that foreign private direct investment promotes growth and overall is not bad for democracy.
10 Gartzke (2007), Mousseau (2009), and Gartzke and Hewitt (2010), are the most prominent quantitative analysts claiming that a capitalist peace trumps a democratic one. Critiques include Russett (2010) and Dafoe (2011). McDonald (2010) finds evidence supporting both influences.
11 Lenin ([1917] 1926), Schumpeter ([1927] 1955). See Cohen (1973) for a good conceptual and empirical commentary. Elliott (2006) is a magisterial look at the Spanish and British empires to the middle of the nineteenth century.
12 These 2000–2009 comparisons are from Perlo-Freeman et al. (2009: 186–188). Of all foreign holdings of US Treasury securities at the end of 2009, 23 percent were by China and 6 percent by oil exporters (www.ustreas.gov/tic/mfh.txt). For contrasting views on the economic prospects for sustaining US hegemony contrast Todd and Delogu (2003) and Mandelbaum (2010) with Norloff (2010).
13 Our model includes only the experience of conflict between nation-states, not that from nonstate terrorism. However, as noted in Chapter 11, such terrorism has accounted for only a tiny fraction of the number of fatalities in state-based warfare.
14 Great Britain had the strongest capability to exert power in the Western Hemisphere, but Canada's vulnerability served as a hostage to British good behavior until the full development of an Anglo-American security community in the twentieth century.
15 Depending on the analysis, however, the ratio of democratic wins to losses is probably much lower than the over 90 percent ratio suggested in Chapter 2, depending on various definitional and analytical choices. Recent contributions to the debate include Downes (2009), Reiter et al. (2009), and Gat (2010: ch. 7).
16 The term accountability needs to be parsed carefully. Democratic leaders who lose costly wars are more likely to be removed from office than are dictatorships, but removed peacefully and allowed a good retirement. Dictators who cannot retain their power are more likely to lose their lives or liberty, which may often provide a stronger incentive (Debs and Goemans 2010).
17 See Reiter and Stam (2003: ch. 7), Valentino et al. (2004), Valentino et al. (2006), Downes (2008), Gat (2010: ch. 7).
18 Work on these complexities includes Gelpi et al. (2005/06), Boettcher and Cobb (2006), Gartner (2008), Baum and Groeling (2009), Gelpi et al. (2009), and Caverley (2009/10).

19 Kreps (2010) suggests, from survey data and case studies, that whereas the "coalition of the willing" in Iraq quickly splintered due to a lack of popular support at home, the institutional ties and elite consensus among NATO members helped sustain the cooperative effort in Afghanistan despite popular opposition.

20 Lasswell put forth this construct in 1937, with his best-known exposition in 1941; see the posthumous collection of his essays by Stanley (1997). The most vivid version of the garrison state is of course George Orwell's *1984*. Friedberg (2000) offers an explanation of why a real garrison state did not develop in the United States.

21 Münkler (2007: 96) says that a "discourse of barbarism is a general feature of empires."

22 Gronke *et al.* (2010) cite public opinion data suggesting that a majority of the American people do not support the use of torture even under extreme threat conditions. Merolla and Zechmeister (2009) claim from experimental data that terrorist threats promote attitudes favorable to authoritarianism and activist foreign policies.

23 See the chilling conclusion to Johnson (2004: 312): "Nemesis, the goddess of retribution and vengeance, the punisher of pride and hubris, waits impatiently for her meeting with us."

REFERENCES

Abbott, K.W., and D. Snidal (1998) "Why States Act Through Formal International Organizations," *Journal of Conflict Resolution* 42(1): 3–32.

Abruzzese, S. (2007) "Iraq War Brings Drop in Black Enlistees," *New York Times* (August 22): 12.

Achen, C. (2005) "Let's Put Garbage-Can Regressions and Garbage-Can Probits Where They Belong," *Conflict Management and Peace Science* 22(4): 327–340.

Ackerman, B. (2010) *The Decline and Fall of the American Republic.* Cambridge, MA: Belknap.

Adler, E. (1998) "Seeds of Peaceful Change: The OSCE's Security-Community Building Model," in E. Adler and M. Barnett (Eds.) *Security Communities.* Cambridge: Cambridge University Press, pp. 119–160.

Adler, E., and M. Barnett (1994) *Pluralistic Security Communities: Past, Present and Future.* Madison, WI: University of Wisconsin, Global Studies Research Program.

Adler, E., and M. Barnett (1998) "A Framework for the Study of Security Communities," in E. Adler and M. Barnett (Eds.) *Security Communities.* Cambridge: Cambridge University Press, pp. 29–66.

Adler, K.P. (1986) "West European and American Public Opinion on Peace, Defence, and Arms Control in a Cross-national Perspective," *International Social Science Journal* 110: 589–600.

Albright, M., and D. Obey (1997) "Does NATO Enlargement Serve US Interests?" *CQ Researcher* 7: 449.

Alesina, A., and R. Perotti (1994) "The Political Economy of Growth: A Critical Survey of the Recent Literature," *World Bank Economic Review* 8(3): 355–371.

Alker, H.R. (1973) "Power in a Schedule Sense," in K.W. Deutsch and A.H. Stoetzel (Eds.) *Mathematical Approaches to Politics.* San Francisco, CA: Jossey-Bass.

Allan, P., and K. Goldmann, Eds. (1992) *The End of the Cold War: Evaluating Theories of International Relations.* Dordrecht: Martinus Nijhoff.

Allison, G.T. (1971) *Essence of Decision: Explaining the Cuban Missile Crisis.* Boston, MA: Little, Brown.

Arat, Z. (1991) *Democracy and Human Rights in Developing Countries.* Boulder, CO: Rienner.

Arbatov, A. (1996) "Eurasia Letter: A Russian–US Security Agenda," *Foreign Policy* 104: 102–117.

Archibugi, D. (1995a) "From the United Nations to Cosmopolitan Democracy," in D. Archibugi and D. Held (Eds.) *Cosmopolitan Democracy: An Agenda for a New World Order.* Cambridge: Polity Press, pp. 121–162.

Archibugi, D. (1995b) "Immanuel Kant, Cosmopolitan Law and Peace," *European Journal of International Relations* 1(4): 429–456.

Arms Control Today (1997) "The Debate over NATO Expansion: A Critique of the Clinton Administration's Responses to Key Questions," *Arms Control Today* 27: 3–12.

Arrighi, G. (1982) "A Crisis of Hegemony," in S. Amin, A.G. Frank, I. Wallerstein, and G. Arrighi (Eds.) *Dynamics of Global Crisis.* New York: Monthly Review Press.

Artner, S.J. (1985) *A Change of Course: The West German Social Democrats and NATO, 1957–1961.* Westport, CT: Greenwood Press.

Asher, J.R. (1997) "Lockheed Martin Buys Russian Rocket Engines," *Aviation Week & Space Technology* 146: 24–25.

Ashley, R.K. (1989) "Living on Borderlines: Man, Poststructuralism, and War', in J. Der Derian and M. Shapiro (Eds.) *International/Intertextual Relations: Postmodern Readings in World Politics.* Lexington, MA: Lexington Books.

Ashley, R.K., and R.B.J. Walker, Eds. (1990) "Speaking the Language of Exile: Dissidence in International Studies," Special Issue of *International Studies Quarterly* 34: 259–416.

Asmus, R.D., R.L. Kugler, and S.F. Larrabee (1996) "What Will NATO Enlargement Cost?" *Survival* 38: 5–26.

Aurswald, D. (2000) *Disarmed Democracies: Domestic Institutions and the Use of Force.* Ann Arbor, MI: University of Michigan Press.

Avant, D. (2006) "The Implications of Marketized Security for IR Theory: The Democratic Peace, Late State Building, and the Nature and Frequency of Conflict," *Perspectives on Politics* 4(3): 507–528.

Aviation Week & Space Technology (1993) "Russian Zhukovsky Facility Shows Flight Test Diversity," *Aviation Week & Space Technology* 138: 66–67.

Axelrod, R. (1984) *The Evolution of Cooperation.* New York: Basic Books.

Bacevich, A. (2010) *Washington Rules: America's Path to Permanent War.* New York: Metropolitan Books.

Bairoch, P. (1976) "Europe's Gross National Product, 1800–1975," *Journal of European Economic History* 5: 273–340.

Bairoch, P. (1982) "International Industrialization Levels from 1750 to 1980," *Journal of European Economic History* 11: 269–333.

Ball, D. (1981) "Can Nuclear War Be Controlled?" *Adelphi Paper* 161.

Baoxiang, Z. (1997) "NATO–Russia Talks over Expansion Remain Deadlocked," *Beijing Review* 40: 8.

Baranovsky, V., and H.-J. Spanger, Eds. (1992) *In From the Cold: Germany, Russia, and the Future of Europe.* Boulder, CO: Westview.

Barbieri, K. (1996) "Economic Interdependence: A Path to Peace or Source of Interstate Conflict?" *Journal of Peace Research* 33(1): 29–49.

Barnett, M. (1995a) "The New UN Politics of Peace," *Global Governance* 1(1): 79–98.

Barnett, M. (1995b) "Partners in Peace? The UN, Regional Organizations, and Peace-keeping," *Review of International Studies* 21(4): 411–433.

Batt, J. (1994) "The International Dimension of Democratisation in Czechoslovakia and Hungary," in G. Pridham, E. Herring, and G. Sanford (Eds.) *Building Democracy? The International Dimension of Democratization in Eastern Europe.* New York: St. Martin's Press, pp. 168–187.

Baum, M., and T. Groeling (2009) *War Stories: The Causes and Consequences of Public Views of War.* Princeton, NJ: Princeton University Press.

Baylis, J. (1992) *The Diplomacy of Pragmatism: Britain and the Formation of NATO, 1942–1949*. London: Macmillan.

Bearce, D.H. (2003) "Grasping the Commercial Institutional Peace," *International Studies Quarterly* 47(3): 347–370.

Beck, N., J.N. Katz, and R. Tucker (1998) "Beyond Ordinary Logit: Taking Time Seriously in Binary Time-Series Cross-Section Models," *American Journal of Political Science* 42(4): 1260–1288.

Beijing Review (1995) "News Briefing by the Chinese Foreign Ministry," *Beijing Review* 38 (September 18): 9.

Beijing Review (1996) "Joint Statement by the People's Republic of China and the Russian Federation," *Beijing Review* 39 (May 13): 6–8.

Bennett, D.S. (2006) "Toward a Continuous Specification of the Democracy–Autocracy Connection," *International Studies Quarterly* 49(2): 313–338.

Bennett, D.S., and A.C. Stam (2004) *The Behavioral Origins of War*. Ann Arbor, MI: University of Michigan Press.

Bercovitch, J. (1991) "International Mediation and Dispute Settlement: Evaluating the Conditions for Successful Mediation," *Negotiation Journal* 7: 17–30.

Bercovitch, J., and J. Langley (1993) "The Nature of Dispute and the Effectiveness of International Mediation," *Journal of Conflict Resolution* 37(4): 670–691.

Berger, P.L., and T. Luckman (1966) *The Social Construction of Reality*. New York: Doubleday.

Bergsten, C.F., T. Horst, and T. Moran (1978) *American Multinationals and American Interests*. Washington, DC: Brookings Institution.

Bernstein, R., and R.H. Munro (1996) *The Coming Conflict with China*. New York: Knopf.

Bertram, E. (1995) "Reinventing Governments: The Promise and Perils of United Nations Peacebuilding," *Journal of Conflict Resolution* 39(3): 387–418.

Betts, R.K. (1987) *Nuclear Blackmail and Nuclear Balance*. Washington, DC: Brookings Institution.

Bhaskar, R. (1978) *A Realist Theory of Science*, 2nd ed. London: Routledge & Kegan Paul.

Biddle, S. (1996) "Victory Misunderstood: What the Gulf War Tells Us About the Future of Conflict," *International Security* 21: 139–179.

Blair, B.G. (1985) *Strategic Command and Control: Redefining the Nuclear Threat*. Washington, DC: Brookings Institution.

Blair, B.G., V. Esin, M. McKenzie, V. Yarnich, and P. Zolotarev (2010) "Smaller and Safer: A New Plan for Nuclear Postures," *Foreign Affairs* 89(5): 9–16.

Blanco, W., and J.T. Roberts, Eds. (1998) *Thucydides, The Peloponnesian War*. New York: Norton.

Blechman, B., and S.S. Kaplan (1978) *Force without War*. Washington, DC: Brookings Institution.

Bliss, H., and B. Russett (1998) "Democratic Trading Partners: The Liberal Connection," *Journal of Politics* 58.

Bobbio, N. (1995) "Democracy and the International System," in D. Archibugi and D. Held (Eds.) *Cosmopolitan Democracy: An Agenda for a New World Order*. Cambridge: Polity Press, pp. 17–41.

Bobrow, D., and R. Kudrle (1976) "Theory, Policy, and Resource Cartels," *Journal of Conflict Resolution* 20: 3–56.

Boegehold, A. (1996) "The Athenian Government in Thucydides," in R. Strassler (ed.) *Thucydides: A Comprehensive Guide to the Peloponnesian War*. New York: Free Press, pp. 577–582.

Boehmer, C. (2008) "A Reassessment of Democratic Pacifism at the Monadic Level of Analysis," *Conflict Management and Peace Science* 25(1): 81–94.

Boehmer, C., E. Gartzke, and T. Nordstrom (2004) "Do Intergovernmental Organizations Promote Peace?" *World Politics* 57(1): 1–38.

Boettcher, W.A. III, and M.D. Cobb (2006) "Echoes of Vietnam? Casualty Framing and Public Perceptions of Success and Failure in Iraq," *Journal of Conflict Resolution* 50(6): 831–854.

Born, H., and H. Hänggi (2005) "Governing the Use of Force under International Auspices: Deficits in Parliamentary Accountability', in *SIPRI Yearbook 2005: Armaments, Disarmament and International Security*. Oxford: Oxford University Press.

Bosgra, S.J. (1969) *Portugal and NATO*. Amsterdam: Angola Committee.

Boulding, K.E. (1978) *Stable Peace*. Austin, TX: University of Texas Press.

Boutros-Ghali, B. (1992) *An Agenda for Peace*. New York: United Nations.

Boutros-Ghali, B. (1995) *An Agenda for Development*. New York: United Nations.

Boutros-Ghali, B. (1996) *An Agenda for Democratization*. New York: United Nations.

Bracken, P. (1983) *The Command and Control of Nuclear Forces*. New Haven, CT: Yale University Press.

Braudel, F. (1984) *The Perspective of the World*. New York: Harper & Row.

Brecher, M. (1993) *Crises in World Politics: Theory and Reality*. Oxford: Pergamon.

Bremer, S. (1992) "Dangerous Dyads: Conditions Affecting the Likelihood of Interstate War, 1816–1965," *Journal of Conflict Resolution* 36: 309–341.

Brilmayer, L. (1994) *American Hegemony: Political Morality in a One-Superpower World*. New Haven, CT: Yale University Press.

Brooks, S.G., and W.C. Wohlforth (2008) *World out of Balance: International Relations and the Challenge of American Primacy*. Princeton, NJ: Princeton University Press.

Brown, M.E. (1995) "The Flawed Logic of NATO Expansion," *Survival* 37: 34–52.

Brzezinski, Z., Ed. (1969) *Dilemmas of Change in Soviet Politics*. New York: Columbia University Press.

Brzezinski, Z. (1996) "Geopolitical Pivot Points," *Washington Quarterly* 19: 209–216.

Bueno de Mesquita, B. (1981) *The War Trap*. New Haven, CT: Yale University Press.

Bueno de Mesquita, B. (1984) "Forecasting Political Decisions," *PS: Political Science and Politics* 17: 226–236.

Bueno de Mesquita, B. (1985) "The War Trap Revisited: A Revised Expected Utility Model," *American Political Science Review* 79: 156–177.

Bueno de Mesquita, B. (1990) "Multilateral Negotiations: A Spatial Analysis of the Arab–Israeli Dispute," *International Organization* 44: 317–340.

Bueno de Mesquita, B. (1993) "The Game of Conflict Interactions: A Research Program," in J. Berger and M. Zelditch (eds.) *Theoretical Research Programs*. Stanford, CA: Stanford University Press.

Bueno de Mesquita, B. (1994) "Political Forecasting: An Expected Utility Method," in B. Bueno de Mesquita and F. Stokman (Eds.) *European Community Decision Making*. New Haven, CT: Yale University Press.

Bueno de Mesquita, B. (1996) "The Benefits of a Social Scientific Approach to Studying International Affairs," in N. Woods (ed.) *Explaining International Affairs Since 1945*. Oxford: Oxford University Press.

Bueno de Mesquita, B., and A.F.K. Organski (1992) "A Mark in Time Saves Nein," *International Political Science Review* 13: 81–100.

Bueno de Mesquita, B., and G.W. Downs (2006) "Intervention and Democracy," *International Organization* 60(3): 627–649.

Bueno de Mesquita, B., and C.-H. Kim (1991) "Prospects for a New Regional Order in Northeast Asia," *Korean Journal of Defense Analysis* 3.

Bueno de Mesquita, B., and D. Lalman (1992) *War and Reason*. New Haven, CT: Yale University Press).

Bueno de Mesquita, B., and G. lusi-Scarborough (1988) "Forecasting the Nature of Political Settlement in Nicaragua," paper for the Conference on Nicaragua: Prospects for a Democratic Outcome, sponsored by the Orkand Corporation, Washington, DC, October.

Bueno de Mesquita, B., and R.M. Siverson (1995) "War and the Survival of Political Leaders: A Comparative Study of Regime Types and Political Accountability," *American Political Science Review* 89: 841–855.

Bueno de Mesquita, B., and A. Smith (2007) "Foreign Aid and Policy Concessions," *Journal of Conflict Resolution* 51(2): 251–284.

Bueno de Mesquita, B., and F. Stokman, Eds. (1994) *European Community Decision Making: Models, Applications and Comparisons*. New Haven, CT: Yale University Press.

Bueno de Mesquita, B., D. Newman, and A. Rahushka (1985) *Forecasting Political Events*. New Haven, CT: Yale University Press.

Bueno de Mesquita, B., R. Siverson, and G. Woller (1992) "War and the Fate of Regimes," *American Political Science Review* 86(3): 638–646.

Bueno de Mesquita, B., A. Smith, R. Siverson, and J. Morrow (2003) *The Logic of Political Survival*. Cambridge, MA: MIT Press.

Bueno de Mesquita, B., J. Morrow, R. Siverson, and A. Smith (2004) "Testing Novel Implications of the Selectorate Theory of War," *World Politics* 56(3): 363–388.

Bull, H. (1977) *The Anarchical Society*. New York: Columbia University Press.

Bunce, V. (1997) "The Visegrad Group: Regional Cooperation and European Integration in Post-Communist Europe," in P. Katzenstein (ed.) *Mitteleuropa: Between Europe and Germany*. Providence, RI: Berghahn Books, pp. 240–284.

Bundy, M. (1984). "The Unimpressive Record of Nuclear Diplomacy," in G. Prins (ed.) *The Nuclear Crisis Reader*. New York: Vantage.

Bundy, M., G. Kennan, R. McNamara, and G. Smith (1982) "Nuclear Weapons and the Atlantic Alliance," *Foreign Affairs* 60(4): 753–768.

Burkhart, R., and M. Lewis-Beck (1994) "Comparative Democracy: The Economic Development Thesis," *American Political Science Review* 88(4): 903–910.

Campbell, C.S. (1974) *From Revolution to Rapprochement: The United States and Great Britain, 1783–1900*. New York: Wiley.

Caporaso, J. (1974) "Methodological Issues in the Measurement of Inequality, Dependence, and Exploitation," in S.J. Rosen and J.R. Kurth (Eds.) *Testing Theories of Economic Imperialism*. Lexington, MA: DC Heath.

Caporaso, J. (1978) "Dependence, Dependency, and Power in the Global System: A Structural and Behavioral Analysis," *International Organization* 32: 13–44.

Caprioli, M., and P. Trumbore (2006) "First Use of Violent Force in Militarized Interstate Disputes, 1980–2001," *Journal of Peace Research* 43(6): 741–749.

Carr, E.H. (1939) *The Twenty Years Crisis, 1919–1939*. London: Macmillan.

Cartledge, P. (1996) "Spartan Institutions in Thucydides," in R. Strassler (ed.) *Thucydides: A Comprehensive Guide to the Peloponnesian War*. New York: Free Press, pp. 589–592.

Caverley, J. (2007) "United States Hegemony and the New Economics of Defense," *Security Studies* 16(4): 597–613.

Caverley, J. (2009/10) "The Myth of Military Myopia," *International Security* 34(3): 119–157.

Cederman, L.-E. (2001) "Back to Kant: Reinterpreting the Democratic Peace as a Macrohistorical Learning Process," *American Political Science Review* 95(1): 15–31.

Cederman, L.-E., and M. Penubarti Rao (2001) "Exploring the Dynamics of the Democratic Peace," *Journal of Conflict Resolution* 45(6): 818–833.

Chan, S. (1995) "Grasping the Peace Dividend: Some Propositions on the Conversion of Swords into Plowshares," *Mershon International Review* 39: 53–95.

Chanda, N. (1993) "The View From Japan," *Far Eastern Economic Review* (December 2): 14.

Charles, D. (1987) *Nuclear Planning in NATO*. Cambridge, MA: Ballinger.

Charlton, M. (1987) *From Deterrence to Defense: The Inside Story of Strategic Policy*. Cambridge, MA: Harvard University Press.

Charney, J.I. (1993) "Universal International Law," *American Journal of International Law* 87: 529–551.

Chernoff, F. (1991) "Ending the Cold War: The Soviet Retreat and the US Military Buildup," *International Affairs* 67: 111–126.

Chernoff, F. (2004) "The Study of Democratic Peace and Progress in International Relations," *International Studies Review* 6(2): 49–78.

Ching, F. (1996) "Sino–Russian Pact a Good Sign," *Far Eastern Economic Review* (May 23): 40–41.

Christensen, T., and J. Snyder (1990) "Chain Gangs and Passed Bucks: Predicting Alliance Patterns in Multipolarity," *International Organization* 44: 137–168.

Chudodeyev, A., P. Felgengauer, and V. Abarinov (1996) "Taiwan Crisis and Russian-Chinese Ties," *The Current Digest of the Post-Soviet Press* 48 (April 10): 10–12.

Cohen, B. (1973) *The Question of Imperialism: The Political Economy of Dominance and Dependence*. New York: Basic Books.

Cohen, R. (1994) "Pacific Unions: A Reappraisal of the Theory that 'Democracies Do Not Go to War With Each Other'," *Review of International Studies* 20: 207–223.

Colas, A. (2007) *Empire*. Cambridge: Polity Press.

Collins, Gen. A.S., Jr. (1982) "Theatre Nuclear Warfare: The Battlefield," in J.F. Reichart and S.R. Sturm (Eds.) *American Defense Policy*, 5th ed. Baltimore, MD: Johns Hopkins University Press.

Collins, R., and D. Waller (1992) "What Theories Predicted the State Breakdowns and the Revolutions of the Soviet Bloc?" *Research in Social Movements, Conflicts, and Change* 14: 31–47.

Commission on Global Governance (1995) *Our Global Neighborhood*. New York: Oxford University Press.

Commodity Yearbook, 1982 (1982). New York: Commodity Research Bureau.

Conybeare, J.A.C. (1984) "Public Goods, Prisoners' Dilemma, and the International Political Economy," *International Studies Quarterly* 28(1): 5–22.

Conybeare, J.A.C. (1994) "The Portfolio Benefits of Free Riding in Military Alliances," *International Studies Quarterly* 38: 405–419.

Cornford, F. (1907) *Thucydides Mythistoricus*. London: Edward Arnold.

Council on Economics and National Security (1981) *Strategic Minerals: A Resource Crisis*. New York: National Strategy Information Center.

Covault, C. (1996) "Mir Assembly Nears Finale," *Aviation Week & Space Technology* 144 (April 29): 29–30.

Covault, C. (1997) "Zenit Explosion Hits Military, Civil Projects," *Aviation Week & Space Technology* 146 (May 26): 34.

Cowhey, P.F. (1993) "Domestic Institutions and the Credibility of International Commitments: Japan and the United States," *International Organization* 47(2): 299–326.

Cox, R. (1983) "Gramsci, Hegemony and International Relations: An Essay in Method," *Millennium: Journal of International Studies* 2(2): 632–675.

Cox, R.W., and H.K. Jacobson (1982) "The United States and World Order: On Structures of World Power and Structural Transformation," paper delivered at the Twelfth World Congress of the International Political Science Association, Rio de Janeiro, August.

Crawford, N. (1994) "A Security Regime among Democracies: Cooperation Among Iroquois Nations," *International Organization* 48: 345–385.

Cronin, A.K., and P.M.Cronin (1996) "The Realistic Engagement of China," *Washington Quarterly* 19: 141–170.

Current Digest of the Post-Soviet Press (1997) "Yeltsin, China's Jiang Call for 'Multipolar' World," *The Current Digest of the Post-Soviet Press* 49 (May 28): 1–5.

Dafoe, A. (2011) "Statistical Critiques of the Democratic Peace: Caveat Emptor," *American Journal of Political Science* 55(2).

Dahl, R.A. (1984) *Modern Political Analysis*, 4th ed. Englewood Cliffs, NJ: Prentice-Hall.

Davis, D. (2007) "Illegal Immigrants: Uncle Sam Wants You." Available at: www. inthese times.com/article/3271/illegal_immigrants_uncle_sam_wants_you/. (Accessed August 15, 2007).

Davis, D.W. (2007) *Negative Liberty: Public Opinion and the Terrorist Attacks on America*. New York: Russell Sage Foundation.

Dean, J. (1997) "The NATO Mistake: Expansion for All the Wrong Reasons," *Washington Monthly* 29 (July–August): 35–38.

Debs, A., and H. Goemans (2010) "Regime Type, the Fate of Leaders, and War," *American Political Science Review* 104(3): 430–445.

Deese, D., and J. Nye, Eds. (1981) *Energy and Security*. Cambridge, MA: Ballinger.

Dembinski, M., and K. Freistein (2005) "Comparing Regional Security Organizations: Is Democracy the Key?" Paper presented at the 1st Annual Conference of the World International Studies Committee, August 24–27, Istanbul.

Dembinski, M., A. Hasenclever, and W. Wagner (2004) "Towards an Executive Peace? The Ambivalent Effects of Inter-Democratic Institutions on Democracy, Peace, and War," *International Politics* 41(3): 543–564.

DeSoto, A., and G. del Castillo (1994) "Obstacles to Peacebuilding," *Foreign Policy* 94: 69–83.

De Soysa, I. (2003) *Foreign Direct Investment, Democracy, and Development: Assessing Contours, Correlates, and Concomitants of Globalization*. London: Routledge.

Dessler, D. (1991) "Beyond Correlations: Toward a Causal Theory of War," *International Studies Quarterly* 35: 337–355.

Dessler, D. (1994) "What International Relations Theorists Can Learn from the Natural Sciences," paper given at the Annual Meeting of the American Political Science Association, New York, September.

Deudney, D. (1995) "The Philadelphian System: Sovereignty, Arms Control, and Balance of Power in the American States-Union, circa 1787–1861," *International Organization* 49(2): 191–228.

Deutsch, K.W. (1963) *The Nerves of Government*. New York: Free Press.

Deutsch, K.W. (1978) *The Analysis of International Relations*, 2nd ed. Englewood Cliffs, NJ: Prentice-Hall.

Deutsch, K.W., and D. Senghaas (1971) "A Framework for a Theory of War and Peace," in A. Lepawsky, E. Buehrigj, and H. Lasswell (Eds.) *The Search for World Order*. New York: Appleton-Century-Crofts.

Deutsch, K.W., S. Burrell, R. Kann, M. Lee, M. Lichterman, R. Lindgren, F. Loewenheim, and R. Van Wagenen (1957) *Political Community and the North Atlantic Area: International Organization in the Light of Historical Experience*. Princeton, NJ: Princeton University Press.

Diehl, P.F., Ed. (1998) *The Dynamics of Enduring Rivalries*. Urbana, IL: University of Illinois Press.

Dixon, W. (1994) "Democracy and the Peaceful Settlement of International Conflict," *American Political Science Review* 88: 14–32.

Doherty, C.J. (1997) "Pact with Russia Eases Way for NATO Expansion," *Congressional Quarterly Weekly Report* (May 17): 1149.

Donno, D. (2008) *Defending Democratic Norms: Regional Intergovernmental Organizations, Domestic Opposition, and Democratization.* Ph.D. dissertation, New Haven, CT: Yale University.

Donohue, L. (2008) *The Cost of Counterterrorism: Power, Politics, and Liberty.* New York: Cambridge University Press.

Doran, C.F. (1977) *Myth, Oil, and Politics.* New York: Free Press.

Dorussen, H., and H. Ward (2008a) "International Organizations and the Kantian Peace: A Network Analysis," *Journal of Conflict Resolution* 52(2): 189–212.

Dorussen, H., and H. Ward (2008b) "Trade Links and the Kantian Peace," paper presented at the annual meeting of the International Studies Association, San Francisco, March.

Dower, J.D. (1986) *War without Mercy: Race & Power in the Pacific War.* New York: Pantheon.

Downes, A.B. (2008) *Targeting Civilians in War.* Ithaca, NY: Cornell University Press.

Downes, A.B. (2009) "How Smart and Tough are Democracies? Reassessing Theories of Democratic Victory in War," *International Security* 33(4): 9–51.

Doyle, M. (1983) "Kant, Liberal Legacies, and Foreign Affairs," *Philosophy and Public Affairs* 12(3): 205–235.

Doyle, M. (1986a) *Empires.* Ithaca, NY: Cornell University Press.

Doyle, M. (1986b) "Liberalism and World Politics," *American Political Science Review* 80: 1151–1170.

Doyle, M. (1997) *Ways of War and Peace.* New York: Norton.

Doyle, M. (2008) *Striking First: Pre-emption and Prevention in International Conflict.* Princeton, NJ: Princeton University Press.

Draper, R. (2007) *Dead Certain: The Presidency of George W. Bush.* New York: Free Press.

Dreyer, J.T. (1996) "Regional Security Issues—Contemporary China: The Consequences of Change," *Journal of International Affairs* 49: 391–411.

Duvall, R., S. Jackson, B. Russett, D. Snidal, and D. Sylvan (1981) "A Formal Model of 'Dependencia' Theory: Structure and Measurement," in R.L. Merritt and B. Russett (Eds.) *From National Development to Global Community.* London: Allen & Unwin.

Easton, D. (1969) "The New Revolution in Political Science," *American Political Science Review* 63: 1051–1061.

Ehrlich, T. (1974) *Cyprus 1958–1967: International Crises and the Role of Law.* Oxford: Oxford University Press.

Eichenberg, R., and R. Stoll (2006) "War President: The Approval Ratings of George W. Bush," *Journal of Conflict Resolution* 50(6): 783–808.

Eilstrup-Sangiovanni, M., and D. Verdier (2005) "European Integration as a Solution to War," *European Journal of International Relations* 11(1): 99–135.

Eland, I. (2004) *The Empire Has No Clothes: US Foreign Policy Exposed.* Oakland, CA: The Independent Institute.

Elias, N. (1982) *The Civilizing Process, Vol. 2, State Formation and Civilization.* Oxford: Basil Blackwell.

Elliott, J.H. (2006) *Empires of the Atlantic World: Britain and Spain in America 1492–1830.* New Haven, CT: Yale University Press.

Ellsberg, D. (1981) "Introduction: Call to Mutiny," in E.P. Thompson and D. Smith (Eds.) *Protest and Survive.* New York: Monthly Review Press.

Elvin, M. (1973) *The Pattern of the Chinese Past.* London: Methuen.

Ember, C.R., M. Ember, and B. Russett (1992) "Peace Between Participatory Polities: A Cross-Cultural Test of the 'Democracies Rarely Fight Each Other' Hypothesis," *World Politics* 44: 573–599.

Encausse, H. d' (1979) *Decline of an Empire: The Soviet Socialist Republics in Revolt*. New York: Harper & Row.

Engardio, P. (1996) "Global Tremors from an Unruly Giant," *Business Week* (March 4): 59–62.

Erlanger, S. (1996) "US Warns Three Nations on Missile Technology Sale: Is China Seeking Soviet Rocket Secrets?" *New York Times* (May 22).

Erlanger, S. (1997) "A War of Numbers Emerges Over Cost of Enlarging NATO," *New York Times* (October 13).

Esty, D. (1997) *Sustaining the Asia Pacific Miracle: Environmental Protection and Economic Integration*. Washington, DC: Institute for International Economics.

Farber, H., and J. Gowa (1997) "Common Interests or Common Politics? Reinterpreting the Democratic Peace," *Journal of Politics* 59(2): 393–417.

Fearon, J.D. (1994) "Domestic Political Audiences and the Escalation of International Disputes," *American Political Science Review* 88(3): 577–593.

Fearon, J.D. (1995) "Rationalist Explanations for War," *International Organization* 49(3): 378–415.

Fearon, J.D., and A. Wendt (2002) "Rationalism v. Constructivism: A Skeptical View," in W. Carlsnaes, T. Risse, and B. Simmons (Eds.) *Handbook of International Relations*. London: Sage, pp. 52–72.

Feder, S. (1995) "Factions and Policon: New Ways to Analyze Politics," *Studies in Intelligence* (recently declassified article in a classified publication), in H.B. Westerfield (ed.) *Inside CIA's Private World: Declassified Articles from the Agency's Internal Journal, 1955–1992*. New Haven, CT: Yale University Press.

Ferejohn, J., and F. Rosenbluth (2008) "Warlike Democracies," *Journal of Conflict Resolution* 52(1): 3–38.

Finnemore, M. (1993) "International Organizations as Teachers of Norms: The United Nations Educational, Scientific, and Cultural Organization and Science Policy," *International Organization* 47(4): 565–597.

Finnemore, M. (1996) *National Interests in International Society*. Ithaca, NY: Cornell University Press.

Finnemore, M., and K. Sikkink (1998) "International Norm Dynamics and Political Change," *International Organization* 52(4): 887–917.

Fischer, D.A.V., and W.C. Potter (1996) "NATO Expansion: The March of Folly," *Moscow News* (April 11): 5.

Fischman, L. (1980) *World Mineral Trends and US Supply Problems*. Washington, DC: Brookings Institution, pp. 500, 512.

Forde, S. (1989) *The Ambition to Rule: Alcibiades and the Politics of Imperialism in Thucydides*. Ithaca, NY: Cornell University Press.

Fordham, B., and C. Sarver (2001) "Militarized Interstate Disputes and United States Uses of Force," *International Studies Quarterly* 45(3): 455–466.

Fordham, B., and T.C. Walker (2005) "Kantian Liberalism, Regime Type, and Military Resource Allocation: Do Democracies Spend Less?" *International Studies Quarterly* 49(1): 141–157.

Foucault, M. (1972) *The Archaeology of Knowledge*. New York: Pantheon.

Friedberg, A. (2000) *In the Shadow of the Garrison State: America's Anti-Statism and its Cold War Grand Strategy*. Princeton, NJ: Princeton University Press.

Frye, J. (1993) *The Helsinki Process: Negotiating Security and Cooperation in Europe*. Washington, DC: National Defense University Press.

Fukuyama, F. (1992) *The End of History and the Last Man*. New York: Free Press.

Fulghum, D. (1996) "China Buys SU-27 Rights from Russia," *Aviation Week & Space Technology* 144 (February 12): 60.

Gaddis, J.L. (1987). *The Long Peace: Inquiries into the History of the Cold War*. New York: Oxford University Press.

Gaddis, J.L. (1992a) *The United States and the End of the Cold War*. New York: Oxford University Press.

Gaddis, J.L. (1992b) "How the Cold War's End Dramatizes the Failure of Political Theory," *Chronicle of Higher Education* 38 (July 22).

Gaddis, J.L. (1992/93) "International Relations Theory and the End of the Cold War," *International Security* 17: 5–58.

Gaddis, J.L. (1997) *We Now Know: Rethinking Cold War History*. New York: Oxford University Press.

Gandhi, J., and A. Przeworski (2006) "Cooperation, Cooptation, and Rebellion under Dictatorships," *Economics and Politics* 18(1): 1–26.

Garfinkel, M. (1994) "Domestic Politics and International Conflict," *American Economic Review* 84: 1294–1309.

Garrett, B., and B.S. Glaser (1995) "Chinese Perspectives on Nuclear Arms Control," *International Security* 20: 43–78.

Gartner, S.S. (2008) "The Multiple Effects of Casualties on Public Support for War: An Experimental Approach," *American Political Science Review* 102(1): 95–106.

Gartzke, E. (2007) "The Capitalist Peace," *American Journal of Political Science* 51(1): 166–191.

Gartzke, E., and J. Hewitt (2010) "International Crises and the Capitalist Peace," *International Interactions* 36(2): 115–145.

Gartzke, E., Q. Li, and C. Boehmer (2001) "Investing in the Peace: Economic Interdependence, and International Conflict," *International Organization* 55(2): 391–438.

Gastil, R.D. (1989) *Freedom in the World: Political Rights and Civil Liberties, 1988–1989*. New York: Freedom House.

Gat, A. (2005) "The Democratic Peace Theory Reframed: The Impact of Modernity," *World Politics* 58(1): 73–100.

Gat, A. (2010) *Victorious and Vulnerable: Why Democracy Won in the 20th Century and How it is Still Imperiled*. Lanham, MD: Rowman & Littlefield.

Gaubatz, K.T. (1996) "Democratic States and Commitment in International Relations," *International Organization* 50(1): 109–139.

Gavin, F.J. (2009/10) "Same as it Ever Was: Nuclear Alarmism, Proliferation, and the Cold War," *International Security* 34(3): 7–37.

Geertz, C. (1973) *The Interpretation of Cultures*. New York: Basic Books.

Geiss, A., L. Brock, and H. Muller, Eds. (2006) *Democratic Wars: The Dark Side of the Democratic Peace*. London: Palgrave.

Gelpi, C., P. Feaver, and J. Reiffler (2005/06) "Success Matters: Casualty Sensitivity and the War in Iraq," *International Security* 30(3): 7–46.

Gelpi, C., P. Feaver, and J. Reifler (2009) *Paying the Human Costs of War: American Public Opinion and Casualties in Military Conflicts*. Princeton, NJ: Princeton University Press.

Gheciu, A. (2005) "Security Institutions as Agents of Socialization? NATO and the 'New Europe'," *International Organization* 59(4): 973–1012.

Ghosn, F., and G. Palmer (2003) Codebook for the Militarized Interstate Dispute Data, Version 3.0. Available at: www.correlatesofwar.org. Accessed June 30, 2006.

Gibler, D.M., and M. Sarkees (2003) Measuring Alliances: The Correlates of War Formal Interstate Alliance Data Set, 1816–2000. Available at: www.correlatesofwar.org. Accessed June 7, 2006.

Gilpin, R. (1975) *US Power and the Multinational Corporation: The Political Economy of Direct Foreign Investment.* New York: Basic Books.

Gilpin, R. (1981) *War and Change in World Politics.* New York: Cambridge University Press.

Gilpin, R. (1988) "The Origin and Prevention of Major Wars," *Journal of Interdisciplinary History* 18(4): 591–613.

Gleditsch, K.S. (2002a) *All International Politics is Local: The Diffusion of Conflict, Integration, and Democratization.* Ann Arbor, MI: University of Michigan Press.

Gleditsch, K.S. (2002b) "Expanded Trade and GDP Data," *Journal of Conflict Resolution* 46(5): 712–724.

Gleditsch, K.S., and M.D. Ward (1997) "Double Take: A Reexamination of Democracy and Autocracy in Modern Polities," *Journal of Conflict Resolution* 41(3): 361–383.

Gleditsch, N.P. (2008) "The Liberal Moment Fifteen Years On," *International Studies Quarterly* 52(4): 691–712.

Gleditsch, N.P., and H. Hegre (1997) "Peace and Democracy: Three Levels of Analysis," *Journal of Conflict Resolution* 41(2): 283–310.

Goemans, H.E. (2000) *War and Punishment: The Causes of War Termination and the First World War.* Princeton, NJ: Princeton University Press.

Goldgeier, J. (1998) "NATO Expansion: The Anatomy of A Decision," *Washington Quarterly* 21: 85–102.

Goldsmith, B. (2003) "Bearing the Defense Burden, 1886–1989," *Journal of Conflict Resolution* 47(5): 551–573.

Goldstein, J. (1998) "International Institutions and Domestic Politics: GATT, WTO, and the Liberalization of International Trade," in A.O. Krueger (ed.) *The WTO as an International Organization.* Chicago, IL: University of Chicago Press, pp. 133–160.

Goodby, J.E. (1998) *Europe Undivided: The New Logic of Peace in US–Russian Relations.* Washington, DC: US Institute of Peace Press.

Graham, T.W. (1987) *Future Fission: Extended Deterrence and American Public Opinion.* Occasional Paper. Cambridge, MA: Harvard University, Center for Science and International Affairs.

Green, D.P., and I. Shapiro (1994) *Pathologies of Rational Choice Theory: A Critique of Applications in Political Science.* New Haven, CT: Yale University Press.

Gronke, P., and D. Rejali, with D. Drenguis, J. Hickes, P. Miller, and B. Nakayama (2010) "US Public Opinion on Torture, 2001–2009," *PS: Political Science and Politics* 43(3): 437–444.

Gruber, L. (2000) *Ruling the World: Power Politics and the Rise of Supranational Institutions.* Princeton, NJ: Princeton University Press.

Gurr, T.R. (1988) "War, Revolution, and the Growth of the Coercive State," *Comparative Political Studies* 21(1): 45–65.

Gurr, T.R. (1993) *Minorities at Risk: A Global View of Ethnopolitical Conflict.* Washington, DC: US Institute of Peace.

Haas, E. (1993) "Collective Conflict Management: Evidence for a New World Order," in T. Weiss (ed.) *Collective Security in a Changing World.* Boulder, CO: Lynne Rienner, pp. 63–117.

Habermas, J. (2007) *The Divided West,* translated by C. Cronin. Cambridge: Polity Press.

Haftel, Y., and A. Thompson (2006) "The Independence of International Organizations: Concepts and Applications," *Journal of Conflict Resolution* 50(2): 253–275.

Halperin, M.H. (1987) *Nuclear Fallacy: Dispelling the Myth of Nuclear Strategy.* Cambridge, MA: Ballinger.

Harries, O. (1993) "The Collapse of the 'West'," *Foreign Affairs* 72: 41–53.

Hart, P.T. (1990) *Two NATO Allies at the Threshold of War: Cyprus, a Firsthand Account of Crisis Management, 1965–1968*. Durham, NC: Duke University Press.

Hasenclever, A., and B. Weiffen (2006) "International Institutions are the Key," *Review of International Studies* 32(4): 563–585.

Hawking, S. (1988) *A Brief History of Time: From the Big Bang to Black Holes*. New York: Bantam.

Hegre, H., J.R. Oneal, and B. Russett (2010) *Trade Does Promote Peace: The Perils of Simultaneous Estimation of the Reciprocal Effects of Trade and Conflict, Journal of Peace Research* 47(6): 763–774.

Held, D. (1995) *Democracy and the Global Order: From the Modern State to Cosmopolitan Governance*. Cambridge: Polity Press.

Helliwell, J.F. (1994) "Empirical Linkages between Democracy and Economic Growth," *British Journal of Political Science* 24(2): 225–248.

Hempel, C. (1965) "The Function of General Laws of History," in C. Hempel (ed.) *Aspects of Scientific Explanation*. New York: The Free Press.

Heng, Y.-K. (2010) "Mirror, Mirror, on the Wall, Who Is the Softest of Them All? Evaluating Japanese and Chinese Strategies in the 'Soft' Power Competition Era," *International Relations of the Asia-Pacific* 10(2): 275–304.

Heston, A., R. Summers, and B. Aten (2009) Penn World Table Version 6.3, Center for International Comparisons of Production, Income and Prices at the University of Pennsylvania, Philadelphia, PA.

High-level Panel on Threats, Challenges, and Change (2004) *A More Secure World: Our Shared Responsibility*. New York: United Nations A/59/565, December 2. Online at http://UN. org/secureworld/report2.pdf. Accessed November 3, 2010.

Hirschfeld, N. (1996) "Trireme Warfare in Thucydides," in R. Strassler (ed.) *Thucydides: A Comprehensive Guide to the Peloponnesian War*. New York: Free Press, pp. 608–613.

Hirschman, A. (1945) *National Power and the Structure of Foreign Trade*. Berkeley, CA: University of California Press.

Hoare, Q., and G.N. Smith, Eds. (1971) *Selections from the Prison Notebooks of Antonio Gramsci*. New York: International Publishers.

Hoffman, D. (2009) *The Dead Hand: The Untold Story of the Cold War Arms Race and Its Dangerous Legacy*. New York: Doubleday.

Hogan, W.W. (1981) "Import Management and Oil Emergencies," in D. Deese and J. Nye (Eds.) *Energy and Security*. Cambridge, MA: Ballinger.

Hollis, M., and S. Smith (1990) *Explaining and Understanding International Relations*. New York: Oxford University Press.

Holloway, N. (1996) "Playing for Keeps," *Far Eastern Economic Review* (February 8): 14–16.

Holloway, N. (1997) "Brothers in Arms: The US Worries about Sino-Russian Military Cooperation," *Far Eastern Economic Review* (March 13): 20–21.

Holloway, N., and C. Bickers (1997) "China's Buying Binge in Moscow's Armory," *World Press Review* 44 (June): 10–11.

Hoopes, T. (1973) *The Devil and John Foster Dulles*. Boston, MA: Little, Brown & Co.

Horgan, J. (1995) "From Complexity to Perplexity," *Scientific American* 272: 104–109.

Horowitz, M., E. Simpson, and A.C. Stam (2007) "Domestic Institutions and Wartime Casualties," Harvard University and Dartmouth College, manuscript.

Houweling, H., and J. Siccama (1988) "Power Transitions as a Cause of War," *Journal of Conflict Resolution* 32: 87–102.

Howell, W., and J. Pevehouse (2007) *While Dangers Gather: Congressional Checks on Presidential War Powers*. Princeton, NJ: Princeton University Press.

Howell, L., J. Vincent, and C. McClelland (1983) "Symposium: Events Data Collections," *International Studies Quarterly* 27(2): 149–177.

Howorth, J. (2007) *Security and Defence Policy in the European Union.* London: Palgrave.

Howorth, J., and A. Menon (2009) "Still Not Pushing Back: Why the European Union is Not Balancing the United States," *Journal of Conflict Resolution* 53(5): 727–744.

Hughes, H., and J. Waelbroeck (1983) "Foreign Trade and Structural Adjustment—Is There a New Protectionism?" in H.-G. Braun, H. Lanmer, W. Leibritz, and H. C. Sherman (Eds.) *The European Economy in the 1980s.* Aldershot: Gower.

Human Security Research Project (2011) *Human Security Report 2009/10.* Oxford: Oxford University Press.

Hunter, S. (1996) "Forging Chains Across Eurasia," *The World Today* 52: 313–316.

Huntington, S. (1996) *The Clash of Civilizations and the Remaking of World Order.* New York: Simon & Schuster.

Hurrell, A. (1998) "An Emerging Security Community in South America?" in E. Adler and M. Barnett (Eds.) *Security Communities.* Cambridge: Cambridge University Press, pp. 228–264.

Hurrell, A., and N. Woods (1995) "Globalisation and Inequality," *Millennium* 24(3): 447–470.

Huth, P. (1988) *Extended Deterrence and the Prevention of War.* New Haven, CT: Yale University Press.

Huth, P. (1990) "The Extended Deterrent Value of Nuclear Weapons," *Journal of Conflict Resolution* 2(4): 270–290.

Huth, P., and T. Allee (2002) *The Democratic Peace and Territorial Conflict in the Twentieth Century.* New York: Cambridge University Press.

Huth, P., and B. Russett (1988) "Deterrence Failure and Crisis Escalation," *International Studies Quarterly* 32(1): 29–45.

Huth, P., and B. Russett (1993) "General Deterrence Between Enduring Rivals: Testing Three Competing Models," *American Political Science Review* 87: 61–73.

Ikenberry, G.J. (1996) "The Myth of Post-Cold War Chaos," *Foreign Affairs* 75(3): 79–91.

Ikenberry, G.J. (2001/2) "American Power and the Empire of Capitalist Democracy," *Review of International Studies* 27(1): 191–212.

Independent Working Group on the Future of the United Nations (1995) *The United Nations in Its Second Half-Century.* New York: Ford Foundation. Online at www.centerfor unreform.org/node/224. Accessed on November 3, 2010.

Jackson, M.O., and M. Morelli (2007) "Political Bias and War," *American Economic Review* 97(4): 1353–1373.

Jaggers, K., and T. Gurr (1995) "Transitions to Democracy: Tracking the Third Wave with Polity III Indicators," *Journal of Peace Research* 33(4): 469–482.

James, P. (1992) "Rational Choice? Crisis Bargaining Over the Meech Lake Accord," paper presented at the Annual Meeting of the Canadian Political Science Association, Charlottetown, Prince Edward Island, June.

Jervis, R. (2005) *American Foreign Policy in a New Era.* New York: Routledge.

Jervis, R. (2006) "The Remaking of a Unipolar World," *Washington Quarterly* 29(3): 7–19.

Jervis, R. (2009) "Unipolarity: A Structural Perspective," *World Politics* 61(1): 188–213.

Johnson, C. (2004) *Nemesis: The Last Days of the American Republic.* New York: Metropolitan Books.

Johnson, C., and E.B. Keehn (1994) "A Disaster in the Making: Rational Choice and Asian Studies," *The National Interest* 36: 14–22.

Johnston, A.I. (1995) "China's New Old Thinking: The Concept of Limited Deterrence," *International Security* 20: 5–42.

Jones, D., S. Bremer, and J.D. Singer (1996) "Militarized Interstate Disputes, 1816–1992: Rationale, Coding Rules, and Empirical Patterns," *Conflict Management and Peace Science* 15(2): 163–213.

Kacowicz, A. (1998) *Zones of Peace in the Third World: South America and West Africa in Comparative Perspective*. Albany, NY: State University of New York Press.

Kagan, D. (1969) *The Outbreak of the Peloponnesian War*. Ithaca, NY: Cornell University Press.

Kagan, R. (2002) "Power and Weakness," *Policy Review* 113: 3–28.

Kahler, M. (2000) "Legalization as Strategy: The Asia-Pacific Case," *International Organization* 54(3): 549–571.

Kant, I. ([1795] 1970) *Perpetual Peace: A Philosophical Sketch* in H. Reiss (ed.) *Kant: Political Writings*. Cambridge: Cambridge University Press.

Kant, I. ([1784] 1991) *Idea for a Universal History with a Cosmopolitan Purpose* in H. Reiss (ed.) *Kant: Political Writings*, 2nd ed. Cambridge: Cambridge University Press.

Karaosmanoglu, A.L. (1991) "The International Context of Democratic Transition in Turkey," in G. Pridham (ed.) *Encouraging Democracy: The International Context of Regime Transition in Southern Europe*. New York: St. Martin's Press, pp. 159–174.

Karpychev, A. (1992) "Russia Wants to Join NATO," *The Current Digest of the Soviet Press* 43 (January 29): 19.

Kaysen, C. (1990) "Is War Obsolete?" *International Security* 14(4): 42–64.

Keat, R., and J. Urry (1982) *Social Theory as Science*. London: Routledge & Kegan Paul.

Keller, J. (2005) "Leadership Style, Regime Type, and Foreign Policy Crisis Behavior: A Contingent Monadic Peace?" *International Studies Quarterly* 49(2): 205–231.

Kelley, C.T. (1995) *Admitting New Members: Can NATO Afford the Costs?* Santa Monica, CA: RAND.

Kennedy, P.M. (1984a) "Why Did the British Empire Last So Long?" in P.M. Kennedy, *Strategy and Diplomacy, 1860–1945*. London: Allen & Unwin.

Kennedy, P.M. (1984b) "The First World War and the International Power System," *International Security* 9(1): 7–40.

Kennedy, P.M. (1987) *The Rise and Fall of the Great Powers*. New York: Random House.

Keohane, R.O. (1983) "Theory of World Politics: Structural Realism and Beyond," in A.W. Finifter (ed.) *Political Science: The State of the Discipline*. Washington, DC: American Political Science Association, pp. 503–540.

Keohane, R.O. (1984a) *After Hegemony: Cooperation and Discord in the World Political System*. Princeton, NJ: Princeton University Press.

Keohane, R.O. (1984b) "The Demand for International Regimes," *International Organization* 36(2): 325–355.

Keohane, R.O., and L. Martin (1995) "The Promise of Institutionalist Theory," *International Security* 20(2): 39–51.

Keohane, R.O., and J. Nye, Eds. (1977) *Power and Interdependence*. Boston, MA: Little, Brown & Co.

Keohane, R.O, A. Moravcsik, and A.-M. Slaughter (2000) "Legalized Dispute Resolution: Interstate and Transnational," *International Organization* 54(3): 457–488.

Keylor, W.R. (1996) *The Twentieth Century World: An International History*, 3rd ed. Oxford: Oxford University Press.

Khalilzad, Z. (1984) "Islamic Iran: Soviet Dilemma," *Problems of Communism* 33(1): 1–20.

Kim, S.Y. (1988) "Ties that Bind: The Role of Trade in International Conflict Processes, 1950–1992," Ph.D. dissertation, Yale University.

Kim, W., and B. Bueno de Mesquita (1995) "How Perceptions Influence the Risk of War," *International Studies Quarterly* 39: 51–65.

Kim, W., and J.D. Morrow (1992) "When do Power Shifts Lead to War?" *American Journal of Political Science* 36: 896–922.

Kindleberger, C. (1973) *The World in Depression, 1929–1939*. Berkeley, CA: University of California Press.

Kindleberger, C. (1976) "Systems of International Economic Organization," in D. Calleo (ed.) *Money and the Coming World Order*. New York: New York University Press.

King, A.H. (1977) *Materials Vulnerability of the United States—An Update*. Carlisle Barracks, PA: US Army War College.

King, G. (2001) "Proper Nouns and Methodological Propriety: Pooling Dyads in International Relations Data," *International Organization* 55(2): 497–507.

King, G., and L. Zeng (2001) "Explaining Rare Events in International Relations," *International Organization* 55(3): 693–715.

King, G., M. Tomz, and J. Wittenberg (2000) "Making the Most of Statistical Analyses: Improving Interpretation and Presentation," *American Journal of Political Science* 44(2): 347–361.

Kinsella, D. (2005) "No Rest for the Democratic Peace," *American Political Science Review* 89(3): 453–458.

Kinsella, D., and B. Russett (2002) "Conflict Emergence and Escalation in Interactive International Dyads," *Journal of Politics* 64(4): 1045–1068.

Kinsella, D., B. Russett, and H. Starr (forthcoming 2012) *World Politics: The Menu for Choice*, 10th ed. Boston, MA: Wadsworth.

Kirchner, E.J., and J. Sperling (1992) *The Federal Republic of Germany and NATO: 40 Years After*. London: Macmillan.

Kitcher, P. (1989) "Explanatory Unification and the Causal Structure of the World," in P. Kitcher and W. Salmon (Eds.) *Scientific Explanation: Vol. XIII*, Minnesota Studies in the Philosophy of Science. Minneapolis, MN: University of Minnesota Press.

Kitfield, J. (1996) "A Larger NATO Means Bigger Headaches?" in K.W. Thompson (ed.) *NATO and the Changing World Order: An Appraisal by Scholars and Policymakers*. Lanham, MD: University Press of America.

Kitfield, J. (1997) "A Larger NATO Means Bigger Headaches?" *National Journal* 29 (July 19): 1467–1469.

Kohut, A., and N. Horrock (1984) "Generally Speaking: Surveying the Military's Top Brass," *Public Opinion* 7(5): 42–45.

Komiya, R., and M. Itoh (1988) "Japan's International Trade and Trade Policy, 1955–1984," in T. Inoguchi and D. Okimoto (Eds.) *The Political Economy of Japan: The Changing International Context*. Stanford, CA: Stanford University Press.

Kondrashov, S. (1997) "Russia, NATO Agree on Act Formalizing Relations," *The Current Digest of the Post-Soviet Press* 49 (June 18): 1–5.

Koretsky, A. (1996) "China Will Build Russian Planes Itself," *Current Digest of the Post-Soviet Press* 48 (March 20): 23–24.

Koslowski, R., and F.V. Kratochwil (1995) "Understanding Change in International Politics: The Soviet Empire's Demise and the International System," in R.N. Lebow and T. Risse-Kappen (Eds.) *International Relations Theory and the End of the Cold War*. New York: Columbia University Press, pp. 127–165.

Kozhemiakin, A.V. (1998) *Expanding the Zone of Peace? Democratization and International Security*. New York: St. Martin's.

Krain, M. (1997) "State-Sponsored Mass Murder: The Onset and Severity of Genocides and Politicides," *Journal of Conflict Resolution* 41: 331–360.

Kramer, B., M. Kalick, and M. Milburn (1983) "Attitudes toward Nuclear Weapons and Nuclear War, 1945–82," *Public Opinion Quarterly* 39(1): 7–24.

Krasner, S. (1974) "Oil Is the Exception," *Foreign Policy* 14: 68–83.

Krasner, S. (1975) "State Power and the Structure of International Trade," *World Politics* 27(3): 317–347.

Krasner, S. (1981) "Transforming International Regimes: What the Third World Wants and Why," *International Studies Quarterly* 25(1): 119–148.

Krasner, S. (1982) "Structural Causes and Regime Consequences: Regimes as Intervening Variables," *International Organization* 36(2): 185–205.

Krasner, S. (1995/96) "Compromising Westphalia," *International Security* 20(3): 115–151.

Kreps, S. (2010) "Elite Consensus as a Determinant of Alliance Cohesion: Why Public Opinion Hardly Matters for NATO-led Operations in Afghanistan," *Foreign Policy Analysis* 6(3): 191–215.

Kriner, D.J. (2010) *After the Rubicon: Congress, Presidents, and the Politics of Waging War*. Chicago, IL: University of Chicago Press.

Kriner, D., and F.X. Shen (2010) *The Casualty Gap: The Causes and Consequences of American Wartime Inequalities*. New York: Oxford University Press.

Kruzel, J. (1994) "More a Chasm Than a Gap, But Do Scholars Want to Bridge It?" *Mershon International Studies Review* 38: 179–181.

Kugler, J. (1984) "Terror without Deterrence," *Journal of Conflict Resolution* 28(3): 470–506.

Kugler, J. (1987) "The Politics of Foreign Debt in Latin America: A Study of the Debtors' Cartel," *International Interactions* 13: 115–144.

Kugler, J., and D. Lemke, Eds. (1996) *Parity and War*. Ann Arbor, MI: University of Michigan Press.

Kugler, J., and D. Lemke (1998) "The Power Transition," in M.I. Midlarsky (ed.) *Handbook of War Studies II*. Ann Arbor, MI: University of Michigan Press.

Kugler, J., L.W. Snider, and W. Longwell (1994) "From Desert Shield to Desert Storm: Success, Strife, or Quagmire?" *Conflict Management and Peace Science* 13: 113–148.

Kugler, R.L. (1996) *Enlarging NATO: The Russia Factor*. Santa Monica, CA: RAND.

Kuhn, T. (1962) *The Structure of Scientific Revolutions*. Chicago, IL: University of Chicago Press.

Kupchan, C. (2010) "NATO's Final Frontier," *Foreign Affairs* 89(3): 100–113.

Lacina, B., and N.P. Gleditsch (2005) "Monitoring Trends in Global Combat: A New Dataset of Battle Deaths," *European Journal of Population* 21(2–3): 145–166.

Lagazio, M., and B. Russett (2004) "A Neural Network Analysis of Militarized Disputes, 1885–1992: Temporal Stability and Causal Complexity," in P. Diehl (ed.) *The Scourge of War: New Extensions on an Old Problem*. Ann Arbor, MI: University of Michigan Press, pp. 28–60.

Laitin, D. (1994) "The Return of the Son of the Bride of the Future of Comparative Politics," *APSA–CP, Newsletter of the American Political Science Association's Organized Section in Comparative Politics* 5: 4.

Lakatos, I. (1970) "Falsification and the Methodology of Scientific Research Programmes," in I. Lakatos and A. Musgrave (Eds.) *Criticism and the Growth of Knowledge*. Cambridge: Cambridge University Press.

Lake, D.A. (1992) "Powerful Pacifists: Democratic States and War," *American Political Science Review* 86: 24–37.

Lake, D.A. (2009) *Hierarchy in International Relations: Authority, Sovereignty, and the New Structure of World Politics*. Ithaca, NY: Cornell University Press.

Landsberg, H.H., and J.H. Tilton (1982) "Nonfuel Minerals," in P.R. Portney (ed.) *Current Issues in Natural Resources Policy*. Washington, DC: Resources for the Future.

Lapid, Y. (1989) "The Third Debate: On the Prospects of International Theory in a Post-Positivist Era," *International Studies Quarterly* 33: 235–254.

Lasswell, H.D. (1941) "The Garrison State," *American Journal of Sociology* 96(4): 455–468.

Lawler, A. (1996) "Russian Deal Bolsters the Space Station—at a Price," *Science* 271 (February 9): 753–754.

Lawyers' Committee on Nuclear Policy (1981, 1984) "Statement on the Illegality of Nuclear Weapons," reprinted in B.H. Weston (ed.) *Toward Nuclear Disarmament and Global Security: A Search for Alternatives.* Boulder, CO: Westview.

Layne, C. (1994) "Kant or Cant: The Myth of Democratic Peace," *International Security* 19: 5–49.

Layne, C. (1995) "On the Democratic Peace," *International Security* 19(4): 175–177.

Layne, C. (2006) "The Unipolar Illusion Revisited: The Coming End of the United States' Unipolar Moment," *International Security* 31(2): 7–41.

Lebow, R.N. (1995) "The Long Peace, the End of the Cold War, and the Failure of Realism," in R.N. Lebow and T. Risse-Kappen (Eds.) *International Relations Theory and the End of the Cold War.* New York: Columbia University Press, pp. 23–56.

Lebow, R.N. (2003) *The Tragic Vision of Politics: Ethics, Interests and Order.* Cambridge: Cambridge University Press.

Leeds, B.A. (1999) "Domestic Political Institutions, Credible Commitments, and International Cooperation," *American Journal of Political Science* 43(4): 979–1002.

Leeds, B.A. (2003) "Do Alliances Deter Aggression? The Influence of Military Alliances on the Initiation of Militarized International Disputes," *American Journal of Political Science* 47(4): 427–439.

Lenin, N. ([1917] 1926) *Imperialism: The Last Stage of Capitalism.* New York: Vanguard.

Leskiw, C.S. (2002) *Sown for Peace? International Organizations and Interstate Conflict.* Ph.D. dissertation, Vanderbilt University, Nashville, TN.

Levy, J.S. (2008) "Preventive War and Democratic Politics," *International Studies Quarterly* 52(1): 1–24.

Levy, J.S., and W.R. Thompson (2010) "Balancing on Land and at Lea: Do States Ally against the Leading Great Power," *International Security* 35(1): 7–43.

Lijphart, A. (1966) *The Trauma of Decolonization: The Dutch and West New Guinea.* New Haven, CT: Yale University Press.

Lintott, A. (1982) *Violence, Civil Strife, and Revolution in the Classical City.* London: Croom Helm.

Lipson, C. (2003) *Reliable Partners: How Democracies Have Made a Separate Peace.* Princeton, NJ: Princeton University Press.

Liptak, A. (2008) "More than 1 in 100 Adults are Now in Prison in US," *New York Times* (February 29): A15.

Liska, G. (1978) *Career of Empire.* Baltimore, MD: Johns Hopkins University Press.

Lockwood, J.S. (1983) *The Soviet View of US Strategic Doctrine: Implications for Decision Making.* New Brunswick, NJ: Transaction Books.

Lorenz, E. (1972) "Predictability: Does the Flap of a Butterfly's Wings in Brazil set off a Tornado in Texas?" paper presented at the Annual Meeting of the American Association for the Advancement of Science, Washington, DC, December.

Loshak, V. (1997) "Army Bigger Threat Than NATO," *Moscow News* (February 13): 2.

Lundestad, G. (1990) *The American "Empire."* Oslo and London: Norwegian University Press and Oxford University Press.

Lyall, J. (2010) "Do Democracies Make Inferior Counterinsurgents?" *International Organization* 64(1): 167–192.

Lyotard, J.-F. (1992) *Post-Modernism and the Social Sciences.* Princeton, NJ: Princeton University Press.

Machiavelli, N. ([1512–1517] 1998) *The Discourses,* Ed. B. Crick. London: Penguin.

MacMillan, J. (1995) "A Kantian Protest against the Peculiar Discourse of the Inter-Liberal State Peace," *Millennium* 24(3): 549–562.

MacMillan, J. (1998) *On Liberal Peace: Democracy, War and International Order*. London: Tauris.

MacMillan, J. (2003) "Beyond the Separate Democratic Peace," *Journal of Peace Research* 40(2): 233–243.

Madison, J. ([1793] 1857) "The Letters of Helvidius," in *The Federalist: Letters on the New Constitution, New Edition*. Hallowell, ME: Masters Smith, pp. 432–459.

Magdoff, H. (1969) *The Age of Imperialism*. New York: Monthly Review Press.

Mahbubani, K. (1993) "The Dangers of Decadence: What the Rest Can Teach the West," *Foreign Affairs* 72: 10–14.

Maier, C.S. (1997) *The Crisis of Communism and the Collapse of East Germany*. Princeton, NJ: Princeton University Press.

Mandelbaum, M. (1995a) "Preserving the New Peace: The Case Against NATO Expansion," *Foreign Affairs* 74: 9–13.

Mandelbaum, M., Ed. (1995b) *The Strategic Quadrangle: Japan, China, Russia and the United States in East Asia*. New York: Council on Foreign Relations.

Mandelbaum, M. (2010) *The Frugal Superpower: American's Global Leadership in a Cash-Strapped Era*. New York: Public Affairs.

Mandell, B. (1992) "The Cyprus Conflict: Explaining Resistance to Resolution," in N. Salem (ed.) *Cyprus: A Regional Conflict and its Resolution*. New York: St. Martin's.

Mann, P. (1997) "Clinton, Senate Duel over NATO Expansion," *Aviation Week & Space Technology* 147 (July 14): 38–39.

Mansfield, E.D., and J.C. Pevehouse (2003) "Institutions, Interdependence, and International Conflict," in G. Schneider, K. Barbieri, and N.P. Gleditsch (Eds.) *Globalization and Armed Conflict*. London: Routledge.

Mansfield, E.D., and J.C. Pevehouse (2006) "Democratization and International Organizations," *International Organization* 60: 137–167.

Mansfield, E.D., and B.M. Pollins, Eds. (2003) *Economic Interdependence and International Conflict: New Perspectives on an Enduring Debate*. Ann Arbor, MI: University of Michigan Press, pp. 233–250.

Mansfield, E.D., and J. Snyder (1995) "Democratization and the Danger of War," *International Security* 20: 5–38.

Mansfield, E.D., and J. Snyder (1996) "The Effects of Democratization on War," *International Security* 20(4): 196–207.

Mansfield, E.D., and J. Snyder (1997) "A Reply to Thompson and Tucker," *Journal of Conflict Resolution* 41(3): 457–461.

Mansfield, E.D., and J. Snyder (2002) "Incomplete Democratization and the Outbreak of Military Disputes," *International Studies Quarterly* 46(4): 529–550.

Mansfield, E.D., and J. Snyder (2005) *Electing to Fight: Why Emerging Democracies Go to War*. Cambridge, MA: MIT Press.

Mansfield, E.D., J.C. Pevehouse, and D.H. Bearce (1999–2000) "Preferential Trading Arrangements and Military Disputes," *Security Studies* 9(1–2): 96–118.

Mansfield, E.D., H. Milner, and B.P. Rosendorf (2002) "Why Democracies Cooperate More: Electoral Control and International Trade Agreements," *International Organization* 56(3): 477–513.

Maoz, Z. (1996) *Domestic Sources of Global Change*. Ann Arbor, MI: University of Michigan Press.

Maoz, Z. (1997) "The Renewed Controversy over the Democratic Peace Result: Rear-Guard Action or Cracks in the Wall?" *International Security* 22(1): 428–454.

Maoz, Z. (1998) "Realist and Cultural Critiques of the Democratic Peace: A Theoretical and Empirical Re-assessment," *International Interactions* 24(1).

Maoz, Z. (2002) Dyadic Militarized Interstate Dispute Dataset Version 1.1. Revised version available as Dydic MID Data v. 3.10 at www.correlatesofwar.org/. Accessed December 22, 2010.

Maoz, Z. (2004) "Pacifism and Fightaholism in International Politics: A Structural History of National and Dyadic Conflict, 1816–1992," *International Studies Review* 6(4): 107–133.

Maoz, Z., and B. Russett (1993) "Normative and Structural Causes of Democratic Peace 1946–1986," *American Political Science Review* 87(3): 624–638.

March, J.G., and J.P. Olsen (1998) "The Institutional Dynamics of International Political Orders," *International Organization* 52(4): 943–969.

Markides, K.C. (1977) *The Rise and Fall of the Cyprus Republic.* New Haven, CT: Yale University Press.

Marshall, M. (2004) *Polity IV Dataset.* Available at: www.bsos.umd.edu0cidcm0polity&. Accessed June 30, 2006.

Martin, L. (1992) *Coercive Cooperation: Explaining Multilateral Economic Sanctions.* Princeton, NJ: Princeton University Press.

Martin, L. (2000) *Democratic Commitments: Legislatures and International Cooperation.* Princeton, NJ: Princeton University Press.

Martin, L., and B. Simmons (1998) "Theories and Empirical Studies of International Institutions," *International Organization* 52(4): 729–758.

Mason, A. (1998) "The End of Cold War Thinking: Change and Learning in Foreign Policy Belief Systems," Ph.D. dissertation, Yale University.

Mastny, V. (1992) *The Helsinki Process and the Reintegration of Europe.* New York: New York University Press.

Matlock, J.F., Jr. (2010) *Superpower Illusions: How Myths and False Ideologies Led America Astray—and How to Return to Reality.* New Haven, CT: Yale University Press.

McCarthy, T. (1999) "On Reconciling Cosmopolitan Unity and National Diversity," *Public Culture* 11(1): 175–208.

MccGwire, M. (1987) *Military Objectives in Soviet Foreign Policy.* Washington, DC: Brookings Institution.

MccGwire, M. (1997) *NATO Expansion and European Security.* London: Brasseys.

McColm, R.B. (1992) *Freedom in the World: Political Rights and Civil Liberties, 1991–1992.* New York: Freedom House.

McDonald, M. (2006) "5 Myths about Turning out the Vote," *Washington Post* (October 29): B03.

McDonald, P.J. (2010) "Capitalism, Commitment, and Peace," *International Interactions* 36(2): 146–168.

McGillivray, F., and A. Smith (2000) "Trust and Cooperation through Agent-Specific Punishments," *International Organization* 54(4): 809–824.

McGillivray, F., and A. Smith (2004) "The Impact of Leadership Turnover on Trading Relations Between States," *International Organization* 58(3): 567–600.

McKeown, T.J. (1983) "Tariffs and Hegemonic Stability Theory," *International Organization* 37(1).

McNamara, R.S. (1983) "The Military Role of Nuclear Weapons," *Foreign Affairs* 62(1): 59–80.

McNeely, C. (1995) *Constructing the Nation-State: International Organization and Prescriptive Action.* Westport, CT: Greenwood.

Mearsheimer, J. (1994/95) "The False Promise of International Institutions," *International Security* 19(3): 5–49.

Mearsheimer, J. (2001) *The Tragedy of Great Power Politics*. New York: Norton.

Mearsheimer, J., and S. Walt (2007) *The Israel Lobby and US Foreign Policy*. New York: Farrar, Straus & Giroux.

Mercer, J. (1995) "Anarchy and Identity," *International Organization* 49(2): 229–252.

Merolla, J.L., and E.J. Zechmeister (2009) *Democracy at Risk: How Terrorist Threats Affect the Public*. Chicago, IL: University of Chicago Press.

Miall, H. (1992) *The Peacemakers: Peaceful Settlement of Disputes since 1945*. New York: St. Martin's.

Miller, J.A., D. Fine, and D. McMichael, Eds. (1981) *The Resource War in 3-D: Dependency, Diplomacy, Defense*. Pittsburgh, PA: World Affairs Council of Pittsburgh.

Miller, R.W. (2008) "Globalizing Justice: The Ethics of Poverty and Power," Ithaca, NY: Cornell University Department of Philosophy, manuscript.

Milner, H.V. (1998) "Regional Economic Co-operation, Global Markets, and Domestic Politics," in W. Coleman and G.R.D. Underhill (Eds.) *Regionalism and Global Economic Integration*. London: Routledge, pp. 19–41.

Minnich, D. (2005) "Veto Players, Electoral Incentives, and International Commitments: The Impact of Domestic Institutions on Intergovernmental Organization Membership," *European Journal of Political Research* 44(2): 295–325.

Mintz, A., and Nehemia Geva (1993) "Why Don't Democracies Fight Each Other?" *Journal of Conflict Resolution* 37: 484–503.

Mitchell, S.M. (2002) "A Kantian System? Democracy and Third-Party Conflict Resolution," *American Journal of Political Science* 46(4): 749–759.

Modelski, G. (1978) "The Long Cycle of Global Politics and the Nation State," *Comparative Studies in Society and History* 20(2): 214–235.

Monk, P. (1996) "China's Power Trip," *Far Eastern Economic Review* (March 21): 28.

Moravcsik, A. (1993) "Preference and Power in the European Community: A Liberal Intergovernmental Approach," *Journal of Common Market Studies* 31(4): 473–524.

Moravcsik, A. (1998) *The Choice for Europe: Social Purpose and State Power from Messina to Maastricht*. Ithaca, NY: Cornell University Press.

Morgan, P.M. (1983) *Deterrence: A Conceptual Analysis*. Beverly Hills, CA: Sage.

Morgenstern, O., K. Knorr, and K.P. Heiss (1973) *Long-Term Projections of Power: Political, Economic, and Military Forecasting*. Cambridge, MA: Ballinger.

Morgenthau, H.J. (1948) *Politics among Nations: The Struggle for Power and Peace*. New York: Knopf.

Morgenthau, H.J. (1960) *Politics among Nations: The Struggle for Power and Peace*, 3rd ed. New York: Knopf.

Morrow, J.D., B. Bueno de Mesquita, and S. Wu (1993) "Forecasting the Risks of Nuclear Proliferation: Taiwan as an Illustration of Method," *Security Studies* 2: 311–331.

Mousseau, M. (2009) "The Social Market Roots of Democratic Peace," *International Security* 33(4): 52–86.

Mousseau, M., H. Hegre, and J.R. Oneal (2003) "How the Wealth of Nations Conditions the Liberal Peace," *European Journal of International Relations* 9(2): 277–314.

Mueller, J. (1986) "Containment and the Decline of the Soviet Empire," paper presented to the Annual Convention of the International Studies Association, Anaheim, California, March.

Mueller, J. (1988a) "The Essential Irrelevance of Nuclear Weapons: Stability in the Postwar World," *International Security* 13(2): 55–90.

Mueller, J. (1988b) *Retreat from Doomsday: The Obsolescence of Major War*. New York: Basic Books.

Mueller, J. (2006) *Overblown: How Politicians and the Terrorism Industry Inflate the National Security Threats, and Why We Believe Them.* New York: Free Press.

Mueller, J. (2009) *Nuclear Alarmism, from Hiroshima to Al-Qaeda.* New York: Oxford University Press.

Muller, E. (1995) "Economic Determinants of Democracy," *American Sociological Review* 60(6): 965–982.

Müller, H. (2004) "The Antimony of Democratic Peace," *International Politics* 41(4): 494–520.

Müller, H., and J. Wolff (2006) "Democratic Peace: Many Data, Little Explanation," in A. Geiss, L. Brock, and H. Müller (Eds.) *Democratic Wars: Looking at the Dark Side of Democratic Peace.* Basingstoke: Palgrave Macmillan, pp. 41–73.

Münkler, H. (2007) *Empires: The Logic of World Dominion from Ancient Rome to the United States,* translated by P. Camiller. Cambridge: Polity Press.

Murdoch, J.C., and T. Sandler (1991) "NATO Burden Sharing and the Forces of Change: Further Observations," *International Studies Quarterly* 35: 109–114.

Murphy, C. (1994) *International Organizations and Industrial Change: Global Governance since 1850.* New York: Oxford University Press.

Myrdal, A. (1976) *The Game of Disarmament: How the United States and the Soviet Union Run the Arms Race.* New York: Pantheon.

Narang, N., and R. Nelson (2009) "Who Are Those Belligerent Democratizers? Reassessing the Impact of Democratization on War," *International Organization* 63(2): 357–379.

Nathan, A.J., and R.S. Ross (1997) *The Great Wall and the Empty Fortress: China's Search for Security.* New York: Norton.

Newman, D., and B. Bridges (1994) "North Korean Nuclear Weapons Policy: An Expected Utility Study," *Pacific Focus* 9: 61–80.

Nincic, M., and D. Nincic (2002) "Race, Gender, and War," *Journal of Peace Research* 39(5): 547–568.

Nincic, M., and P. Wallensteen, Eds. (1984) *Dilemmas of Economic Coercion: Sanctions in World Politics.* New York: Praeger.

Niu, W.Y., and W. Harris (1996) "China: The Forecast of Its Environmental Situation in the 21st Century," *Journal of Environmental Management* 47: 101–115.

Nolan, P. (1996) "Large Firms and Industrial Reform in Former Planned Economies: The Case of China," *Cambridge Journal of Economics* 20: 1–28.

Nordhaus, W. (2010) *The Economics of an Integrated World Oil Market.* Occasional paper. New Haven, CT: Yale University Economics Dept.

Nordhaus, W., J.R. Oneal, and B. Russett (2010) *The Effects of the Security Environment on Military Expenditures: Pooled Analyses of 159 Countries, 1950–2000.* Working Paper, Yale University Leitner Program, New Haven, CT. Available at: www.yale.edu/leitner/papers.html. Accessed November 3, 2010.

Norloff, C. (2010) *America's Global Advantage: US Hegemony and International Cooperation.* New York: Cambridge University Press.

Nye, J.S. (1997–1998) "China's Re-emergence and the Future of the Asia Pacific," *Survival* 39: 65–79.

Nye, J.S. (2003) *The Paradox of American Power: Why the World's Only Superpower Can't Go it Alone.* New York: Oxford University Press.

O'Neill, B. (1997) "Power and Satisfaction in the Security Council," in B. Russett (ed.) *The Once and Future Security Council.* New York: St. Martin's.

O'Toole, F., and E. Strobl (1995) "Compulsory Voting and Government Spending," *Economics and Politics* 7(3): 271–280.

Ober, J. (1989) *Mass and Elite in Democratic Athens: Rhetoric Ideology, and the Power of the People.* Princeton, NJ: Princeton University Press.

Ober, J. (1998) *Political Dissent in Democratic Athens: Intellectual Critics of Popular Rule.* Princeton, NJ: Princeton University Press.

Ober, J. (2008) *Democracy and Knowledge: Innovation and Learning in Classical Athens.* Princeton, NJ: Princeton University Press.

OECD (2008) *Growing Unequal? Income Distribution and Poverty in OECD Countries.* Paris: OECD.

Olson, M. (1971) *The Logic of Collective Action: Public Goods and the Theory of Groups.* Cambridge, MA: Harvard University Press.

Olson, M., and R. Zeckhauser (1966) "An Economic Theory of Alliances," *Review of Economics and Statistics* 48(3): 269–279.

Oneal, J.R. (1990) "The Theory of Collective Action and Burden Sharing in NATO," *International Organization* 44: 379–402.

Oneal, J.R. (2006) "Confirming the Liberal Peace with Analyses of Directed Dyads, 1885–2001," in H. Starr (ed.) *Approaches, Levels and Methods of Analysis in International Politics: Crossing Boundaries.* New York: Palgrave Macmillan.

Oneal, J.R., and P.F. Diehl (1994) "The Theory of Collective Action and NATO Defense Burdens: New Empirical Tests," *Political Research Quarterly* 47: 373–396.

Oneal, J.R., and B. Russett (1997) "The Classical Liberals Were Right: Democracy, Interdependence, and Conflict, 1950–85," *International Studies Quarterly* 41(2): 267–293.

Oneal, J.R., and B. Russett (1999) "The Kantian Peace: The Pacific Benefits of Democracy, Interdependence, and International Organizations, 1885–1992," *World Politics* 52(1): 1–37.

Oneal, J.R., and B. Russett (2005) "Rule of Three, Let It Be? When More Really is Better," *Conflict Management and Peace Science* 22(4): 293–310.

Oneal, J.R., and B. Russett (2006) "Seeking Peace in a Post-Cold War World of Hegemony and Terrorism," in B. Russett, *Purpose and Policy in the Global Community.* New York: Palgrave Macmillan, pp. 231–252.

Oneal, J.R., and J. Tir (2006) "Does the Diversionary Use of Force Threaten the Democratic Peace? Assessing the Effect of Economic Growth on Interstate Conflict, 1921–2001," *International Studies Quarterly* 50(4): 755–779.

Oneal, J.R., and H.C. Whatley (1996) "The Effect of Alliance Membership on National Defense Burdens, 1953–88: A Test of Mancur Olson's Theory of Collective Action," *International Interactions* 22(2): 105–122.

Oneal, J.R., F. Oneal, Z. Maoz, and B. Russett (1996) "The Liberal Peace: Interdependence, Democracy, and International Conflict, 1950–1986," *Journal of Peace Research* 32.

Oneal, J.R., B. Russett, and M. Berbaum (2003) "Causes of Peace: Democracy, Interdependence, and International Organizations, 1985–1992," *International Studies Quarterly* 47(3): 371–393.

Oppenheimer, J. (1979) "Collective Goods and Alliances: A Reassessment," *Journal of Conflict Resolution* 23(3): 387–407.

Organski, A.F.K. (1958) *World Politics.* New York: Knopf.

Organski, A.F.K., and B. Bueno de Mesquita (1993) "Forecasting the 1992 French Referendum," in R. Morgan, J. Lorentzen, and A.Leander (Eds.) *New Diplomacy in the Post-Cold War World.* New York: St Martin's Press.

Organski, A.F.K., and S. Eldersveld (1994) "Modelling the EC: Conclusion," in B. Bueno de Mesquita and F. Stokman (Eds.) *European Community Decision Making: Models, Applications and Comparisons.* New Haven, CT: Yale University Press.

Organski, A.F.K., and J. Kugler (1980) *The War Ledger*. Chicago, IL: University of Chicago Press.

Organski, A.F.K., and C. Organski (1961) *Population and World Power*. New York: Knopf.

Owen, J. (1994) "How Liberalism Produces Democratic Peace," *International Security* 19: 87–125.

Oye, K.A. (1979) "The Domain of Choice," in K.A. Oye, D. Rothchild, and R.J. Lieber (Eds.) *Eagle Entangled: US Foreign Policy in a Complex World*. New York: Longman.

Oye, K.A. (1995) "Explaining the End of the Cold War: Morphological and Behavioral Adaptations to the Nuclear Peace?" in R.N. Lebow and T. Risse-Kappen (Eds.) *International Relations Theory and the End of the Cold War*. New York: Columbia University Press, pp. 57–84.

Park, W. (1986) *Defending the West: A History of NATO*. Boulder, CO: Westview Press.

Patrick, H., and H. Rosovsky (1983) "The End of Eras? Japan and the Western World in the 1970–1980," paper delivered at the Japan Political Economy Research Conference, Honolulu, July.

Paul, T.V. (2009) *The Tradition of Non-Use of Nuclear Weapons*. Stanford, CA: Stanford University Press.

Paus, E. (1994) "Economic Growth Through Neoliberal Restructuring? Insights from the Chilean Experience," *Journal of the Developing Areas* 29: 31–56.

Payne, R. (2007) "Neorealists as Critical Theorists: The Purpose of Foreign Policy Debate," *Perspectives on Politics* 5(3): 503–514.

Peceny, M., and C. Beer (2002) "Dictatorial Peace?" *American Political Science Review* 96(1): 15–26.

Perkins, B. (1968) *The Great Rapprochement: England and the United States, 1885–1914*. New York: Atheneum.

Perlo-Freeman, S. (2009) "Arms Production," *SIPRI Yearbook 2009: Armaments, Disarmament and International Security*. Oxford: Oxford University Press.

Perlo-Freeman, S., O. Ismail, and C. Solmirano (2010) "Military Expenditure," in Stockholm International Peace Research Institute, *SIPRI Yearbook 2010: Armaments, Disarmament and International Security*. Oxford: Oxford University Press.

Persada, V. (1992) "From Cold War to Security," *The Current Digest of the Soviet Press* 43 (January 22): 21–22.

Peters, D., and W. Wagner (2009) "Revisiting Reversed Causality: External Threat and the Parliamentary Control of Military Missions in Democracies," paper presented at the meeting of the International Studies Association, New York, February.

Pevehouse, J. (2005) *Democracy from Above: Regional Organizations and Democratization*. Cambridge: Cambridge University Press.

Pevehouse, J., and R. Buhr (2005) "Democracy and Legalism in Regional Trade Organizations," paper presented at the 63rd Annual Meeting of the Midwest Political Science Association, Chicago, April.

Pevehouse, J., and B. Russett (2006) "Democratic Intergovernmental Organizations Promote Peace," *International Organization* 60(4): 969–1000.

Pevehouse, J., T. Nordstrom, and K. Warnke (2004) "Intergovernmental Organizations 1815–2000: A New Correlates of War 2 Data Set," *Conflict Management and Peace Science* 21(2): 101–120.

Phillips, D. (2004) "Turkey's Dreams of Accession," *Foreign Affairs* 83(5): 86–97.

Posen, B. (1984) *The Sources of Military Doctrine: France, Britain and Germany between the World Wars*. Ithaca, NY: Cornell University Press.

Posen, B. (2006) "European Union Security and Defense Policy: Response to Unipolarity?" *Security Studies* 15(2): 149–186.

Powell, R. (1991) "Absolute and Relative Gains in International Relations Theory," *American Political Science Review* 85(1): 1303–1320.

Pratt, M. (2001) "The Maritime Boundary Dispute Between Honduras and Nicaragua in the Caribbean Sea," *Boundary and Security Bulletin* 9(2): 108–116.

Pritchard, D., Ed. (2010) *War, Democracy, and Culture in Classical Athens*. New York: Cambridge University Press.

Przeworski, A., and F. Limongi (1993) "Political Regimes and Economic Growth," *Journal of Economic Perspectives* 7(3): 51–70.

Przeworski, A., and F. Limongi (1997) "Modernization: Theories and Facts," *World Politics* 49(2): 155–183.

Przeworski, A., M. Alvarez, J.A. Cheibub, and F. Limongi (1996) "What Makes Democracies Endure?" *Journal of Democracy* 7(1): 39–55.

Puchala, D.J. (1991) "Woe to the Orphans of the Scientific Revolution," in R. Rothstein (ed.) *The Evolution of Theory in International Relations*. Columbia, SC: University of South Carolina Press.

Pushkov, A.K. (1997) "Don't Isolate Us: A Russian View of NATO Expansion," *The National Interest* 47: 58–62.

Putnam, R. (1988) "Diplomacy and Domestic Politics: The Logic of Two–Level Games," *International Organization* 42(3): 427–462.

Qingshan, T. (1992) *The Making of US China Policy: From Normalization to the Post-Cold War Era*. Boulder, CO: Lynne Rienner.

Quester, G. (1987) *The Future of Nuclear Deterrence*. Lexington, MA: Lexington Books.

Quine, W.V. (1961) "Two Dogmas of Empiricism," in W.V. Quine (ed.) *From a Logical Point of View*. New York: Random House.

Quine, W.V. (1992) *Pursuit of Truth*, rev. ed. Cambridge, MA: Harvard University Press.

Rasler, K., and W.R. Thompson (1983) "Global Wars, Public Debts, and the Long Cycle," *World Politics* 36(1): 489–516.

Rasler, K., and W.R. Thompson (1988) "Longitudinal Change in Defense Burdens, Capital Formation, and Economic Growth," *Journal of Conflict Resolution* 32(1): 61–86.

Ratner, S. (1995) *The New UN Peacekeeping. Building Peace in Lands of Conflict after the Cold War*. New York: St. Martin's.

Ray, J.L. (1993) "Wars Between Democracies: Rare, or Non–Existent?" *International Interactions* 18: 251–276.

Ray, J.L. (1995a) *Global Politics*, 6th ed. Boston, MA: Houghton Mifflin.

Ray, J.L. (1995b) *Democracy and International Conflict*. Columbia, SC: University of South Carolina Press.

Ray, J.L. (1995c) "Promise or Peril? Neorealism, Neoliberalism, and the Future of International Politics," in C. Kegley Jr. (ed.) *Controversies in International Relations Theory*. New York: St Martin's Press.

Ray, J.L. (2005) "Constructing Multivariate Analyses (of Dangerous Dyads)" *Conflict Management and Peace Science* 22(4): 277–292.

Ray, J.L., and J.D. Singer (1973) "Measuring the Concentration of Power in the International System," *Sociological Methods and Research* 1(4): 403–437.

Raymond, G.A. (1994) "Democracies, Disputes, and Third-Party Intermediaries," *Journal of Conflict Resolution* 38: 24–42.

Raymond, G.A. (1996) "Demosthenes and Democracies: Regime-Types and Arbitration Outcomes," *International Interactions* 22(1): 1–20.

Reed, W. (2000) "A Unified Statistical Model of Conflict Onset and Escalation," *American Journal of Political Science* 44(1): 84–93.

Reichhardt, T. (1996) "US Deal Buys into Mir to Keep Russia On Board International Station Project," *Nature* 379 (February 8): 476–477.

Reisman, W.M. (1993) "The Constitutional Crisis in the United Nations," *American Journal of International Law* 87(1): 83–100.

Reiter, D., and A.C. Stam (2002) *Democracies at War*. Princeton, NJ: Princeton University Press.

Reiter, D., and A.C. Stam (2003) "Identifying the Culprit: Democracy, Dictatorship, and Dispute Initiation," *American Political Science Review* 97(2): 333–337.

Reiter, D., and A.C. Stam (2007) "Democracy and War Outcomes: Extending the Debate," Emory University and University of Michigan, manuscript.

Reiter, D., A.C. Stam, and A.B. Downes (2009) "Correspondence: Another Skirmish in the Battle over Democracies and War," *International Security* 34(2): 194–204.

Renwick, R. (1981) *Economic Sanctions*. Cambridge, MA: Harvard Center for International Affairs.

Repko, S. (1996) "We'll Never Be Allies," *The Current Digest of the Post-Soviet Press* 48 (August 21): 21–22.

Reuveny, R., and Q. Li (2003) "The Joint Democracy-Dyadic Conflict Nexus: A Simultaneous Equations Model," *International Studies Quarterly* 47(3): 325–346.

Reuveny, R., and W.R. Thompson (2004) *Growth, Trade, and Systemic Leadership*. Ann Arbor, MI: University of Michigan Press.

Rich, B. (1994) *Mortgaging the Earth: The World Bank, Environmental Impoverishment, and the Crisis of Development*. Boston, MA: Beacon.

Richardson, N. (1981) "Economic Dependence and Foreign Policy Compliance: Bringing Measurement Closer to Conception," in C. Kegley and P. McGowan (Eds.) *The Political Economy of Foreign Policy Behavior*. Beverly Hills, CA: Sage.

Risse, T. (2003) "Beyond Iraq: The Crisis of the Transatlantic Security Community," *Die Friedens-Warte* 78: 175.

Risse-Kappen, T. (1995) *Cooperation among Democracies: Norms, Transnational Relations, and the European Influence on US Foreign Policy*. Princeton, NJ: Princeton University Press.

Robinson, E. (2001) "Reading and Misreading the Ancient Evidence for Democratic Peace," *Journal of Peace Research* 38(5): 593–608.

Rock, S.R. (1989) *Why Peace Breaks Out: Great Power Rapprochement in Historical Perspective*. Chapel Hill, NC: University of North Carolina Press.

Rosato, S. (2003) "The Flawed Logic of Democratic Peace Theory," *American Political Science Review* 97(4): 585–602.

Rosato, S. (2005) "Explaining the Democratic Peace," *American Political Science Review* 99(3): 467–472.

Rosecrance, R. (1976) "Introduction," in R. Rosecrance (ed.) *America as an Ordinary Country*. Ithaca, NY: Cornell University Press.

Rosen, S.P. (2007) *War and Human Nature*. Princeton, NJ: Princeton University Press.

Rosenau, J.N. (1994) "Signals, Signposts and Symptoms: Anticipating and Explaining Major Historical Breakpoints," paper given at the Annual Meeting of the American Political Science Association, New York, September.

Rosenau, P.M. (1992) *Post-Modernism and the Social Sciences*. Princeton, NJ: Princeton University Press.

Rosenberg, A. (1992) *Economics–Mathematical Politics or Science of Diminishing Returns?* Chicago, IL: University of Chicago Press.

Rousseau, D. (2005) *Democracy and War: Institutions, Norms, and the Evolution of International Conflict.* Stanford, CA: Stanford University Press.

Rousseau, D., C. Gelpi, D. Reiter, and P. Huth (1996) "Assessing the Dyadic Nature of the Democratic Peace, 1918–1988," *American Political Science Review* 89(3): 512–533.

Roy, D. (1994) "Hegemon on the Horizon? China's Threat to East Asian Security," *International Security* 19: 149–168.

Ruggie, J.G. (1980) "Review of Stephen Krasner, *Defending the National Interest,*" *American Political Science Review* 74(1): 296–299.

Ruggie, J.G. (1988) *Constructing the World Polity: Essays on International Institutionalization.* New York: Routledge.

Ruggie, J.G. (1992) "Multilateralism: The Anatomy of an Institution," *International Organization* 46(3): 561–598.

Ruggie, J.G. (1996) *Winning the Peace: America and World Order in the New Era.* New York: Columbia University Press.

Rummel, R.J. (1975) *The Dynamic Psychological Field: Vol. 1, Understanding Conflict and War.* New York: Sage.

Rummel, R.J. (1994) *Death by Government.* New Brunswick, NJ: Transaction.

Rummel, R.J. (1997) *Power Kills: Democracy as a Method of Nonviolence.* New Brunswick, NJ: Transaction.

Rupert, M.E., and D.P. Rapkin (1985) "The Erosion of US Leadership Capabilities," in P. Johnson and W.R. Thompson (Eds.) *Rhythms in International Politics and Economics.* New York: Praeger, pp. 155–180.

Russett, B. (1963) *Community and Contention: Britain and America in the Twentieth Century.* Cambridge, MA: MIT Press.

Russett, B. (1967) "Pearl Harbor: Deterrence Theory and Decision," *Journal of Peace Research* 2: 89–105.

Russett, B. (1970) *What Price Vigilance: The Burdens of National Defense.* New Haven, CT: Yale University Press.

Russett, B. (1972) *No Clear and Present Danger: A Skeptical View of the United States Entry into World War II.* New York: Harper & Row.

Russett, B. (1982) "Causes of Peace," in C.M. Stephenson (ed.) *Alternative Methods for International Security.* Washington, DC: University Press of America.

Russett, B. (1983) *The Prisoners of Insecurity: Nuclear Deterrence, the Arms Race, and Arms Control.* New York: Freeman.

Russett, B. (1985) "The Mysterious Case of Vanishing Hegemony; or, Is Mark Twain Really Dead?" *International Organization* 39(2): 207–231.

Russett, B. (1988) "Extended Deterrence with Nuclear Weapons: How Necessary, How Acceptable?" *Review of Politics* 50: 282–302.

Russett, B. (1989) "Democracy and Peace," in B. Russett, H. Starr and R. Stoll (Eds.) *Choices in World Politics.* New York: Freeman.

Russett, B. (1993) *Grasping the Democratic Peace: Principles for a Post-Cold War World.* Princeton, NJ: Princeton University Press.

Russett, B. (1995) "The Democratic Peace: And Yet It Moves," *International Security* 19: 164–177.

Russett, B. (1996) "Counterfactuals about War and Its Absence," in P. Tetlock and A. Belkin (Eds.) *Counterfactuals in International Relations.* Princeton, NJ: Princeton University Press.

Russett, B. (1997a) "Ten Balances for Weighing UN Reform Proposals," in B. Russett (ed.) *The Once and Future Security Council.* New York: St. Martin's.

Russett, B. (1997b) *No Clear and Present Danger: A Skeptical View of the United States Entry into World War II,* Twenty-Fifth Anniversary Edition. Boulder, CO: Westview.

Russett, B., Ed. (1997c) *The Once and Future Security Council.* New York, St. Martin's.

Russett, B. (2005) "Bushwhacking the Democratic Peace," *International Studies Perspectives* 6(4): 395–408.

Russett, B. (2006) "Review of Mansfield and Snyder, 'Electing to Fight: Why Emerging Democracies Go to War'," *Political Science Quarterly* 121(4): 701–703.

Russett, B. (2010) "Capitalism or Democracy? Not So Fast," *International Interactions* 36(2): 198–205.

Russett, B., and D.R. DeLuca (1983) "Theater Nuclear Forces: Public Opinion in Western Europe," *Political Science Quarterly* 99(2): 179–196.

Russett, B., and E. Hanson (1975) *Interest and Ideology: The Foreign Policy Beliefs of American Businessmen.* New York: Freeman.

Russett, B., and J.R. Oneal (2001) *Triangulating Peace: Democracy, Interdependence, and International Organizations.* New York: Norton.

Russett, B., and J.L. Ray (1995) "Why the Democratic-Peace Proposition Lives," *Review of International Studies* 21: 319–323.

Russett, B., and H. Starr (1981) *World Politics: The Menu for Choice,* 1st ed. New York: Freeman.

Russett, B., and H. Starr (1989) *World Politics: The Menu for Choice,* 3rd ed. New York: Freeman.

Russett, B., J.R. Oneal, and D. Davis (1998) "The Third Leg of the Kantian Tripod for Peace: International Organizations and Militarized Disputes, 1950–1985," *International Organization* 52(3): 441–467.

Salmon, M. (1989) "Explanation in the Social Sciences," in P. Kitcher and W. Salmon (Eds.) *Scientific Explanation: Vol. XIII,* Minnesota Studies in the Philosophy of Science. Minneapolis, MN: University of Minnesota Press.

Sanders, D. (1990) *Losing an Empire, Finding a Role.* London: Macmillan.

Sandler, T. (1993) "The Economic Theory of Alliances: A Survey," *Journal of Conflict Resolution* 37: 446–483.

Saunders, E. (forthcoming 2011) *Leaders at War: How Presidents Shape Military Interventions.* Ithaca, NY: Cornell University Press.

Saxonhouse, A. (2006) "Rule among Equals: Reflections from Ancient Athens on Leadership and Responsibility," paper presented at the conference on Statesmen and Demogogues: Democratic Leadership in Political Thought, New Haven, CT, Yale University, April 1.

Saywell, T. (1997) "Fishing for Trouble: Asia's Fish Stocks are Dwindling Because of Over-Exploitation and Pollution," *Far Eastern Economic Review* (March 13): 50–52.

Schafer, M., and S.G. Walker (2006) "Democratic Leaders and the Democratic Peace: The Operational Codes of Tony Blair and Bill Clinton," *International Studies Quarterly* 50(3): 561–583.

Schelling, T.C. (1966). *Arms and Influence.* New Haven, CT: Yale University Press.

Schelling, T.C. (2005) *An Astonishing Sixty Years: The Legacy of Hiroshima.* Available at: http://nobelprize.org/nobel_prizes/economics/laureates/2005/schelling-lecture.html. Accessed November 3, 2010.

Scheve, K., and D. Stasasavage (2010) "The Conscription of Wealth: Mass Warfare and the Demand for Progressive Taxation," *International Organization* 64(4): 530–561.

Schneider, G., K. Barbieri, and N.P. Gleditsch, Eds. (2003) *Globalization and Armed Conflict.* London: Routledge.

Schroeder, P. (1994) *The Transformation of European Politics, 1763–1848.* Oxford: Oxford University Press.

Schultz, G., W. Perry, H. Kissinger, and S. Nunn (2007) "A World Free of Nuclear Weapons," *Wall Street Journal* (January 4): A15.

Schultz, K. (2001) *Democracy and Coercive Diplomacy.* Stanford, CA: Stanford University Press.

Schultz, K., and B. Weingast (1994) "The Democratic Advantage: The Institutional Sources of State Powers in International Competition," paper given at the Annual Meeting of the American Political Science Association, September.

Schultz, K. and B. Weingast (2003) "The Democratic Advantage: Institutional Foundations of Financial Power in International Competition," *International Organization* 57(1): 3–42.

Schumpeter, J. ([1927] 1955) *Imperialism and Social Classes.* Cleveland, OH: World Publishing Company.

Schweller, R.L. (1994) "Bandwagoning for Profit: Bringing the Revisionist State Back In," *International Security* 19: 72–107.

Scott, W. (1997) "Lockheed Martin, Energomash Development of RD-180 on Track," *Aviation Week & Space Technology* 146 (April 7): 40–41.

Sechser, T., and E. Saunders (2010) "The Army You Have: The Determinants of Military Mechanization," *International Studies Quarterly* 54(2): 481–511.

Segal, G. (1996) "East Asia and the 'Constrainment' of China," *International Security* 20: 107–135.

Sen, A. (1981) *Poverty and Famine.* New York: Oxford University Press.

Senese, P. (1997) "Between Disputes and War: The Effect of Joint Democracy on Interstate Conflict Escalation," *Journal of Politics* 59(1): 1–27.

Shambaugh, D. (1996) "Containment or Engagement of China? Calculating Beijing's Responses," *International Security* 21: 180–209.

Shannon, V., and J. Keller (2007) "Leadership Style and International Norm Violation: The Case of the Iraq War," *Foreign Policy Analysis* 3(1): 79–104.

Shapiro, I., and A. Wendt (1992) "The Difference that Realism Makes," *Politics and Society* 20: 197–223.

Shaw, T., Ed. (1993) *The Trireme Project: Operational Experience, 1987–90: Lessons Learnt.* Bloomington, IN: Oxbow.

Shenon, P. (1998) "Pentagon Report Plays Down Cost of Expanding NATO," *New York Times* (February 21).

Shepherd, W.G. (1986) *The Ultimate Deterrent: Foundations of US–USSR Security under Stable Competition.* New York: Praeger.

Shinkarenko, P., and T. Malkina (1996) "Yeltsin Visit Marks Closer Russia–China Ties," *Current Digest of the Post–Soviet Press* 48 (May 22): 6–9.

Signorino, C., and J.M. Ritter (1999) "Tau-B or not Tau-B: Measuring the Similarity of Foreign Policy Positions," *International Studies Quarterly* 43(1): 115–144.

Simon, S. (1996) "Alternative Visions of Security in Northeast Asia," *Journal of Northeast Asian Studies* 15: 77–99.

Singer, J.D. (1961) "The Level-of-Analysis Problem in International Relations," *World Politics* 14: 77–92.

Singer, J.D. (1987) "Reconstructing the Correlates of War Dataset on Material Capabilities of States, 1816–1985," *International Interactions* 14(2): 115–132.

Singer, J.D. (1994a) "Prediction Versus Explanation as Standards of Scientific Progress," paper given at the Annual Meeting of the American Political Science Association, New York City, September.

Singer, J.D. (1994b) "The Evolution of Anarchy vs. the Evolution of Cooperation," *Politics and Life Sciences* 13: 26–28.

Singer, J.D., and M. Small (1976) "The War-Proneness of Democratic Regimes, 1815–1965," *Jerusalem Journal of Conflict Resolution* 1(1): 50–69.

Singer, J.D., and M. Small (1993) "National Material Capabilities Dataset. Study No. 9903," Ann Arbor, MI: Inter-University Consortium for Political and Social Research.

Singer, M.R. (1972) *Weak States in a World of Powers: The Dynamics of International Relationships.* New York: Free Press.

Siverson, R. (1995) "Democracies and War Participation: In Defense of the Institutional Constraints Argument," *European Journal of International Relations* 1(4): 481–489.

Siverson, R., and J. Emmons (1991) "Birds of a Feather: Democratic Political Systems and Alliance Choices," *Journal of Conflict Resolution* 35: 285–306.

Slaughter, A.M. (1992) "Law among Liberal States: Liberal Internationalism and the Act of State Doctrine," *Columbia Law Review* 92: 1907–1996.

Slaughter, A.M. (1995) "International Law in a World of Liberal States," *European Journal of International Law* 6: 503–538.

Small, M., and J.D. Singer (1982) *Resort to Arms.* Beverly Hills, CA: Sage.

Smil, V. (1997) "China's Environment and Security: Simple Myths and Complex Realities," *SAIS Review* 17: 107–126.

Snidal, D. (1979) "Public Goods, Property Rights, and Political Organization," *International Studies Quarterly* 23(4): 532–566.

Snidal, D. (1985) "The Limits of Hegemonic Stability Theory," *International Organization* 39(4): 579–614.

Snyder, J. (1990) "Averting Anarchy in the New Europe," *International Security* 14: 5–41.

Snyder, J. (1994) "Russian Backwardness and the Future of Europe," *Daedalus* 123: 179–202.

Spiro, D. (1994) "The Insignificance of the Liberal Peace," *International Security* 19: 50–86.

Stam, A. (1996) *Win, Lose, or Draw: Domestic Politics and the Crucible of War.* Ann Arbor, MI: University of Michigan Press.

Stanley, A. (1995) "Russia's New Rulers Govern, and Live, in Neo-Soviet Style," *New York Times* (May 23): Section 1, pp. 1, 4.

Stanley, J., Ed. (1997) *Essays on the Garrison State/Harold Lasswell.* New Brunswick, NJ: Transaction.

Starr, H. (1992) "Democracy and War: Choice, Learning and Security Communities," *Journal of Peace Research* 29: 207–214.

Starr, H., and C. Lindborg (2003) "Democratic Dominoes Revisited: The Hazards of Governmental Transitions, 1974–1996," *Journal of Conflict Resolution* 47(4): 490–519.

Stein, A.A. (1982) "Coordination and Collaboration: Regimes in an Anarchic World," *International Organization* 36(2): 324.

Stein, A.A. (1984) "The Hegemon's Dilemma: Great Britain, the United States, and the International Economic Order," *International Organization* 38(2): 355–386.

Stein, A.A. (1989) "Governments, Economies, Interdependence, and International Cooperation," in P. Tetlock, J.L. Husbands, R. Jervis, P.C. Stern, and C. Tilly (Eds.) *Behavior, Society, and International Conflict, Vol. 3.* Oxford: Oxford University Press, pp. 244–254.

Steinbruner, J. (1981–82) "Nuclear Decapitation," *Foreign Policy* 45: 16–28.

Stepan, A., and C. Skatch (1993) "Constitutional Frameworks and Democratic Consolidation: Parliamentarism vs Presidentialism," *World Politics* 46(1): 1–22.

Stiglitz, J., and L. Bilmes (2008) *The Three Trillion Dollar War: The True Cost of the Iraq Conflict.* New York: Norton.

Stone Sweet, A., and T. Brunell (1998) "Constructing a Supranational Constitution: Dispute Resolution and Governance in the European Community," *American Political Science Review* 92(1): 63–82.

Strang, D., and P.M.Y. Chang (1993) "The International Labor Organization and the Welfare State: Institutional Effects on National Welfare Spending, 1960–80," *International Organization* 47(2): 235–262.

Strange, S. (1982a) "*Cave! Hic Dragones*: A Critique of Regime Analysis," *International Organization* 36(2): 299–324.

Strange, S. (1982b) "Still an Extraordinary Power: America's Role in a Global Monetary System," in R.E. Lombra and W.E. Witte (Eds.) *Political Economy of International and Domestic Monetary Relations*. Ames, IA: University of Iowa Press.

Strange, S. (1985) "Protectionism and World Politics," *International Organization* 39(2): 242.

Strassler, R., Ed. (1996) *Thucydides: A Comprehensive Guide to the Peloponnesian War*. New York: Free Press.

Suplee, C. (1995) "Computer Program May Give Insight to How Societies Evolve," *Washington Post*, May (reprinted in the *Tampa Tribune*, May 5, 1995).

Suprowicz, B. (1981) *How to Avoid Strategic Materials Shortages*. New York: Wiley.

Sylvan, D., and S. Majeski (2009) *US Foreign Policy in Perspective: Clients, Enemies and Empire*. New York: Routledge.

Tannenwald, N. (2008) *The Nuclear Taboo: The United States and the Non-Use of Nuclear Weapons Since 1945*. New York: Cambridge University Press.

Tetlock, P.E. (2005) *Expert Political Judgment: How Good Is It? How Can We Know?* Princeton, NJ: Princeton University Press.

Tetlock, P.E, and A. Belkin, Eds. (1996) *Counterfactual Thought Experiments in World Politics: Logical, Methodological, and Psychological Perspectives*. Princeton, NJ: Princeton University Press.

Thies, W. (2009) *Why NATO Endures*. New York: Cambridge University Press.

Thomas, G.M., J.W. Meyer, F.O. Ramirez, and J. Boli (1987) *Institutional Structure: Constituting State, Society, and the Individual*. Newbury Park, CA: Sage.

Thompson, W.R., and R. Tucker (1997a) "A Tale of Two Democratic Peace Critiques," *Journal of Conflict Resolution* 41(3): 428–454.

Thompson, W.R., and R. Tucker (1997b) "Bewitched, Bothered, and Bewildered," *Journal of Conflict Resolution* 41(3): 462–477.

Thucydides (1972) *History of the Peloponnesian War*, translated by R. Warner. London: Penguin.

Tilly, C. (1990) *Coercion, Capital, and European States, A.D. 990–1990*. Oxford: Basil Blackwell.

Tilton, J.E. (1977) *The Future of Non-Fuel Metals*. Washington, DC: Brookings Institution.

Tilton, J.E., and H.H. Landsberg (1983) "Nonfuel Minerals—The Fear of Shortages and the Search for Policies," in E.N. Castle and K.A. Price (Eds.) *US Interests and Global Natural Resources*. Washington, DC: Resources for the Future.

Todd, E., and C.J. Delogu (2003) *After the Empire: The Breakdown of the American Order*. New York: Columbia University Press.

Tsebelis, G. (2002) *Veto Players: How Political Institutions Work*. Princeton, NJ: Princeton University Press.

Turner, S. (1997) *Caging the Nuclear Genie: An American Challenge for Global Security*. Boulder, CO: Westview.

Tyler, P.E. (1996) "China To Buy 72 Advanced Fighter Planes from Russia," *New York Times* (February 7).

US ACDA (US Arms Control and Disarmament Agency) (1997) *World Military Expenditures and Arms Transfers, 1996*. Washington, DC: US Government Printing Office.

US Bureau of the Census (1975) *Historical Statistics of the United States: Colonial Times to 1970*. Washington, DC: Government Printing Office.

USCC (1983) *The Challenge of Peace: God's Promise and Our Response.* Washington, DC: United States Catholic Conference.

US Congress, Office of Technology Assessment (1976) *An Assessment of Alternative Economic Stockpiling Policies.* Washington, DC: GPO, pp. 275–276.

US Congress, Office of Technology Assessment (1982) *Cobalt: Policy Options for a Strategic Mineral.* Washington, DC: GPO, p. 9.

US Congress, Office of Technology Assessment (1983) *Strategic and Critical Nonfuel Minerals: Problems and Policy Alternatives.* Washington, DC: GPO.

US Department of Commerce, Bureau of the Census (1981) *Statistical Abstract of the United States, 1981.* Washington, DC: GPO.

Valentino, B., P. Huth, and D. Balch-Lindsay (2004) "Draining the Sea: Mass Killing and Guerilla Warfare," *International Organization* 58(2): 375–407.

Valentino, B., P. Huth, and S. Croco (2006) "Covenants without the Sword: International Law and the Protection of Civilians in Times of War," *World Politics* 58(3): 339–377.

Van Belle, D. (2000) *Press Freedom and Global Politics.* Westport, CT: Praeger.

Van Wagenen, R. (1952) *Research in the International Organization Field: Some Notes on a Possible Focus.* Princeton, NJ: Center for Research on World Political Institutions.

Van Wagenen, R. (1965) "The Concept of Community and the Future of the United Nations," *International Organization* 19(3): 812–827.

Vasquez, J. (1993) *The War Puzzle.* Cambridge: Cambridge University Press.

Vasquez, J. (1994) "The Promises and Pitfalls of Post-Modernist Approaches to International Politics," paper given at the Annual Meeting of the International Studies Association, Washington, DC, March 30.

Verdier, D. (1994) *Democracy and International Trade: Britain, France, and the United States, 1860–1990.* Princeton, NJ: Princeton University Press.

Vernon, R. (1983) *Two Hungry Giants: The United States and Japan in the Quest for Oil and Ores.* Cambridge, MA: Harvard University Press.

Voeten, E., and P.R. Brewer (2006) "Public Opinion, the War in Iraq, and Presidential Accountability," *Journal of Conflict Resolution* 50(6): 809–830.

Vreeland, J.R. (2003) *The IMF and Economic Development.* New York: Cambridge University Press.

Vreeland, J.R. (2008) "The Effect of Political Regime on Civil War: Unpacking Autocracy," *Journal of Conflict Resolution* 52(3): 401–425.

Waever, O. (1998) "Insecurity, Security, and Asecurity in the West European Non-war Community," in E. Adler and M. Barnett (Eds.) *Security Communities.* Cambridge: Cambridge University Press.

Wagner, W. (2006) "Explaining Variation in Parliamentary Control of Government Use of Force," paper presented at the Central and East European International Studies Association meeting, Tartu, Estonia, June.

Waldrop, M. (1992) *Complexity: The Emerging Science at the Edge of Order and Chaos.* New York: Simon & Schuster.

Wallensteen, P. (1984) "Universalism vs. Particularism: On the Limits of Major Power Order," *Journal of Peace Research* 21(3): 243–257.

Wallensteen, P., and M. Sollenberg (1995) "The End of International War: Armed Conflict 1989–95," *Journal of Peace Research* 33(3): 353–370.

Walt, S.M. (1987) *The Origins of Alliances.* Ithaca, NY: Cornell University Press.

Walt, S.M. (2005) *Taming American Power: The Global Response to US Primacy.* New York: Norton.

Waltz, K. (1979) *Theory of International Politics.* Reading, MA: Addison-Wesley.

Ward, M.D., and K.S. Gleditsch (1998) "Democratizing for Peace," *American Political Science Review* 92: 51–62.

Ward, M.D., D.R. Davis, and S. Chan (1993) "Military Spending and Economic Growth in Taiwan," *Armed Forces & Society* 19: 533–550.

Ward, M.D., D.R. Davis, and C.L. Lofdahl (1995) "A Century of Tradeoffs: Defense and Growth in Japan and the United States," *International Studies Quarterly* 39: 27–50.

Weart, S. (1994) "Peace Among Democracies and Oligarchic Republics," *Journal of Peace Research* 31: 229–316.

Weart, S. (1998) *Never at War: Why Democracies Will Not Fight One Another*. New Haven, CT: Yale University Press.

Weede, E. (1983) "Extended Deterrence by Superpower Alliance," *Journal of Conflict Resolution* 27(2): 231–253.

Weede, E. (1989) "Extended Deterrence, Superpower Control, and Militarized Interstate Disputes," *Journal of Peace Research* 26(1): 7–17.

Weede, E. (1992) "Some Simple Calculations on Democracy and War," *Journal of Peace Research* 29(4): 377–383.

Weede, E. (1995) "Economic Policy and International Security: Rent-Seeking, Free Trade, and Democratic Peace," *European Journal of International Relations* 1(4): 519–537.

Weede, E. (2005) *Balance of Power, Globalization, and the Capitalist Peace*. Berlin: Liberal Verlag GmbH.

Weeks, J. (2008) "Autocratic Audience Costs: Regime Type and Signaling Resolve," *International Organization* 62(1): 35–64.

Weiss, T.G. and L. Gordenker, Eds. (1996) *Non-Governmental Organizations, the United Nations, and Global Governance*. Boulder, CO: Lynne Rienner.

Welch, D.A. (2003) "Why International Relations Theorists Should Stop Reading Thucydides," *Review of International Studies* 29(3): 301–319.

Wendt, A. (1987) "The Agent-Structure Problem in International Relations Theory," *International Organization* 41: 335–368.

Wendt, A. (1994) "Collective Identity Formation and the International State," *American Political Science Review* 88: 384–398.

Wendt, A. (1999) *Social Theory of International Politics*. Cambridge: Cambridge University Press.

Whitehead, L. (1994) "East-Central Europe in Comparative Perspective," in G. Pridham, E. Herring, and G. Sanford (Eds.) *Building Democracy? The International Dimension of Democratization in Eastern Europe*. New York: St. Martin's, pp. 32–59.

Willets, P., Ed. (1996) *The Conscience of the World: The Influence of Non-Governmental Organizations in the UN System*. Washington, DC: Brookings Institution.

Wohlforth, W. (1994/95) "Realism and the End of the Cold War," *International Security* 19: 91–129.

Wohlforth, W. (1999) "The Stability of a Unipolar World," *International Security* 24(1): 5–41.

Woodruff, P., Ed. (1993) *Thucydides on Justice Power and Human Nature: Selections from the History of the Peloponnesian War*. Indianapolis, IN: Hackett.

Woods, K., J. Lacey, and W. Murray (2006) "Saddam's Delusions: The View from the Inside," *Foreign Affairs* 85(3): 2–26.

World Armaments and Disarmament (1985) *World Armaments and Disarmament: SIPRI Yearbook, 1985*. London: Taylor & Francis.

Wright, B., and J. Williams (1982) "The Roles of Public and Private Storage in Managing Oil Import Disruptions," *Bell Journal of Economics* 13: 341–353.

Wu, S., and B. Bueno de Mesquita (1994) "Assessing the Dispute in the South China Sea: A Model of China's Security Decision Making," *International Studies Quarterly* 38: 379–403.

Yankelovich, D., and J. Doble (1984) "The Public Mood," *Foreign Affairs* 63(1): 33–46.
Yanov, A. (1997) "Russian Liberals and NATO," *Moscow News* (January 3): 1–2.
Yurong, C. (1995) "Russia Distances Itself from the West," *Beijing Review* 38 (April 3): 22–5.
Zacher, M. (1992) "The Decaying Pillars of the Westphalian System," in J. Rosenau and E.-O. Czempiel (Eds.) *Governance without Government: Order and Change in World Politics.* Cambridge: Cambridge University Press, pp. 58–101.
Zartman, I.W., Ed. (1995) *Collapsed States: The Disintegration and Restoration of Legitimate Authority.* Boulder, CO: Lynne Rienner.
Zelikow, P., and C. Rice (1995) *Germany Unified and Europe Transformed: A Study in Statecraft.* Cambridge, MA: Harvard University Press.
Zhilin, A. (1996) "Rodionov to NATO: Don't Bait a Wounded Bear," *Moscow News* (December 26): 1–2.
Zurn, M., and J. Checkel (2005) "Getting Socialized to Build Bridges: Constructivism and Rationalism, Europe and the Nation-State," *International Organization* 59(4): 1045–1079.

INDEX

Page numbers in *italic* type indicate illustrations

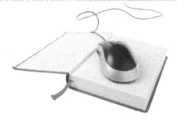
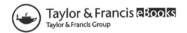

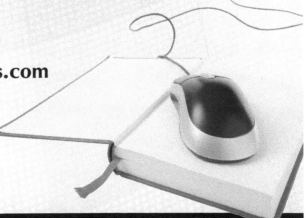

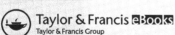

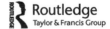

Milton Keynes UK
Ingram Content Group UK Ltd.
UKHW040444071024
449327UK00020B/991